Aging and the Auditory System: Anatomy, Physiology, and Psychophysics

Aging and the Auditory System: Anatomy, Physiology, and Psychophysics

James F. Willott, Ph.D.
Department of Psychology
Northern Illinois University
DeKalb, Illinois

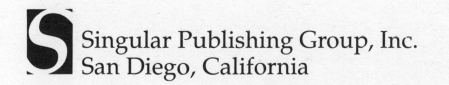
Singular Publishing Group, Inc.
San Diego, California

Cover: Spiral ganglion cells of the cochlea are the links between the ear and the brain. The cover pictures show a series of photomicrographs of ganglion cells of aging C57BL/6J mice from young (top row) to old (bottom row). The loss of ganglion cells with age is obvious, especially near the base of the cochlea (left column). A similar pattern of degeneration occurs in many aging people, resulting in presbycusis. From Willott, J. F. and Bross, L. S. (1990). Morphology of the octopus cell area of the cochlear nucleus in young and aging C57BL/6J and CBA/J mice. *Journal of Comparative Neurology 300*, 61-81. Reprinted with permission.

Singular Publishing Group, Inc.
4284 41st Street
San Diego, California 92105

©**1991 by Singular Publishing Group, Inc**.

Library of Congress Cataloging-in-Publication Data

Willott, James F.
     Aging and the auditory system: anatomy, physiology, and psychophysics / James F. Willott.
     p. cm.
     Includes bibliographical references and index.
     ISBN 1-879105-11-X
     1. Presbycusis. 2. Ear--Aging. I. Title.
     [DNLM: 1. Aging--physiology. 2. Ear--pathology. 3. Ear--physiopathology. 4. Presbycusis.
     5. Psychophysics. WV 270 W739a]
     RF291.5.A35W55 1991
     617.8--dc20
     DNLM/DLC
     for Library of Congress   91-4817
                                       CIP

ISBN 1-879105-11-X

Printed in the United States of America

CONTENTS

Dedication

To three former mentors, each of whom led me in a new, exciting direction:

Dr. J. Donald Harris, Dr. Irving Wagman, and Dr. Kenneth Henry

FOREWORD

Anyone who has worked very long in the area of auditory aging knows the frustrations arising from the host of covarying factors affecting auditory function in the elderly individual. The commingled effects of progressive hearing sensitivity loss at the auditory periphery, declining cognitive abilities, and changes in other dimensions of brain function challenge the designer of both cross-sectional and longitudinal studies to a degree seldom appreciated by the casual observer. In my view, one of the principal virtues of this book is the perspective with which author Willott has highlighted and dissected this major obstacle to the unequivocal interpretation of a wide variety of research findings.

The student of aging will find, in this impressive volume, a sound, scholarly summary of virtually every facet of auditory function in aging, combined with a fresh and forthright approach to the interpretation of the frequently confusing and often contradictory research data. With broad sweeps of his talented pen, Willott leads us through the animal experiments, the extensive literature on physiologic changes, and finally the fascinating, and often perplexing psychophysical literature on auditory aging in humans.

Many disciplines have been involved in the study of auditory aging; psychology, audiology, physiology, and gerontology. Typically, investigators in these various fields have tended to view the problem from their own narrow perspectives. This book, however, effectively transcends these sometimes arbitrary boundaries. It shows, for example, the possible relevance of animal studies of CNS changes in understanding the complex changes in speech understanding of elderly humans. Similarly, it highlights the interweaving themes of specifically-auditory and generalized cognitive changes and how they may impact on human performance.

Certainly this book can be read and studied at many levels. If you are interested in some particular aspect of auditory aging, and you would like to know what the literature says about it, you will find a relatively complete answer here. But, more importantly, if you would like to know how people in other disciplines think about auditory aging, what areas you may have in common with them, and what areas need further cross-disciplinary fertilization, you will find that too in this eminently readable book. It covers just about everything you have ever wanted to know about the effect of age on auditory function.

James Jerger

PREFACE

I decided to write this book to fill a void. Whereas excellent works have appeared on the pathology of presbycusis, clinical audiometry and presbycusis, speech perception by the elderly, and various communicative aspects of aging, no monographs have focused on aging and the auditory system per se.

The book has three goals: (a) to present the most exhaustive bibliographic review of the literature on aging and the auditory system to date, (b) to report and interpret findings accurately and objectively from as many studies as possible, and (c) to evaluate the current "state of the art."

To accomplish the first goal I cited all of the relevant work I could find. I used primary sources whenever possible, but some citations (e.g., in sources or languages that were not accessible) were from secondary sources or abstracts, as indicated. Despite my efforts to be inclusive, it is likely that some pieces were missed, and I apologize to the authors.

The second goal (reporting and interpreting findings) was a real challenge since the research comes from many disciplines such as pathology, neuroanatomy, psychophysics, and audiology, to name several. My own background and training are broadbased, but I was well aware of the need to get expert help. I was fortunate to get some of the best help available. After writing a relatively complete version of the manuscript, all or parts were reviewed by several eminent scholars who have made major contributions over the years, Drs. Martin Feldman, James Jerger, and John Mills. I also received expert help from an audiologist who has not been on the scene as long, Dr. Sharon Sandridge, and from an exceptional graduate student, Sandy McFadden. Many other scholars provided input (sometimes unwittingly) on a smaller scale, in informal discussions or correspondence. These include Drs. Joseph Hawkins, Remy Pujol, Donald Caspary, Lindsay Aitkin, Jody Ryan, Michael McGinn, Elizabeth Keithley, Larry Erway, and others. I also validated many ideas in discussions with top European researchers at the European Communities Workshop on hearing in the aged in Helsingor, Denmark, 1989. After all of this consultation, the number of mistakes that slipped by should not be too great.

In reviewing the literature, I did not exclude pieces of work simply because they had shortcomings or equivocal findings. Such an endeavor would be presumptuous and would make for a rather thin book.

Research on the incredibly complex auditory system, using human and animal subjects whose performance and abilities differ as a function of age *and* hearing impairment, almost always falls short of making conclusive findings that are unequivocal or unconfounded in some way. I have made a number of critical comments concerning specific studies, but more emphasis has been placed on *general* research considerations and problems. In doing this I drew on the insights of numerous authors. Because various authors have made similar observations about research difficulties, it was often impossible to make specific attributions concerning these general issues.

The third goal, interpreting the state of the art, is the most subjective. I viewed the implications and future directions of the research from a perspective that is my own, and may differ significantly from that of others. Various audiologists, psychologists, otolaryngologists, and others may give the findings a different emphasis or importance than I have.

I owe thanks to the National Institute on Aging for supporting my training and research on aging and the auditory system over the years, to Lori Bross who provided outstanding technical assistance in the preparation of the book and, above all, to my wife Niki for her patience and support.

CHAPTER 1

Introduction

Many older people have difficulty hearing. Sounds go undetected, words must be repeated, and problems arise in dealing with the acoustic world. Perhaps this is to be expected since hearing is a multistage process requiring high quality representation of sound by the ear, undistorted neural messages carried into the brain by the auditory nerve, accurate processing of the information by the central auditory system, and cognitive competence to deal with the information provided by the auditory system. Disruption of any of these processes with age would have the potential to cause problems with auditory perception. Thus, an understanding of the relationship between aging and auditory perception must take into account factors that might degrade the neural messages sent from the ear to the brain, as well as factors that affect the brain and its ability to process the ear's neural message. The primary goal of this book is to review and synthesize research that has addressed these issues.

PRESBYCUSIS

The terms "presbycusis" and "presbyacusis" are typically used to describe the decline of hearing associated with aging. Although "presbyacusis" is etymologically more accurate, "presbycusis" has gained wide acceptance. There has been a historical tendency (e.g., Roosa, 1885; Zwaardemaker, 1893) to think of presbycusis in terms of elevations of audiometric thresholds. However, the auditory system supports not only the detection of sounds at threshold levels, but also the perception of suprathreshold aspects of sound (loudness, location, etc.), speech, and signals in noise. The effects of aging on these perceptual abilities are certainly of the utmost importance and must be implicit in the term "presbycusis."

In addition to involving a variety of perceptual deficits, presbycusis can arise from several forms of auditory system pathology or dysfunction, both peripheral and central. "Presbycusis," then, refers to *a variety of hearing disorders* that affect the elderly. Whenever possible, the term "presbycusis" should be modified by relevant histopathological, physiological, or psychophysical information concerning the cause(s) of the hearing disorder.

There has been some criticism regarding the use of presbycusis as a "wastebasket" diagnosis of hearing loss (Paparella, 1978). For instance, Lowell and Paparella (1977) pointed out that "presbycusis" is often used as a label for the condition, in older people, of bilateral high-frequency hearing loss often with disproportionate loss of speech recognition, with no

previous history of ear or severe systemic disease, and with gradual onset and a progressive course. However, Lowell and Paparella have argued, familial, genetic, or other etiologies can present a similar pattern of symptoms. They state that presbycusis should refer to "hearing loss simply resulting from the processes of normal aging" (p.1715).

Kryter (1983) has also addressed the confounding of age-related hearing loss by other influences. He argued for use of the terms "presbycusis," "sociocusis," and "nosocusis" to differentiate among hearing loss due to aging, moderate noise exposure or other environmental insults, and common otological maladies, respectively. Sociocusis and nosocusis are not necessarily maladies of the elderly but, like genetic syndromes, could be mistaken for hearing deficits due to aging per se.

The notion that the term "presbycusis" should be reserved for hearing impairment that cannot be accounted for by factors other than aging has validity. However, attempting to completely divorce presbycusis from the effects of genes and the environment is counterproductive. The most fundamental correlates of aging are the extended passage of time and accrual of life experiences, including biological and acoustic ones. When we talk about hearing impairment and *aging*, the process of aging should be viewed as encompassing the effects of endogenous factors (biological changes in cells, tissue, or systems) *and* exogenous factors (changes in the auditory system due to inevitable environmental insults). There can be no aging in the real world without at least some exposure to noise, chemicals, and illnesses that could be detrimental to the auditory system, and the influences of these factors may be fundamental aspects of presbycusis.

The likelihood that various exogenous and endogenous factors often contribute to presbycusis does not imply that noise-induced hearing loss, diseases, or other extraordinary ototraumatic events are not often primary causes of hearing impairment in people, young or old. Such etiological factors often occur outside of the context of aging and should be distinguished from presbycusis when they can be identified. Examples would include industrial or military exposure to traumatizing noise, malignancies affecting the auditory system, physical head trauma, and numerous other factors that are not "ordinary" concomitants of living to an old age.

From the above considerations, a working definition of the term "presbycusis" can be formulated. *Presbycusis refers to the decline of hearing associated with various types of auditory system dysfunction (peripheral and/or central) that accompany aging and cannot be ac-*

counted for by extraordinary ototraumatic, genetic, or pathological conditions. The term "presbycusis" implies deficits not only in absolute thresholds but in auditory perception, as well.

In restricting the definition of presbycusis to problems associated with the *auditory system*, the assumption is made that the tasks of the auditory system include detection, discrimination, and recognition of sounds, words, phrases, and sentences. Cognitive and linguistic processes may sometimes play a role in these auditory tasks, and their involvement will be discussed when germane (e.g., Chapter 10). *Comprehension and memory* of speech and other complex material rely on cognitive and psycholinguistic processes that undoubtedly encompass areas of the brain largely beyond the auditory system. These topics, while of tremendous importance, are not primarily auditory and will not be addressed here.

CAVEATS REGARDING THE INTERPRETATION OF RESEARCH ON PRESBYCUSIS

As the literature on aging and the auditory system is reviewed, it will become evident that interpretation of research findings is sometimes clouded by inconsistencies between studies or shortcomings in some of the work. While these issues will be discussed in later chapters when appropriate, it is not possible to do so in every case. Thus, several caveats should be mentioned at the outset. (a) The definition of "old" and "young" can differ significantly among studies so that "old" may refer to people in their 50's in one study, and people in their 70's in another; likewise, "young" can mean children, very young adults, or young middle-aged. These differences can influence findings significantly. (b) The criteria used to choose subjects for experiments or surveys differ and are sometimes not clearly stated. Subjects are typically screened in some way, and this varies across studies. (c) The severity of hearing loss that constitutes "presbycusis" varies within the literature according to criteria adopted by individual researchers or clinicians and/or by the audiometric standards they employ. In the eyes of some researchers, the degree of auditory dysfunction defining presbycusis is necessarily more severe than what is "normal for age." However, when an elderly person's hearing is "normal for age," he or she still exhibits a substantial loss of hearing relative to younger persons (see Chapter 8). These "normal" elderly people would be classified as having presbycusis if one's criterion were a certain degree of threshold elevation (e.g., 25 dB) compared to the norms for young listeners. Thus, comparison of studies may be affected by

working criteria defining presbycusis. (d) By the same token, the comparability of "normal" hearing old and young subjects is problematic. Older subjects typically have greater hearing loss than young subjects, even when they fall within a normal range or are "normal for their age." Nevertheless, the assumption is often made that the use of "normal-hearing" subjects controls for the effects of hearing loss—an assumption that is often not valid. (e) A number of factors, such as period or cohort effects, can affect *cross sectional studies* of aging, which make up the vast majority of the research studies. Depending on the occurrence of wars, industrialization, dietary practices, etc., different-aged people being tested at the same time may have rather different histories; likewise, comparison of like-aged subjects by studies conducted in different decades or different geographical regions may be confounded. (f) "Types" of presbycusis are typically identified with respect to the presumed or suspected underlying histopathology or pathophysiology (e.g., neural, conductive, etc.). Consequently, the term "presbycusis" tends to become associated with the presumed underlying cause, rather then with the perceptual *hearing* impairment per se. This is particularly true with research on animal models (in which hearing impairment usually must be inferred from histopathology or pathophysiology), "central" presbycusis (in which the perceptual impact of age-related changes in the brain is unclear), or post-mortem cases (in which the subject cannot be tested for hearing). For instance, post-mortem histopathological changes in the cochlea are often used as evidence of some form of pre-mortem peripheral presbycusis, even though audiometric data may not be not available.

Although these and other problems exist in the literature, it has been the author's philosophy to review most of the available research. An attempt has been made to alert the reader to the shortcomings that exist and to interpret the data as accurately as possible.

THE PREVALENCE OF PRESBYCUSIS

Hearing disorders are among the most common health problems of the elderly, as demonstrated by a number of epidemiological surveys such as those summarized in Figures 1-1 through 1-6. Despite quantitative differences in the data, several conclusions can be made from these representative studies. First, it is clear that the prevalence of hearing problems increases substantially with age; at least 25 percent (and perhaps over 50 percent) of septuagenarians have clinically significant degrees of hearing loss that can be detected by routine audiometric methods (the percentages vary

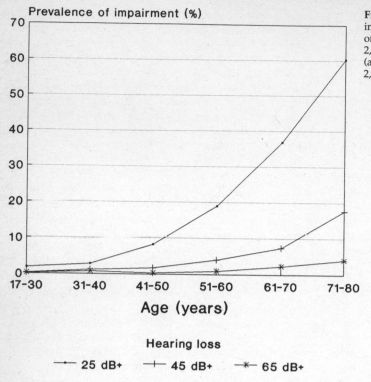

Prevalence of impairment (%)

Better ear

Figure 1-1. Prevalence of hearing impairment in Great Britain as a function of the average threshold for 500, 1,000, 2,000, and 4,000 Hz in the better ear (adapted from Davis, 1989). Sample was 2,662 audiograms.

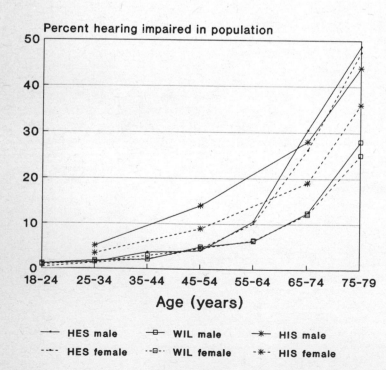

Figure 1-2. Three epidemiological studies (adapted from Davis, 1983). Hearing impairment = better ear >25 dB HL at 500, 1,000, and 2,000 Hz (HES); >35 dB HL, ISO, 1964 (WIL); positive answers to questionnaire (HIS). HES = Health Examination Survey, a sample of about 7,000 in the U.S.A. from 1960-62; WIL = a study by Wilkins (1947) of about 31,000 people in the United Kingdom; HIS = Health Interview Survey conducted in 1971 on 134,000 people selected from 44,000 households in the U.S.A.

Figure 1-3. Hearing impairment: age by frequency (adapted from NCHS, 1980). Hearing impairment = could not hear tones at 31 dB or more at least 50 percent of the time (air conduction).

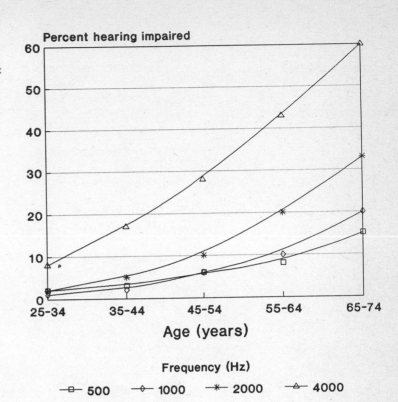

Figure 1-4. Distribution of threshold elevations by frequency in an older population (adapted from Parving, et al., 1983). Sample was 206 Danish men.

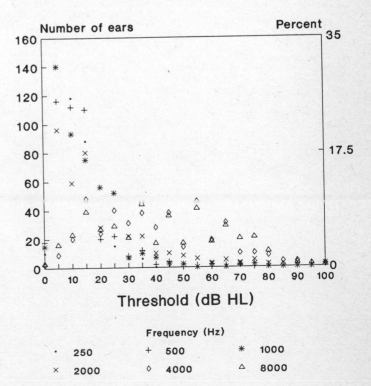

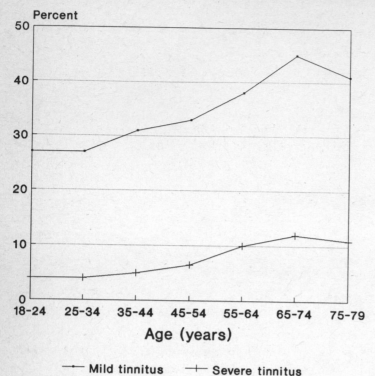

Figure 1-5. Prevalence of tinnitus in the USA (adapted from Leske, 1981).

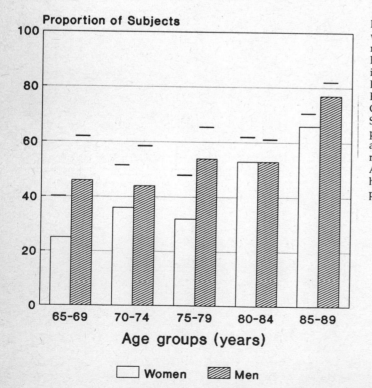

Figure 1-6. The proportion of men and women reporting a hearing problem in response to the question, "Do you have a hearing problem now?" Horizontal bars indicate 95 percent confidence intervals. From the Framingham Heart Study, Framingham, Massachusetts (Gates, Cooper, Kannel, and Miller, 1990). Subjects self-reporting hearing problems performed significantly more poorly on average pure tone threshold (PTA), word recognition (Central Institute for the Deaf Auditory Test W-22), and AMA handicap scores than those denying a problem.

depending on the criterion of hearing loss, testing methods, etc.). It is likely that an even higher prevalence of hearing problems would be detected in the elderly if it were practical for surveys to employ more rigorous methods (e.g., high frequency audiometry or tests using degraded speech). Second, many individuals develop hearing problems well before "old age;" the incidence curves begin to rise during the third and fourth decades (Figs. 1-1 to 1-3). Thus, the notion that presbycusis is an affliction of the elderly needs to be qualified. Although hearing problems are more widespread and, in general, worse in the elderly population, age-related hearing problems may begin in young adulthood or middle age. Third, the prevalence of hearing problems increases with aging to a greater extent in males than in females (Fig. 1-2; 1-6). Finally, with regard to pure tone audiometric hearing loss, most people are more severely affected at high tone frequencies than at low tone frequencies (Figs. 1-3, 1-4).

While epidemiological surveys have tended to focus on thresholds, other hearing disorders are also common in the aging population. Some epidemiological data have been obtained with regard to tinnitus, or "ringing in the ear." Tinnitus is often a manifestation of presbycusis, although its prevalence is difficult to pin down. As reviewed by Milne (1976), Sheldon (1948) determined that tinnitus was reported by 17.8 percent of people over 65 years of age; the data of Hobson and Pemberton (1955) indicated that 37.5 percent of men over 65 and 38.5 percent of women over 60 suffered from tinnitus; in a study by Hinchcliffe (1961), 37 percent of older men and women, aged 65-74, reported tinnitus; the 1960-62 United States Health Survey indicated that 41 to 45 percent of older people suffered from tinnitus. In randomly selected Swedish subjects tested by Axelsson (1991), 24 percent of males and 17 percent of females in their 60's reported that they suffered from tinnitus "always" or "often." One variable that may contribute to the range of tinnitus reported in these surveys is the degree of hearing loss. In a sample of individuals aged 60 to 90, conducted by Milne (1976), 19.2 percent of men and 15.3 percent of women reported experiencing tinnitus. The subjects reporting tinnitus had higher thresholds at 1000 and 4000 Hz than those subjects not reporting tinnitus. In the Framingham Heart Study (Gates, Cooper, Kannel, and Miller, 1990), tinnitus was reported by 14 percent of women and 21 percent of men over 65, and was more common in those reporting a hearing problem (26 percent) than in those not reporting a problem (10 percent). Another source of variance among surveys might be the severity criteria for inclusion of cases. Figure 1-5 presents age functions for tinnitus derived by Leske (1981) that makes this point well. Yet another factor may be the degree of annoyance; older patients with tinnitus may suffer less than young patients (von Wedel, von Wedel, and Zorowska, 1991). This could account for several observations that the prevalence of tinnitus peaks in older middle age and then declines (Reed, 1960; Hazell, 1979). Tinnitus is clearly a significant problem in many elderly people, but it appears to be influenced by a number of variables.

It will be demonstrated throughout this book that presbycusis encompasses a variety of auditory perceptual problems besides threshold elevations and tinnitus. Unfortunately, most of these are difficult to routinely measure in large numbers of individuals and have not been subjected to epidemiological analysis.

ORGANIZATION OF THE BOOK

Our discussion of presbycusis begins with a review of anatomical and physiological correlates of aging, progressing from the outer ear and middle ear (Chapter 2) to the inner ear (Chapters 3 and 4). The etiology of peripheral presbycusis is discussed in Chapter 5 before moving on to the central auditory system (Chapter 6). Chapter 7 addresses the relationship between aging and measures of hearing that have both clinical and theoretical relevance, the acoustic reflex, evoked responses, and otoacoustic emissions. Chapters 8 and 9 review the literature on human psychophysics for non-speech and speech stimuli, respectively. In Chapter 10, material from the previous chapters is synthesized to depict our current understanding of the processes underlying perceptual deficits in the elderly.

CHAPTER 2

Aging and the Outer and Middle Ear

THE OUTER EAR

The outer ear consists of the pinna and the external auditory meatus (ear canal), bounded by the eardrum. Thus, the ability of changes in air pressure (i.e., sound) to effect movements of the eardrum is related to the condition of the outer ear. The pinnae and canals also modify sounds by enhancing the intensity of some frequencies through resonance and by deflecting high-frequency sounds (i.e., producing a "sound shadow"). Because the relative positions of the sound source and ears influence these effects, the outer ear is important for sound localization.

Maurer and Rupp (1979) summarized some changes that may occur in the outer ear of elderly people: (a) hardened and sometimes long-standing wax deposits, of which older people are often unaware (perhaps because of decreased tactile sensation); (b) hair growth in and around the ear canal, especially in males; and (c) prolapsed ear canal, impairing air conduction, especially for high frequencies (Chandler, 1964). There may also be changes in the physical properties of the skin, including atrophy, loss of elasticity, dehydration (Fowler, 1944), and enlargement of the pinnae (Tsai, Fong-Shyong, and Tsa-Jung, 1958), which might affect acoustical properties of the ear.

These changes probably do not affect hearing greatly in most elderly people. However, they could alter the amplitude or resonance characteristics of sound transmitted to the eardrum or change sound shadows used in spatial localization. Thus, their contributions to age-related hearing problems may sometimes be significant (Maurer and Rupp, 1979).

EAR CANAL COLLAPSE

The supporting cartilage of the ear canal often undergoes a degree of atrophy in the elderly (Babbitt, 1947). Pressure from earphones may cause the ear canals to collapse during audiometric testing in some individuals, producing an artifactual elevation of thresholds (Ventry, Chaiklin and Boyle, 1961). Randolph and Schow (1983) evaluated the prevalence of collapsing ear canals, noting that the literature indicated a general trend toward greater prevalence in the elderly (Hildyard and Valentine, 1962; Schow and Goldbaum, 1980). In subjects aged 60 to 79 years, threshold shifts suggestive of collapse were found in over one-third of those tested. Threshold shifts of 15

dB at several frequencies were typical, suggesting that serious measurement errors (including air-bone gaps misconstrued as middle ear conductive losses) may be common in audiometric studies of presbycusis.

THE EARDRUM

Thinning of the eardrum was observed by Zanzucchi (1938) in histological sections of patients aged 51 to 75 years. From clinical observations, Fowler (1944) noted that the eardrum of elderly people was often thinner than normal, sometimes markedly so; however, he felt that thinning alone was not associated with hearing loss. Rosenwasser (1964) also indicated that thinning of the eardrum was concomitant of aging, and Crowe, Guild, and Polvogt (1934) saw destruction of portions of the eardrum in some of their older patients. Recently, Ruah et al. (1991) observed a tendency for thinning of the eardrum in histological material obtained from several elderly patients. The range of thickness shifted downward in several parts of the eardrum including the pars flaccida, posterior quadrant of the pars tensa, and the umbo. Vascularity of the eardrum also decreased in the old subjects. Finally, fibroblasts decreased with aging, and thin elastic fibers in the tissue disappeared and were replaced by thicker fibers that were granular or fragmented. The authors concluded that, with aging, the eardrum "becomes thinner, less vascular, less cellular, more rigid, and less elastic" (p. 54).

Whereas thinning of the eardrum may typically accompany aging, thickening and scarring of the eardrum have also been reported in older patients (Corso, 1963; Crowe, et al., 1934; Hansen, 1973; Leisti, 1949; Nixon, Glorig, and High, 1962). Given the vulnerability of the eardrum to damage "from the outside" and its exposure to middle ear infections "from the inside," it is not surprising that different types of change are observed in the elderly.

THE MIDDLE EAR

The primary structural feature of the air-filled middle ear is the chain of ossicles (malleus, incus, and stapes) that mechanically connects the eardrum to the oval window of the cochlea. Airborne changes in sound pressure between the outer and middle ear cause the eardrum to move, setting the ossicular chain in motion and, ultimately, displacing the fluid-filled compartments of the cochlea. Two muscle systems, the tensor tympani and stapedius, can alter the mechanical efficiency of the chain. The middle ear muscles are reflexively activated by loud sound, presumably to protect the cochlea from over-stimulation. The Eustachian tube connects the middle ear and nasal passages (i.e., outside the middle ear) to allow for equalization of air pressure required for effective performance of the system.

Impairment of the mechanical transmission of sound energy from the outer ear to the cochlea is referred to as conductive hearing loss. Conductive losses can arise from numerous causes, such as middle ear infections and alterations in the physical properties of the ossicular chain. Routine audiometry can be used to identify conductive losses by comparing air- and bone-conduction thresholds. Air conducted sound stimulates the cochlea indirectly, via the middle ear system, whereas bone conducted sound bypasses the middle ear to stimulate the cochlea. A conductive loss is indicated when the air conduction thresholds are significantly higher than the bone conduction thresholds (an air-bone gap).

Since aging is associated with changes in many of the body's joints and muscles, it is reasonable to suppose that the middle ear system may likewise become less effective with age, even in the absence of otosclerosis (discussed below) or other frank pathological conditions. Thus, it is not surprising that a possible role of the middle ear in presbycusis has been assumed for many years (e.g., Politzer, 1926), although its importance has often been underestimated (Davis, 1970) or dismissed (Saxen, 1952). Some European workers in the 1950s proposed middle ear involvement in presbycusis (Proctor, 1960). For instance, Kobrak (1952) and Gatti (1956) suggested that age-related changes in the ossicular chain (e.g., hypotonus of the middle ear muscles) might occur, interfering with the protecting function of the middle ear reflexes and contributing to the pathogenesis of presbycusis.

More recently, Glorig and Davis (1961) argued for *conductive presbycusis* as a major diagnostic category of presbycusis. In an audiometric study of individuals with histories that excluded major noise exposure, an unexpectedly large difference (about 40 dB at 4 kHz) was found between high frequency air- and bone-conduction thresholds (an air-bone gap); thresholds were better for bone conduction, indicating significant conductive impairment (Fig. 2-1). Nixon, Glorig, and High (1962) suggested that changes in the tympanic membrane or loss of mechanical integrity of the ossicles could cause dissipation of sound energy, contributing to this high-frequency gap.

Goodhill (1969) proposed that bilateral malleal fixation, causing conductive hearing loss, can be one cause of presbycusis. He presented a case history of an older patient whose presbycusis was dramatically improved following middle ear surgery to mobilize the malleus. Goodhill suggested that middle ear conductive problems, in the absence of otosclerosis, may be more significant in presbycusis than is typically assumed.

Despite some evidence and the reasonable supposition that aging will affect the joints and muscles of the middle ear, there has been disagreement in the literature with regard to the importance of conductive presbycusis. The disagreement revolves around two indications of conductive loss, the existence of an audiometric air-bone gap in the elderly and changes in the acoustic properties (immitance) of the middle ear system (impedance, admittance, susceptance, compliance).

THE AIR-BONE GAP CONTROVERSY

A high-frequency air-bone gap, such as that reported by Glorig and Davis (1961), can result from several conditions, including constriction of the ear canal, cerumen occlusion in the ear canal, ear canal collapse, mechanical change in the middle ear system (eardrum and/or ossicular chain), and interest variability by the subject during testing (Marshall, Martinez, and Schlaman, 1983). It is conceivable that any of these variables might increase the likelihood of air-bone gaps in the elderly. However, the occurrence of significant air-bone gaps in the elderly has received equivocal support in the literature (Marshall, 1981; Thompson, Sills, Recke, and Bui, 1979).

Klotz and Kilbane (1962), and Sataloff, Vassalo, and Menduke (1965) observed no significant differences in air- and bone-conduction thresholds in the elderly. Goetzinger et al. (1961) selected subjects with good hearing and implied that significant air-bone gaps did not occur: "bone-conduction thresholds had indicated that the shifts in hearing level were perceptive" (p. 666). However, they presented no data on the air-bone gap.

In contrast to these findings, Milne (1977) did report an air-bone gap for high frequencies in subjects aged 62 to 90 years, albeit less pronounced than that of Glorig and Davis (1961). Longitudinal retesting showed no further progression of the gap as a function of aging per se; however, the size of the air-bone gap at high frequencies increased in individuals if hearing loss at those frequencies increased. Rosen (1966) and colleagues studied hearing in the Mabaan tribe of the

Figure 2-1. The audiometric air bone gap (adapted from Glorig and Davis, 1961). "Threshold shift" refers to the difference in the air- and bone-conduction audiograms with the young subjects as a reference.

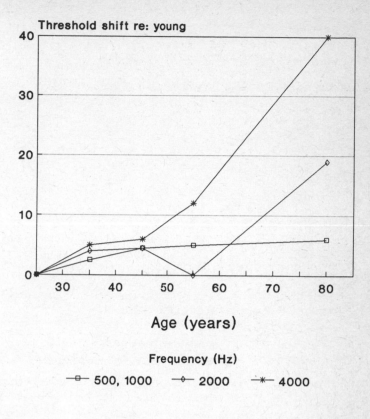

Sudan (a group with little exposure to noise) and discovered an air-bone gap at 4 kHz. The gap increased from zero in their 10 to 29 year group to more than 10 dB in their 70 year-plus group. This gap, while clear, was also a good deal less pronounced than that reported by Glorig and Davis (1961).

Miller and Ort (1965) presented data on a population of residents in a home for the aged, with no screening for "normal" audiograms (Fig. 2-2). They found air-bone gaps of more than 10 dB in more than 20 percent of their 65 to 99-year-olds, with the greatest gap (about 19 dB) occurring for 4 kHz tones (compared to about 14 dB for 250, 500, 1,000, and 2,000 Hz). The great majority of the subjects, however, had high frequency threshold elevations with little or no air-bone gap, indicating sensorineural rather than conductive losses.

Sataloff et al. (1965) cited various problems with bone conduction audiometry as possible contributors to the discrepant findings among studies of the air-bone gap. These include placement and pressure of the oscillator, impedance of the head, occlusion effects, airborne sound from the bone vibrator, etc., implying that the air-bone gap in presbycusis may be an experimental artifact. In this regard, a study by Melrose,

Welsh, and Luterman (1963) is instructive. They tested men aged 74 to 89, screened for unusually good health, using tones as high as 4 kHz, and found very similar mean air- and bone-conduction thresholds. However, "over 20 percent of the bone conduction responses were *less* acute than the air conduction thresholds" (p. 268), suggesting technical problems with air-bone threshold comparisons in the elderly (because, theoretically, hearing by bone conduction can never be worse than by air conduction). Marshall (1983) suggested that another problem may have been that some studies (e.g., Nixon et al., 1962) averaged air-conduction across both ears as a reference for bone conduction thresholds, and this could inflate the apparent air-bone gap for the better ear.

A potential valid source of variance may be the procedures used to screen subjects for inclusion in research studies. At least some studies finding no air-bone gap may have selected their test subjects in a manner that would work against finding an air-bone gap. In the Klotz and Kilbane (1962) study, "no [subject] was included in the final study ... if his air-bone gap suggested the presence of a conductive or partly conductive hearing loss" (p. 278). Miller and Ort's (1965) finding of air-bone gaps in a fairly

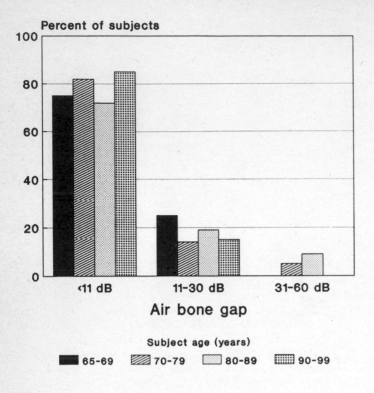

Percent of subjects

Figure 2-2. The audiometric air bone gap (adapted from Miller and Ort, 1965). An air-bone gap of less than 11 dB was considered to be clinically insignificant.

Air bone gap

Subject age (years)

■ 65-69   ▨ 70-79   ▨ 80-89   ▦ 90-99

65-69, N = 12; 70-79, N = 44;
80-89, N = 43; 90-99, N = 13

large proportion of unscreened subjects supports the notion that a significant number of subjects with air-bone gaps are removed from study by screening procedures.

Another relevant variable that may influence the air-bone gap is dietary fat and, presumably, associated circulatory changes. Rosen (1966) described work done in Helsinki on hospitalized patients given a "control" diet high in fat (the normal Finnish diet) and a group given an "experimental" diet low in fat (see also Chapter 5). The 4kHz air-bone gap in 40 to 59-year-old patients was less than 5 dB in the experimental group compared to more than 10 dB in the controls.

Marshall, Martinez, and Schlaman (1983) set out to clarify the air-bone gap controversy. They tested subjects in the third to seventh decade who had no history of recurrent outer or middle ear disease and had tympanogram peak-pressures within normal limits. They defined a high frequency air-bone gap as being at least 15 dB at 4000 Hz. The mean air-bone gap was small at all frequencies tested, and there was no indication of an age effect in the means, standard deviations, or scatterplot. The percentage of subjects with air-bone gaps occurring at 4000 Hz but not at 500 Hz

rose from three percent in young subjects to six percent in the oldest group. Marshall and colleagues then selected eight subjects over 50 with high-frequency air-bone gaps for further testing. The probable cause of the gaps in three of these subjects was cerumen occlusion; four subjects appeared to have mechanical changes of the middle ear system, as indicated by immittance measures; no cause was apparent in one subject. Thus, the findings of Marshall and colleagues indicate that air-bone gaps occur in elderly individuals who have been otologically screened, but the prevalence is only on the order of five percent.

To summarize, there is good evidence of an increasing air-bone gap in a proportion of older persons, particularly at higher frequencies (e.g., 4 kHz). However, the prevalence may only be about five percent in screened subjects. Those studies finding a low incidence of air-bone gaps may have selected for subjects without conductive problems. Thus, in the general population the prevalence of air-bone gaps is likely to be somewhat higher than five percent. High-frequency air-bone gaps might result from several conditions, including cerumen occlusion of the ear canal or mechanical alterations of the ossicular chain.

ACOUSTIC IMMITANCE OF THE MIDDLE EAR

If the ability of the middle ear to transmit sound to the cochlea (i.e., the immitance of the middle ear) were to change with aging, conductive presbycusis might result. Although histological evidence of age-related physical change exists (see below), the literature is, again, in disagreement regarding the effects of aging on immitance measures: acoustic admittance (the ease of energy transmission, sometimes including measures of conductance and susceptance), compliance (the ease with which the structures may be moved), and impedance (resistance to the flow of energy). Jerger, Jerger, and Mauldin (1972) (Fig. 2-3), Alberti and Kristensen (1972), and Blood and Greenberg (1976; 1977) found that compliance *decreases* (i.e., impedance increases) beyond 50 to 60 years. In contrast, Sweitzer (1964, cited by Thompson, et al., 1979) and Beattie and Leamy (1975) found *increased* compliance with aging. Finally, Nerbonne et al. (1978), Osterhammel and Osterhammel (1979a), Thompson, Sills, Recke, and Bui (1979), and Wilson (1981) found *no significant age effect* on acoustic properties of the middle ear. There were some trends in the latter studies, but they did not coincide: Wilson (1981) found a non-significant trend for older subjects to have higher admittance. In con-

trast, the Osterhammels' (1979a) data suggest a downward trend in compliance in older subjects (Fig. 2-5), although the variance in the data (shown as standard errors of the mean) was quite high. One aspect of all of these studies is that the immitance values do not stray far (if at all) from the normal clinical range.

Thompson and colleagues (1979) suggest several possible explanations for the widely discrepant conclusions of these studies, including differences in instrumentation and calibration, subject age groups, or experimental design. As seen in Figure 2-4, the frequency used to measure immitance may affect the age function. Subtle methodological flaws may also influence the data. For instance Marshall (1981) pointed out that the Beattie and Leamy study used only males in their old group, and both males and females in their young comparison group; some studies have found that females, in general, have lower acoustic admittance than men, possibly confounding the findings.

Another potentially confounding factor is that age-related changes in immitance may not be a simple function of age across the life span. The data of Jerger et al. (1972) showed an increase in static compliance between the second and fourth decades, followed by a gradual decrease in later years (Fig. 2-3). The Osterhammels' (1979a) findings (Fig. 2-5) also suggest a non-linear age function for compliance. It might

Figure 2-3. Static compliance of the middle ear (adapted from Jerger et al., 1972).

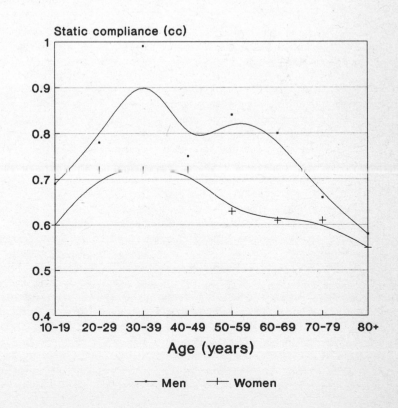

make a substantial difference in an experiment's findings depending on the age of the "young" and "old" subject groups that are being compared.

To summarize, the acoustic properties of the aging middle ear appear to vary a great deal among individuals, and no consistent or pronounced trends have emerged from the literature. The way that subjects are selected for research studies also makes it difficult to assess the prevalence of abnormal middle ear immittance in the elderly. As was the case with the air-bone gap studies, selection criteria for experimental subjects has used normal-hearing subjects with no signs of middle ear impairments, such as air-bone gaps (e.g., Thompson et al., 1979; Wilson, 1981; Osterhammel and Osterhammel, 1979a). Thus, if a portion of older listeners in the general population were to exhibit age-related changes in middle ear immittance, they would be excluded from these studies, making it less likely that significant age effects would be found. As an alternative research strategy, it might prove interesting to select older listeners who *do* exhibit immittance changes and determine if there are any factors other than aging (e.g., history of infection or trauma) that caused these changes. Then, one could determine what proportion of middle ear conductive hearing loss fits the definition of presbycusis (Chapter 1).

HISTOPATHOLOGY OF THE MIDDLE EAR

Crowe, Guild, and Polvogt (1934) performed a histopathological study that included many older patients with high-frequency hearing loss. They divided these and other subjects on the basis of histopathology of the middle and inner ears compared to a control group with normal hearing. Middle ear pathology was not common in older patients, with more than 90 percent showing no evidence of abnormal degrees of middle ear pathology. Histological changes that were found in older subjects included fibrous adhesions on the stapes and fibrous tissue surrounding portions of the ossicular chain.

The ossicles of subjects who had no clinical or pathological evidence of a specific ear disease were described by Belal (1975). Belal saw an increased diameter of the Haversian systems (the basic unit of structure in compact bone) and cavities of varying size and shape indicative of osteoporosis, replacement of bone structure by fibrous tissue, increased number of fat cells in the bone marrow, and thickening of the intraosseous blood vessels and reduced lumina. Since these

changes were not associated with significant hearing loss or an air-bone gap, they apparently had little effect on hearing.

The ossicular joints were evaluated histologically by Harty (1953), who provided evidence that aging is accompanied by fragmentation of the capsule of ossicular joints. Rosenwasser (1964) observed ossicular atrophy, ossification of the malleoincudal joint, and calcification of joint cartilage. Hansen (1973) found "severe osteitic lesions" in 2 of 12 elderly patients who also had cochlear pathology. Gussen (1968) observed calcification in the cartilage at the stapediovestibular joint (where stapes contacts oval window) in all of her temporal bone specimens from people older than 30 years.

Etholm and Belal (1974) and Belal (1975) found signs of arthritic change in the middle ear that began before age 30 and increased with age. The earliest changes consisted of fraying of the articular cartilage and the appearance of vacuoles in the ground substance. This was followed by thinning and calcification of the cartilage, atrophy and hyalinization of the elastic capsule surrounding the articular border of the cartilage, and atrophy of the articular disc. In individuals over 70, complete fusion of the space between bone joints could occur. They devised the histopathological classification scheme shown in Table 2-1. Grade 3 classifications were observed in the incudomalleal joint in 20 percent of subjects under age 30, rose to 66 percent in subjects aged 30 to 70, and reached 81.6 percent in subjects over 70. For the incudostapedial joint, the percentages of grade 3 classification in these three age groups were zero, 36 percent, and 68 percent, respectively. Grade 1 classifications were not observed in either joint in any subjects older than 70 years.

In the study of Etholm and Belal, audiometric data were available for 32 subjects. The details of the testing were not presented, but there was apparently no air-bone gap in 31 of the subjects, indicating that the histological changes found (Table 2-1) did not cause conductive hearing loss. However, this study did not rule out the possibility of high-frequency conductive losses.

Belal (1975) observed some age-related increases in the amounts of endomysium (the sheath of fibrils surrounding muscle fibers) and perimysium (the connective tissue demarcating muscle fiber fascicles) in the stapedius muscle and fatty tissue around the tensor tympani muscle fibers. These changes were apparently minor and were found irrespective of the degree of hearing loss.

To summarize, alterations of the ossicular tissue and arthritic changes seem to be rather common in aging middle ears. However, a relationship between

Figure 2-4. Middle ear immitance measured with 220 and 660 Hz tones (adapted from Thompson et al., 1979). 100 percent equals the mean value of young subjects.

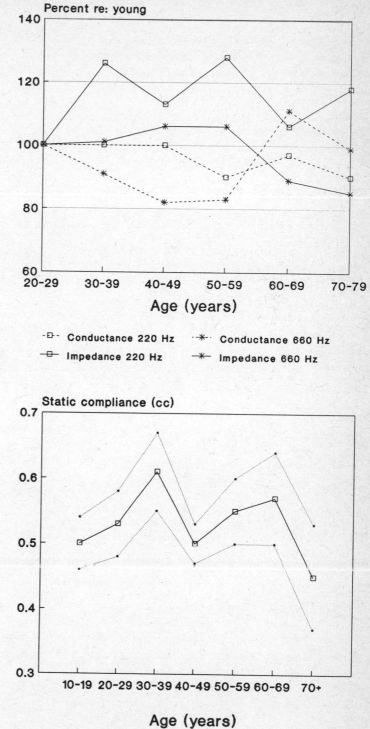

Figure 2-5. Static compliance of the middle ear (adapted from Osterhammel and Osterhammel, 1979a).

TABLE 2-1. HISTOPATHOLOGICAL GRADING OF ARTHRITIS OF ETHOLM AND BELAL (1974)

Grade	Capsule	Articular Cartilage	Arthritic Changes Disc	Joint-space
I (mild)		fraying, vacuolation, fibrillation		
II (moderate)	hyalinization	thinning, calcification	hyaline deposits	narrowing
III (severe)	calcification	diffuse calcification	calcium deposits	obliteration

such observations and conductive hearing loss has not been shown.

THE EUSTACHIAN TUBE

One potential source of middle ear dysfunction in the elderly is impaired function of the Eustachian tube, the mechanism by which middle ear pressure is maintained. Age-related decline of muscle function that opens the Eustacian tube (e.g., during swallowing) might be expected to hamper its ability to equalize pressure, thereby contributing to presbycusis. With this possibility in mind, Chermak and Moore (1981) and Newman and Spitzer (1981) evaluated Eustachian tube functioning in the elderly using tympanometric measurement of middle ear pressure. Neither study found a significant age effect in response (middle ear pressure change after swallowing) to a given test condition (alteration in ear canal pressure). However, Newman and Spitser obtained a statistical interaction between age and tympanometric condition, which, the authors suggest, might indicate an aging influence on Eustachian tube efficiency. They presented subjects with both increased and decreased air pressure conditions. Middle ear pressure of both young and old subjects shifted in the expected direction for each condition, but the magnitude of the shifts was reduced in the older subjects.

Belal's (1975) histological study found some age-related changes in the Eustachian tube, mostly in its cartilaginous portion. The number of cilia were reduced and goblet cells had disappeared, the tunica propria (lining) had a "less evident" lymphoid layer, and elastic fibers were fragmented and reduced in number, and there was some calcification of cartilage.

However, these changes were found in subjects that had no history of hearing impairment. An earlier study by Terracol, Corone, and Guerrier (1949) concluded that calcification of Eustachian tube cartilage occurred in older patients but was not as frequent as in other cartilaginous tissues.

Taking the studies together, age-related changes in the Eustachian tube do not seem to be a major contributor to presbycusis.

MIDDLE EAR DISEASES IN THE ELDERLY

Otosclerosis is a fairly common otologic disease with a strong genetic component (Konigsmark, 1971) and an insidious onset, usually appearing during adulthood. Konigsmark (1971) summarized the characteristics of otosclerosis as follows: (a) autosomal dominant genetic transmission; (b) gradual onset of hearing loss in the middle decades of life; (c) slow progressive, conductive, or mixed (conductive plus sensorineural[1]) bilateral hearing loss of varying severity; (d) normal vestibular responses. Threshold elevations tend to occur at low, as well as high frequencies (Linthicum et al., 1975) but may be greatest at the higher frequencies (Schuknecht, 1974).

An otosclerotic lesion consists of a focal spongy overgrowth of bone containing numerous small blood vessels. The lesion typically attacks the cochlear capsule near the oval window and may spread toward the round window and up the basal turn of the cochlea. A "bridge formation" can be observed between the stapes footplate and oval window, which can be entirely covered by otosclerotic bone (Konigsmark, 1971; Ruedi and Spoendlin, 1966).

---

[1] Because otoscerosis often involves sensorineural pathology, it does not fit snugly into the present chapter on the middle ear. Nevertheless, its initial site of action is typically the middle ear conductive mechanism, so it has been included in this chapter. Sensorineural aspects of otosclerosis are discussed in Chapter 5.

Otosclerosis is usually manifested first as a conductive disorder prior to old age (Lindsay, 1985) and often progresses to include sensorineural involvement, particularly in older adults. For instance, a study by Jorgensen and Kristensen (1967) found the highest incidence of histological otosclerosis (i.e., not necessarily manifested clinically) in subjects aged 60 to 80 years (18 percent of temporal bones) and 80 to 100 years (10 percent of temporal bones); no subjects under 20 years in this sample had signs of otosclerosis. It is appropriate, therefore, to include this disease in a discussion of aging and the auditory system.

Other middle ear diseases, such as acute, recurrent, or chronic *otitis media* do not appear to be especially prevalent in the elderly (Corcoran and Axline, 1982). Furthermore, histopathological changes in the middle ear mucosa are typically more severe in children than in older individuals for the same types of otitis media (Yoon et al., 1990). However, according to Rosenwasser (1964), when acute otitis media does occur after age 60, the relative prevalence of mastoiditis and other complications is sharply increased.

CONCLUSIONS

The importance of middle ear conductive disorders in presbycusis is often minimized. Statements such as, "it is ... generally accepted that the middle ear, despite its arthritic joint changes, does not contribute to hearing loss in the aged" (Anderson and Meyerhoff, 1982, p. 357) are common in the literature. The evidence supports the conclusion that the majority of elderly listeners show few, if any, signs of conductive loss if they have been screened for middle ear disorders. However, it is likely that a significantly larger proportion of the general, unscreened population of elderly listeners is affected by conductive problems.

CHAPTER 3

Histopathology of the Human Inner Ear and Its Relationship to Presbycusis

The mechanical motion of the middle ear ossicles against the oval window of the cochlea leads to the next step in the process of hearing: the transduction of mechanical activity into neural responses to be relayed to the brain. For normal hearing to occur, the various functional components of the inner ear (sensory, neural, vascular, supporting, synaptic, mechanical, etc.) must function in an interactive, interdependent manner. In theory, aging could be associated with malfunction of virtually any of these components, resulting in disruption of physiological processes to cause presbycusis. In this chapter, the literature on the aging human cochlea is reviewed, to be followed in Chapter 4 by an examination of related research on non-human animals. The etiology of inner ear presbycusis is discussed in Chapter 5.

Research on the aging human inner ear has relied heavily upon the analysis of post-mortem histopathological material, since most other anatomical and physiological methods cannot be practically or ethically employed with humans. Consequently, presbycusis associated with inner ear disorders has been conceptualized in terms of the specific forms of histopathology thought to be responsible for hearing impairment. The most influential organizational scheme has been that of Schuknecht (1964, 1974), which distinguishes between pathology of the organ of Corti *(sensory presbycusis)*, spiral ganglion cells and their processes *(neural presbycusis)*, the stria vascularis *(strial presbycusis)*, and the basilar membrane, spiral ligament and other structures related to cochlear mechanics *(mechanical, or cochlear conductive presbycusis)*. The work of other researchers indicates that presbycusis associated with inner ear vascular pathology *(vascular presbycusis)* and the combined pathology of different cochlear tissue *(sensorineural presbycusis)* should be added to the list, as well. To mesh with this conceptual framework, the ensuing discussion is organized according to these six types of histopathology, followed by an assessment of the validity of six associated types of presbycusis.

RESEARCH CONSIDERATIONS

Several caveats should be mentioned in dealing with human histological material from autopsies.

With human temporal bones from autopsy, pathology might be more likely than it would be in the overall population, since the diseases that caused the death of the patient may be responsible for some of the changes seen (Hansen, 1973; Johnsson and Hawkins, 1972a).

Peripheral pathology in the elderly may include the influence of superimposed conditions, such as noise-induced or ototoxic pathology (see Chapters 4 and 5).

Post-mortem autolytic changes can cause artifacts in histological material, particularly in the organ of Corti (Schuknecht, 1974). According to Soucek, Michaels, and Frohlich (1987) outer hair cells (OHCs) are well preserved if they are perfused with fixative within a day of death. Inner hair cells (IHCs), on the other hand, may demonstrate significant autolysis if they are not fixed within 10 hours of death. Bagger-Sjoback and Engstrom (1985) obtained fixation suitable for electron microscopy within 6 hours of death; however, after 12 hours, reliability of results was poor. Unfortunately, histological material is often obtained at longer post-mortem intervals than these.

Most researchers are aware of these potential problems and take care to minimize them or to qualify conclusions appropriately. Thus, a great deal of valid histopathological data has been obtained from post-mortem human tissue.

AGE-RELATED HISTOPATHOLOGY OF THE ORGAN OF CORTI

BACKGROUND

The organ of Corti is the site of transduction of mechanical to neural energy. Destruction or impairment of organ of Corti tissue would be expected to interfere with the transduction process to produce a loss of sensitivity to sounds.

The organ of Corti sits atop the basilar membrane and is comprised of the sensory cells (OHCs and IHCs), tectorial membrane, and supporting cells (inner and outer pillar cells, cells of Hensen, Deiters, among others). The inner and outer hair cells appear to comprise two rather different systems with different functional roles. IHCs are the major, if not sole, site of transduction of mechanical energy (displacement of the basilar membrane) to neural activity (action potentials to the brain via the eighth nerve). OHCs appear to alter the sensitivity of the cochlea, perhaps acting more as effectors than as sensory receptor cells. Loss of IHCs in a region of the cochlea would be expected to eliminate that region's participation in hearing; loss of OHCs would have a less devastating effect on cochlear input to the brain, but might alter properties of the cochlea (e.g., mechanics) in ways that would significantly elevate thresholds.

The integrity of *Reissner's membrane* is important to the fluid environment of the organ of Corti and stria vascularis (see below), separating the endolymph in contact with these structures from the perilymph of the scala vestibuli.

Stereocilia have a number of structural features that are probably important for efficient performance of sensory cells, including their number, length (which varies according to position on individual hair cells and baso-apical location of the hair cells), attachment to the tectorial membrane (at least for tall outer hair cell stereocilia), the charged stereocilia coat, cross-link connections among neighboring stereocilia, and the protein structure of the stereocilia and cuticular plate, which includes the contractile protein actin (Nielsen and Slepecky, 1986). Age-related changes in stereocilia (e.g., fusion, distortion) would presumably affect at least some functional properties of stereocilia and, consequently, the process of sensory transduction.

The *tectorial membrane* plays an integral role in cochlear function because it is a determinant of stereocilia motion. Movement of the basilar and tectorial membranes causes a shearing action of stereocilia that leads to the transduction of mechanical to neural energy.

HISTOPATHOLOGY

DEGENERATION OF THE ORGAN OF CORTI

A number of studies have reported degenerative changes in the organ of Corti of aging people (Table 3-1). In an early publication, von Fieandt and Saxen (1937) reported flattening and compression of the organ of Corti, reduced numbers of sensory cells, deformity of supporting cells, and, in advanced cases, replacement of the organ of Corti by an epithelial layer. Although some authors have suggested that these early observations may have been tainted by post-mortem artifact (Lange, 1937; Fernandez, 1958; Hansen and Reske-Nielsen, 1965), more recent reports (e.g., Bredberg, 1968) have described a general loss of structural integrity or "collapse" of the organ of Corti in cochleas of elderly persons. There is little doubt that pathology of the organ of Corti is common in the elderly (Table 3-1).

TABLE 3-1. STUDIES SHOWING AGE-RELATED ORGAN OF CORTI ATROPHY

Fabinyi (1931): basal losses often found, but correlation with aging was unclear

Crowe et al. (1934): characteristic of "abrupt high tone" loss; most frequently found by middle age

von Fieandt and Saxon (1937): interpreted as secondary to angiosclerotic degeneration

Schuknecht (1964, 1967, 1974, 1989): one of the four major types of presbycusis

Hansen and Reske-Nielsen (1965): flattening of organ of Corti (may be post-mortem artifact)

Bredberg (1968): IHC loss confined to cochlear base; OHC loss throughout, especially at base and apex

Johnsson and Hawkins (1972a, 1979): often seen; usually accompanying but preceding neural degeneration

Johnsson (1974): loss of sensory cells was accompanied by neural loss

Belal (1975): OHC loss was greater than IHC loss

Suga and Lindsay (1976): often saw "diffuse senile atrophy" of the organ of Corti

Soucek et al. (1987): felt sensory degeneration was the primary lesion of presbycusis

Engstrom et al. (1987): all subjects over 50 had some loss of OHCs and IHCs

Gleeson and Felix (1987): scanning EM showed loss of hair cells and build-up of lipofuscin

Wright et al. (1987): loss of inner and outer hair cells in normal hearing (for age) older people

Zallone et al. (1987): supporting cells are key to secondary sensorineural degeneration

---

The loss of hair cells is in general most severe in the basal region of the cochlea (e.g., Crowe et al., 1934; Schuknecht, 1974; 1989). However, Bredberg (1968) identified two other patterns of sensory cell degeneration that were not necessarily related to the baso-apical location. These patterns, occurring in about one third of his patients, involved either the loss of OHCs over a fairly wide area (5 to 10 mm) or a severe loss of both outer and inner hair cells over a distance of less than 5 mm.

Another factor determining the severity of age-related degeneration of OHCs is the row in which they are located. Degeneration of the outer row of OHCs is often more severe than in the other rows (Bredberg, 1968; Schuknecht, 1974; Soucek et al., 1987).

After degeneration of both outer and inner hair cells, the reticular lamina, which supports the upper end of the hair cells, heals over (Johnsson and Hawkins, 1972a). Apparently, the phalangeal processes of Deiters cells (which support the OHCs) grow together and cover the gap left by the missing hair cells, producing "phalangeal scars" (Johnsson and Hawkins, 1979).

According to Schuknecht (1974), sensory changes usually begin in middle age (but often before the third decade) and may accelerate in later years. Lesions generally continue to be most severe in the basal region of the cochlea.

OTHER HISTOPATHOLOGICAL CHANGES

Age-related changes less severe than total degeneration of hair cells have been described. "*Giant stereocilia*," the result of adhesion and enlargement of adjacent stereocilia, have been observed in hair cells of

elderly people by several groups of researchers. Engstrom and colleagues (1987) found fused or modified stereocilia in many inner and outer hair cells of older subjects (compare Fig. 3-1 A and B). Giant stereocilia were observed by Soucek and colleagues (1987) in OHCs of the apical and middle coils, but not in the basal cochlea. A smaller number of giant stereocilia were observed in IHCs throughout the cochlea. In a study by Gleeson and Felix (1987), the cochleas of three subjects aged 47, 70, and 84 years were evaluated with light- and electron-microscopy. Giant stereocilia were observed on hair cells of each of their subjects, especially on the OHCs. However, the largest number of giant stereocilia were seen on OHCs of their youngest (47-year-old) subject, who had nor-

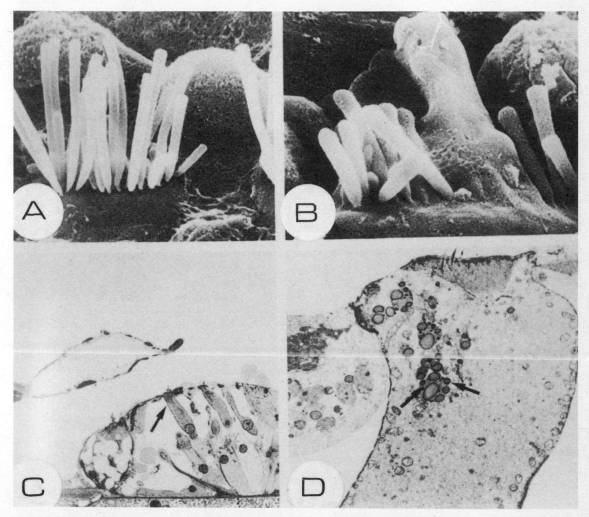

Figure 3-1. Micrographs of human cochleas. A. Scanning EM of a normal looking IHC in the apical turn of a 64-year-old woman. B. An IHC with fused cilia from the basal turn of an elderly man. C. Light micrograph of the organ of Corti; arrow points to lipofuscin in an OHC. D. Transmission EM showing the upper portion of an OHC; arrow indicates lipofuscin. From Engstrom, B., Hillerdal, M., & Laurell, G. (1987) Selected pathological findings in the human cochlea. *Acta Otolaryngology Supplement* 436:110–116, with permission.

mal hearing for his age. Thus, the functional significance of giant stereocilia and their relationship to aging remain unclear.

The *tectorial membrane* appears to fare relatively well during aging, at least at the light microscopic level. Bredberg (1968) reported that the tectorial membrane covered the organ of Corti in all cochleas studied. In areas of complete organ of Corti degeneration the tectorial membrane was never observed to be displaced from its normal position. In the material of Suga and Lindsay (1976) degeneration of the stria, hair cells and supporting cells—even when severe—was not associated with atrophy of the tectorial membrane. Of course, once OHCs have degenerated, the role of the tectorial membrane is presumably moot.

A few studies have noted changes in *Reissner's membrane*, but severe damage appears to be rare. Reissner's membrane can become vacuolized in older cochleas (Johnsson, 1973), and in a few cases studied by Jorgensen (1961) it had become adhered to a portion of the stria vascularis superiorly. Similar findings were reported by von Fieandt and Saxen (1937). The effects of age on this tissue warrants further scrutiny, because atrophy of Reissner's membrane could have significant consequences regarding presbycusis. Mixing of perilymph from the scala vestibuli and the endolymph of the scala media might disrupt the electrical potentials generated by the endolymph system and interfere with the functioning of the organ of Corti, or even cause secondary damage to cochlear tissue (Duvall, 1968; Lawrence, 1966).

OUTER VERSUS INNER HAIR CELL DAMAGE

Differences in the spatial pattern of OHC and IHC loss along the baso-apical dimension are often the case in older ears. The data summarized in Figure 3-2 were obtained from a population with varying degrees of high-frequency hearing loss studied by Bredberg (1968). IHC loss is largely restricted to the basal cochlea, whereas OHC loss occurs in the apex and, to a lesser extent, the middle cochlea. A similar pattern was observed in subjects with normal hearing for their age by Wright and colleagues (1987)(Figs. 3-3 and 3-4): IHC loss with aging was restricted to the cochlear base, whereas OHC losses occurred in both base and apex. A consistent finding in the study by Johnsson and Hawkins (1972a) was severe to complete loss of OHCs (with only mild nerve degeneration) in the upper apical turn.

If the total number of hair cells is counted without respect to location along the basilar membrane, age-related degeneration of OHCs is typically more severe than degeneration of IHCs (compare Figs. 3-3 and 3-4). In the study of Bredberg (1968), shown in Figure 3-5,

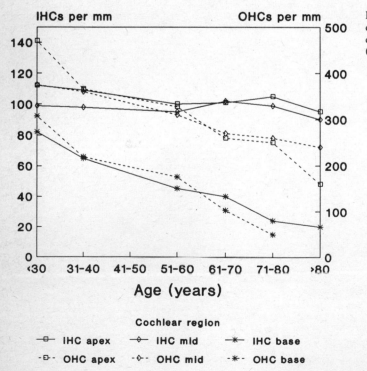

Figure 3-2. Density of hair cells per mm by cochlear region in subjects with varying degrees of high frequency hearing loss (adapted from Bredberg, 1968).

Figure 3-3. Number of inner hair cells in subjects with hearing "normal for age" (adapted from Wright et al., 1987). See also Figure 3-4.

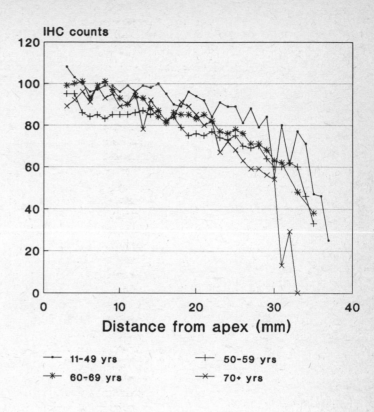

Figure 3-4. Number of outer hair cells in subjects with hearing "normal for age" (adapted from Wright et al., 1987). See also Figure 3-3.

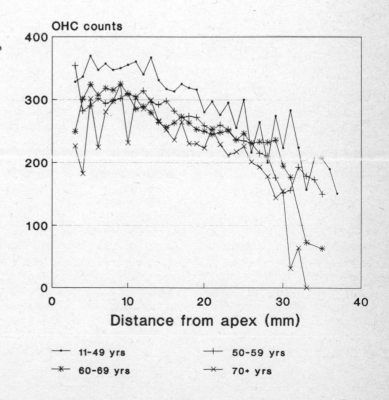

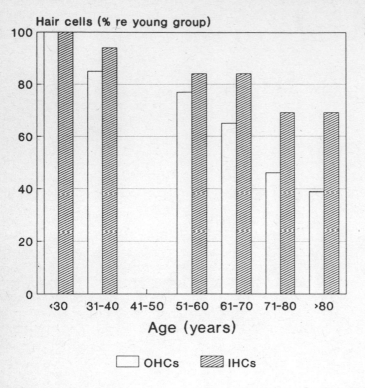

Figure 3-5. Loss of inner and outer hair cells (adapted from Bredberg, 1968).

OHCs decreased from more than 12,000 before age 30 to less than 6,000 by age 70. IHCs decreased from about 3,000 to about 2,000. All available audiometric data indicated high frequency threshold elevations in the elderly subjects of this study.

Soucek, Michaels, and Frohlich (1987) obtained surface preparations of the organ of Corti from subjects who had demonstrated severe high-frequency loss and some low-frequency loss prior to death. The number of OHCs in the inner row decreased from about 120-200 cells per mm in subjects less than 1 year-old to 0-100 cells per mm in subjects older than 65; the outer-row OHCs decreased from about 120-140 per mm to 0-80. IHC counts were near zero in the basal coil of some cochleas of elderly patients, with only moderate losses in the middle and apical turns.

It is clear that IHCs and OHCs can degenerate independently and that OHCs are typically more vulnerable to damage. Both types of hair cells are particularly susceptible in the basal region of the cochlea, but OHC damage is likely to be found in the apical and mid-cochlear regions as well.

RELATIONSHIP OF HISTOPATHOLOGY TO HEARING IMPAIRMENT

The organ of Corti of older people typically has some degree of pathology, even in the absence of presbycusis. Seven of 15 subjects in the "control" group (middle-aged individuals with "good" hearing to at least 8192 Hz) of Crowe and colleagues (1934) showed organ of Corti pathology in the most basal 2-3 mm of the cochlea. Belal (1975) found atrophy of the organ of Corti in the first half of the basal cochlear turn in older patients with "normal" hearing.

Hair cell counts were obtained by Wright and coworkers (1987) from people whose audiometric thresholds were within normal limits for their age (i.e., showed some elevation relative to young listeners; see Chapter 8) prior to their death. As shown in Figures 3-3 and 3-4, there was an age-related decrease in the number of hair cells in this population, with the loss of OHCs being somewhat more pronounced than the loss of IHCs. Decreased numbers of both types of hair cells were most pronounced within about 10 mm of the cochlear base, with lesser OHC losses occurring near the apex as well. These findings suggested to the authors that the loss of hair cells, particularly OHCs, is responsible for the "normal" decline of hearing with aging.

Bredberg (1968) determined that a loss of up to 40 percent of apical OHCs (250-720 Hz region of the cochlea) could occur with less than 15 dB hearing loss; even a 50 to 75 percent loss of OHCs here was associated with losses less than 40 dB. In contrast, relatively small losses near the cochlear base were associated with greater threshold elevations (e.g., 25 percent loss led to 20-30 dB elevations; 50 percent loss led to 50-75 dB elevations). Bredberg did not find a correspondence between the degree of IHC loss and threshold elevations.

The examples of histopathology in patients diagnosed as having sensory presbycusis, presented by Schuknecht and colleagues (Gacek and Schuknecht, 1969; Schuknecht, 1964; 1974; 1989), typically show losses in excess of 50 percent within the basal 10 mm of

the organ of Corti and, in some cases, less severe losses of sensory cells in more apical regions (Fig. 3-6).

Belal (1975) presented data on six elderly patients with clinically significant high-frequency threshold elevations and, apparently, good speech recognition. Two had complete atrophy of both inner and outer hair cells extending 15 mm (of a total length of 33 mm) from the cochlear base; the remaining four had a near total loss of OHCs to 9-12 mm from the base, with less severe loss of IHCs. (One case had no loss of IHCs.)

In summary, a substantial hair cell loss in the basal few mm of the cochlea can occur in aging individuals with little effect on audiometric thresholds at frequencies usually tested (e.g., 8 kHz or less). However, the ubiquitous pathology of hair cells in the extreme cochlear base suggests that high frequency losses probably occur in virtually all older people (see Chapter 8). A loss of about 20 percent of hair cells throughout the cochlea appears to result in minimal significant hearing loss ("normal for age"). More severe loss of hair cells, particularly OHCs, extending 10 mm or more from the base of the cochlea, is likely to produce significant presbycusis at high frequencies.

Figure 3-6. Sensory presbycusis, audiogram and histopathology (adapted from Nadol, 1981). mm on abscissa refers to distance from cochlear base.

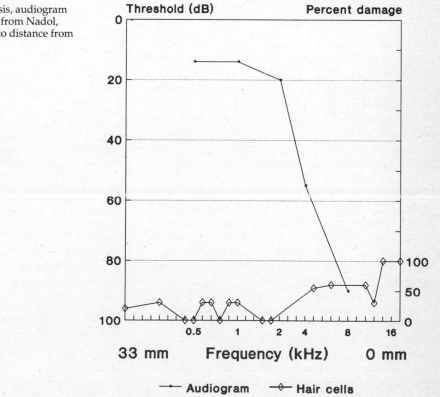

AGE-RELATED HISTOPATHOLOGY OF THE SPIRAL GANGLION CELLS AND THEIR PROCESSES

BACKGROUND

The cell bodies of the cochlear neurons (spiral ganglion cells) are located in the central core of the cochlea (modiolus). Their peripheral dendritic processes pass through the osseous spiral lamina to the organ of Corti where they innervate the hair cells. The majority of ganglion cells are Type I, with peripheral processes that follow a fairly direct radial course to synapse with IHCs. Peripheral processes of smaller Type II ganglion cells take a spiral course, branching to synapse with a number of OHCs. Centrally-directed axons of the ganglion cells transmit sensory information via the auditory portion of the eighth nerve to the central auditory system for further processing. Degeneration or reduction in the number of ganglion cells would presumably alter the auditory information entering the brain.

Efferents to the IHCs (inner spiral fibers) travel in the inner spiral bundle to synapse with the radial dendrites. Efferents to the OHCs cross the tunnel of Corti and synapse directly on the hair cells. Efferent fibers permit nerve impulses originating in the central nervous system to influence cochlear physiology. Although the precise function of the efferent system(s) is unclear, it may influence the functional state of the cochlea, perhaps by affecting the process of synaptic transmission between sensory cells and afferent terminals (e.g., inhibition), by causing contraction of hair cells, and/or by other means. A loss of efferents would presumably alter the transduction process in denervated regions.

HISTOPATHOLOGY

Studies demonstrating neural histopathology are summarized in Table 3-2. As is the case with sensory cells, the age-related loss of ganglion cells and their processes is typically greatest near the base of the cochlea. For instance, Saxen (1952) found losses in excess of 50 percent in the basal cochlea with little loss more apically. Crowe and coworkers (1934) reported a prevalence of neural degeneration in the basal cochlea in their older patients whose hearing loss extended

TABLE 3-2. STUDIES SHOWING AGE-RELATED LOSS OF GANGLION CELL/NERVE FIBERS

Early reports (Habermann, 1891; Bruhl, 1905; Manasse, 1906)[**]

Fabinyi (1931): virtually all patients over 60 had ganglion cell/nerve degeneration but only half had organ of Corti or strial atrophy

Guild et al. (1931): greatest and most consistent losses in the cochlear base

Crowe et al. (1934): characteristic of "gradual high-tone loss" group

von Fieandt and Saxen (1937): "senile atrophy of the spiral ganglion"

Saxen (1952):"senile atrophy of the ganglion cochleare" is an independent and self-contained disease; the organ of Corti often appears normal.

Rasmussen (1940): small loss of eighth nerve fibers with age

Altmann (1955)[*]: ganglion cell atrophy not necessarily associated with hair cell loss.

Fleischer (1956): basal loss as early as third or fourth decade; most consistent correlate of aging

Jorgensen (1961):loss of ganglion cells in cochlear base, progressing with age

Schuknecht (1964, 1974, 1989): one of the four types of presbycusis

Hansen and Reske-Nielsen (1965): ganglion cell loss in basal cochlea

Makishima (1967): basal losses were the most consistent histopathological correlate of aging

Nomura and Kirikae (1967,68): some efferent fibers survive radial fiber loss

Bredberg (1968): losses in cochlear base and patchy degeneration

Krmpotic-Nemanic (1971): caused by ossification and cuffing of fiber bundles

Johnsson and Hawkins (1972a): pure neural presbycusis seen in only a few cases; usually preceded by sensory cell atrophy

Johnsson (1974): "pure" neural presbycusis seen in only five percent of cases

Belal (1975):severe ganglion cell loss in patients with poor speech recognition

Nomura (1976): radial fibers survive efferents

Suga and Lindsay (1976): only change seen in about half of their cases

Otte et al. (1978): ganglion cell loss correlated with speech recognition and other variables

Nadol (1979):various ultrastructural degenerative changes in ganglion cells and dendrites prior to loss of cochlear neurons

Pauler et al. (1986): primary degeneration of ganglion cells; correlation of loss in 15-22 mm segment and speech recognition

Engstrom et al. (1987): some loss of fibers in all subjects over 50, especially in cochlear base

Suzuka and Schuknecht (1988): small but significant loss of ganglion cells with normal hearing

Spoendlin and Schrott (1989, 1990): loss and pathology of eighth nerve fibers

Johnsson et al. (1990): patchy degeneration; greater degeneration of peripheral dendritic processes

[*]cited by Rosen et al. (1964)
[**]cited by Bredberg (1968)

across high frequencies.[1] In a sample of post-mortem material from older patients (mean 79 years) with confirmed high-frequency threshold elevations, Hansen (1973) found that the number of ganglion cells was normal or slightly reduced in the middle and apical portion of the cochlea, but severely reduced in the base. There is often a complete loss of nerve fibers in the most basal 2-3 mm of the cochlea of older subjects (Bredberg, 1968).

"Patchy" degeneration, not confined to the cochlear base, is also observed in elderly people. Indeed, Johnsson and Hawkins (1972a) felt that patchy degeneration of nerve fibers might be characteristic of "pure" neural presbycusis. Bredberg (1968) also observed cases of patchy losses of nerve fibers in the osseous spiral lamina. In about one-fourth of his cases, small circumscribed regions of neural degeneration were seen near the habenula perforata (perforations in the osseous spiral lamina through which nerve fibers pass). A similar observation was made by Johnsson, Felix, Gleeson, and Pollak (1990).

Nadol (1979), using electron microscopy, described a number of degenerative changes in ganglion cells and their dendrites in two case studies in which the hair cells were intact and the audiogram indicated a sharp loss of high frequency sensitivity. In one case, the number of afferent synapses per OHC was lower (1.3) than that of a normal ear (3.7); in 31 percent of the OHCs, no synapses were found, compared to 9 percent in the young ear. The afferent fibers were reduced in number and had abnormal features (e.g., vacuoles). Fewer myelinated fibers were seen in the basal 14 mm of the cochlea, and some had disorganized myelin sheaths. In the second case, the density of myelinated fibers was also reduced in the osseous spiral lamina in the base of the cochlea, and disorganization of myelin sheaths was again observed. The processes of supporting cells contained vacuoles but were otherwise normal.

Another consideration is the *ganglion cell type*. Type I and Type II ganglion cells have been differentiated in various mammalian species. Type I cells are large and myelinated and synapse with IHCs; Type II cells are small and unmyelinated and synapse with OHCs. In humans, unlike other mammals, the vast majority of spiral ganglion cell bodies, large and small, are unmyelinated (Arnold, 1987; Ota and Kimura, 1980; Spoendlin and Schrott, 1989). Interestingly, more myelinated ganglion cells are seen in older individuals: either unmyelinated cells become myelinated or

more myelinated cells are found due to a loss in unmyelinated cells (Arnold, 1987; Ota and Kimura, 1980). Some attempts to identify Type I and II cells in elderly human material have not met with success (Pauler et al., 1986). However, Spoendlin and Schrott (1989) were able to quantify Type I and II cells in two elderly patients. Compared to young, normal hearing adults, one patient, whose pathology was primarily neural, had a substantial loss of Type I cells but little loss of Type II cells. In the other patient, whose pathology was primarily in the organ of Corti, a modest loss of Type I cells was seen in the basal cochlea, but again, there was little loss of Type II cells. In these two cases, Type II cells were minimally involved.

CAN DEGENERATION OF GANGLION CELLS OCCUR INDEPENDENTLY OF ORGAN OF CORTI PATHOLOGY?

A key issue in understanding the effects of aging on the atrophy of spiral ganglion cells is whether it occurs as a primary aspect of aging or as a secondary response to organ of Corti degeneration. A number of studies have found regions of ganglion cell loss without corresponding hair cell loss, suggesting that neural degeneration can occur before and/or independently of sensory cell loss.

In the study of Crowe et al. (1934), a group of older subjects with high-frequency hearing loss and normal middle ears had damage to the organ of Corti that was generally only slightly more severe than in their normal-hearing control group, but they all had significant cochlear neural atrophy. In some cases, only a few normal-looking nerve fibers remained in the osseous spiral lamina, yet the organ of Corti remained normal. Fleischer (1956) saw loss of ganglion cells in the basal cochlea beginning in the third and fourth decades of life and concluded that this was the primary cause of presbycusis. In one pair of cochleas from Bredberg's (1968) study, pronounced nerve fiber degeneration was not associated with corresponding loss of sensory cells. Citron, Dix, Hallpike, and Hood (1963) observed normal organ of Corti histology in young patients with severe (e.g., 80 percent) loss of ganglion cells. In the material of Johnsson and Hawkins (1972a), temporal bones in five percent of their patients (all over 50) showed severe, mostly patchy, loss of nerve fibers in all cochlear turns, without severe hair cell loss. Suga and Lindsay (1976) found atrophy of the spiral

---

[1] The classic study of Crowe et al. (1934) provided a thorough histopathological analysis that included many elderly patients with hearing loss for high frequencies, which they labeled "gradual high tone loss" cases. Because this term is a bit ambiguous, we shall refer to these subjects as being older and having high-frequency hearing loss. This group is to be distinguished from their patients described as having "abrupt high tone loss." This group had a more sharply defined loss of high-frequency sensitivity and was primarily comprised of non-elderly adults, and will not be discussed further.

ganglion to be the most prominent histopathological change in their material; about one half of their cases showed no apparent change in the organ of Corti or stria vascularis. In summary, an impressive amount of evidence supports the occurrence of age-related atrophy of spiral ganglion cells, in many cases independent of damage to the organ of Corti.

A corollary issue is whether degenerative processes at once affect the entire ganglion cell (cell body and processes) or a particular part of the cell (cell body, peripheral or central processes). In theory, age-related pathology to any component of the cell could lead secondarily to degeneration of the entire ganglion cell. Spoendlin (1984) concluded from experimental animal work that the loss of ganglion cells can be caused by damage to the afferent dendritic processes contacting IHCs or by damage to the eighth nerve. The afferent terminals are susceptible to hypoxia and other insults, suggesting that age-related physiological events that can affect these dendrites might cause ganglion cell damage, while sensory cells remain intact. On the other hand, retrograde degeneration of ganglion cells is also induced by nerve damage central to the ganglion: transection of the eighth nerve in experimental animals results in degeneration of the ganglion cells with about five percent surviving; if the blood supply is left intact, the organ of Corti survives (Neff, 1947; Schuknecht, 1953). It is feasible that a similar sequence of degeneration could occur during aging since age-related vascular or bone pathology in the internal auditory meatus might damage eighth nerve fibers (see Chapter 5). It is also conceivable that age-related degeneration of post-synaptic neurons in the cochlear nucleus (the target of ganglion cell axons) could result in retrograde damage (see Chapter 8).

In a recently reported study, Felix, Johnsson, Gleeson, and Pollak (1990) found evidence for primary degeneration of peripheral, rather than central processes of ganglion cells (see below). Whether the loss of peripheral processes would have been followed by atrophy of the cell bodies in these cases is unknown. However, it is apparently not inevitable. Examination of pathological temporal bones (none of which were diagnosed as presbycusis) by Suzuka and Schuknecht (1988) indicated that ganglion cell bodies could survive for years despite dendritic damage. This conclusion was supported in a case reported by Nadol (1990) as well.

In summary, evidence indicates that the loss of spiral ganglion cells often occurs as a primary correlate of aging in humans. In theory, age-related pathology could affect a particular part of the ganglion cells—the cell body, peripheral dendritic processes, or eighth nerve fibers—with secondary degeneration of the remaining portions occurring. In any event, the loss of IHCs (not to mention OHCs) is not a prerequisite for age-related pathology of ganglion cells.

EFFERENT FIBERS

The fate of spiral versus radial fibers has been addressed by Johnsson and Hawkins (1972a), who examined spiral fibers within the osseous spiral lamina. Although they felt that the spiral fibers might be afferent, evidence from studies using stains for acetylcholinesterase (AChE) that are presumed to stain efferents indicate that spiral fibers within the osseous spiral lamina are indeed efferent (Ishii, Murakami, and Balogh, 1967; Nomura and Kirikae, 1967). Johnsson and Hawkins (1972a) observed that, when extensive portions of the cochlea atrophied, degeneration of myelinated intralaminar spiral fibers also occurred; when degeneration was confined to the lower third of the basal turn, spiral fibers usually remained, even though radial fibers had degenerated. Bredberg (1968) observed that, where degeneration of radial fibers was extensive, spiral fibers also tended to disappear. However, in at least one case, spiral fibers were seen in a region of total loss of radial fibers and degeneration of the organ of Corti.

Studies by Ishii and collaborators (1967a) and Nomura and Kirikae (1967; 1968) identified efferent fibers as staining positively for AchE. The cases presented in the first study appeared to have ample, presumably normal, amounts of AchE-positive fibers despite advanced age. In cases with substantial neural losses in the basal cochlea, Nomura and Kirikae were able to visualize individual efferent fibers that apparently survived despite a massive loss of afferents (Fig. 3-7). On the other hand, Nomura (1976) presented two elderly cases in which the efferent fibers were absent while some radial afferents were still present.

HOW DOES THE ROBUSTNESS OF AFFERENT AND EFFERENT SYSTEMS COMPARE?

The data suggest that the efferent system may be somewhat more robust than the afferent system in the face of aging, at least in some cases. Observations on human cochleas, just reviewed, indicate that efferent fibers can outlast degenerated afferents in the aging cochlea. Work on animal models (reviewed in Chapter 4) has shown that the loss of efferents in the basal cochlea of old guinea pigs is minimal (Covell and Rogers, 1957); putative efferent neurotransmitters may not change with age in rats (Hoffman, Jones-King, and Altschuler, 1988); and efferent terminals remain despite severe atrophy of the organ of Corti of old C57

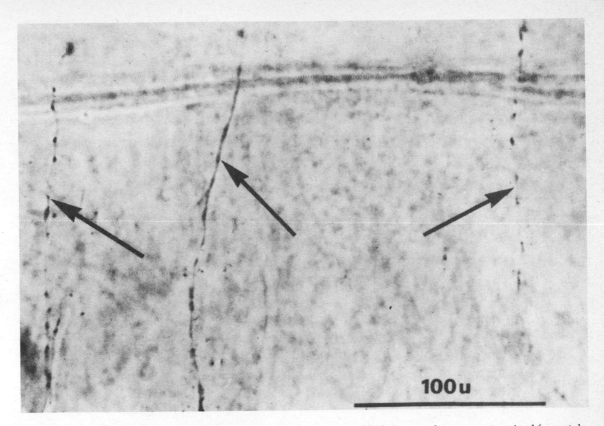

Figure 3-7. Efferent fibers in the spiral lamina of the organ of Corti in an elderly person; phase contrast, stained for acetyl cholinesterase. From Nomura, Y. & Kirikae, I. (1967) Presbycusis: A histological-histochemical study of the human cochlea. *Acta Otolaryngology 66:* 17–24, with permission.

mice (Willott and Pujol, unpublished data). In this regard, Billett and colleagues (1989) showed that efferent terminals in the inner spiral bundle (those involved with the IHC system) were less vulnerable to ischemia than afferents.

These observations of the resiliency of efferent fibers are by no means conclusive, but they have interesting implications. The efferent system is believed to inhibit the afferent system (e.g., Wiederhold, 1986). If the inhibitory efferent system were more robust in the face of aging than the excitatory afferent system, a net reduction of input to the central auditory system would result. This would augment the hearing loss due to atrophy of the afferent system and could explain some instances in which the histopathology does not seem severe enough to account for hearing loss. What is particularly exciting about this possibility is that attenuation of the (now stronger) efferent system (e.g., by pharmacological agents) might be able to restore some lost sensitivity to sounds. While this is speculation, the question of the fate of afferent versus efferent systems during aging may prove to be important.

THE AUDITORY NERVE

The auditory division of the eighth cranial nerve provides the link between the cochlea and the central auditory system. Its axons originate in the spiral ganglion cells.

Most studies of aging spiral ganglion cells have focused on the cochlea, and little information is available on the eighth nerve. Rasmussen (1940) identified an average of 32,500 fibers in the cochlear nerve of subjects aged 2 to 26 years and 30,300 in specimens in the age range of 44 to 60 years. This reduction of seven percent was accompanied by a reduction of five percent in the vestibular portion of the nerve. Spoendlin and Schrott (1989; 1990) counted nerve fibers in the human auditory nerve. They noted a decrease in fibers of elderly patients with sensorineural impairment, with about 24,000 (+/- 2000) fibers remaining. Unusually thin, pathological axons were prevalent in these cases as well.

As the eighth nerve enters the brain it can be divided into two parts, a peripheral part containing Schwann cells and a central part containing glia. Hansen (1973) and Hansen and Reske-Nielsen (1965) found pathology of myelin sheaths and axons in the peripheral part to be comparable to that seen in the basal spiral ganglion. Degeneration in the glial part was more severe. Myelin sheaths and axons of some nerve fibers were swollen, and oligodendrocytes, which provide the myelinated sheaths, were reduced in number and pyknotic.

These observations suggest that further damage to the axons of spiral ganglion cells might occur after they have left the cochlea, which could result in a greater degree of central denervation than is indicated by pathology of the spiral ganglion. However, the opposite type of relationship was observed by Felix, Johnsson, Gleeson, and Pollak (1990). In a sample of temporal bones with different types of cochlear pathology, they always observed a greater loss of peripheral dendritic processes compared to central processes of ganglion cells. The differences were on the order of 20-30 percent and more. In contrast to this work, Spoendlin and Schrott (1990) found that the loss of peripheral processes was only slightly greater (10 percent at best) than the loss of central processes in patients with sensorineural pathology. The reason for the differences in the magnitude of peripheral versus central degeneration in these studies is unclear. However, they provide no evidence for exaggerated damage to the central processes (auditory nerve fibers).

RELATIONSHIP OF HISTOPATHOLOGY TO HEARING LOSS

CONDITION OF THE SPIRAL GANGLION IN THE BASAL REGION OF THE COCHLEA

The early data of Crowe and co-workers (1934) revealed neural degeneration extending 5-7 mm up from the base of the cochlea (probably affecting frequencies of 8 kHz and up) in 8 of 15 "control" (normal hearing) subjects, as shown in three representative cases in Figure 3-8. Only 2 "control" ears in this study had no loss of ganglion cells. In "normal" ears of individuals aged 12 to 40 years (no clinical or pathological evidence of specific ear disease), Belal (1975) found atrophy of 10 to 25 percent of ganglion cells in the most basal 3 mm of the cochlear duct (total length of 33 mm); by age 75, this degree of atrophy extended to about 15 mm (probably affecting frequencies of 2 kHz and up). In the basal 3-5 mm, atrophy of 25 to 50 percent appeared by age 52 with little further increase through 75 years.

Many of the older subjects with high-frequency hearing losses examined by Crowe and colleagues (1934) had ganglion cell loss involving all or most of the entire basal half (15 mm) of the cochlea, with losses typically on the order of 50 percent or more in the basal 10 mm. The majority of these had a minimal loss of

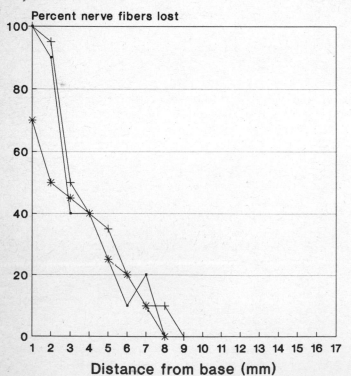

Percent nerve fibers lost

Distance from base (mm)

Figure 3-8. Loss of nerve fibers in the basal cochlea of normal hearing people (adapted from Crowe et al., 1934).

sensory cells. The examples of neural presbycusis presented by Schuknecht and colleagues (e.g., Schuknecht, 1974) show loss of ganglion cells to be on the order of 80 to 100 percent in the basal 10 mm of the cochlea, with less severe losses extending apically, sometimes encompassing all coils (Fig. 3-9, A,B).

Figure 3-9 A,B. Neural presbycusis, audiogram and histopathology (adapted from Nadol, 1981). mm on abscissa refers to distance from cochlear base.

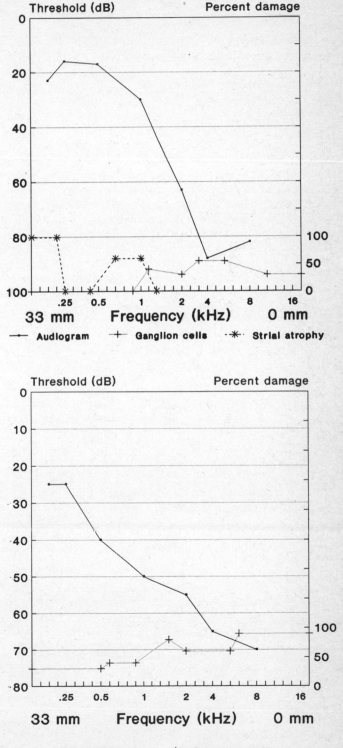

It appears from these studies that severe ganglion cell loss (greater than 50 percent) in the basal 10 mm of the cochlea is associated with significant impairment of high frequencies. When ganglion cell atrophy is restricted to the basal 3-5 mm, hearing loss is not clinically significant for the frequencies routinely tested (e.g., 8 kHz or less).

RELATIONSHIP BETWEEN THE TOTAL NUMBER OF SURVIVING GANGLION CELLS AND PURE TONE THRESHOLDS

In the absence of hearing impairment, the loss of ganglion cells may not be severe, and at least two studies have concluded that aging is not necessarily accompanied by a loss of ganglion cells. However, these "negative" findings must be qualified. In the first study, Pollak, Felix and Schrott (1987) counted ganglion cells in five normal-hearing patients aged 38 to 82 and found no relationship of *overall* counts to age. Nevertheless, the basal cochlear quartile had a mean count of 3,683 in the 38- and 40-year-old patients compared to 1,668 in the 54- to 82-year-olds. The second study (Hinojosa, Seligsohn, and Lerner; 1985) was also on

patients with audiograms that were normal for their age. No relationship was evident between age and the number of ganglion cells present in the base or elsewhere. However, only two of the 16 subjects were over 60 years of age (63 and 68), making it difficult to generalize these findings.

In a much larger sample of subjects who had normal hearing for their age, Suzuka and Schuknecht (1988) demonstrated a clear trend toward a decrease in ganglion cells with aging. As seen in Figure 3-10, the number of ganglion cells decreased by about 20 percent from the fourth to the eighth and ninth decades. In this subject population ganglion cell losses did not differ markedly in degree from base to apex. The results of the study by Suzuka and Schuknecht indicate that, when ganglion cell losses are on the order of only 20 percent, hearing is normal for the age group.

Otte et al. (1978) compared the number of ganglion cells as a function of age and otological diagnosis. In a population in which most individuals had some type of hearing loss, age was associated with a gradual decline from over 30 thousand cells in young adults to under 20 thousand in octogenarians (Fig. 3-11). When the data were arranged according to diagnosis (Fig. 3-12), patients diagnosed as having neural presbycusis

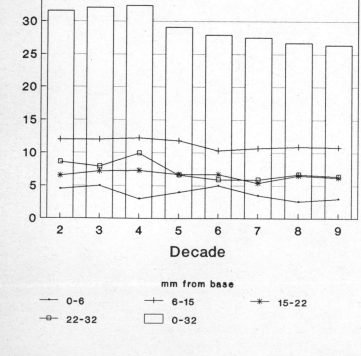

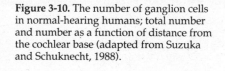

Figure 3-10. The number of ganglion cells in normal-hearing humans; total number and number as a function of distance from the cochlear base (adapted from Suzuka and Schuknecht, 1988).

Figure 3-11. Number of spiral ganglion cells as a function of age (adapted from Otte et al., 1978).

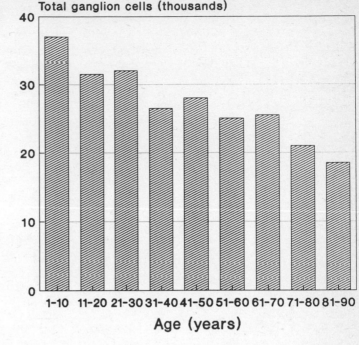

Figure 3-12. Number of spiral ganglion cells for different conditions of cochlear pathology (adapted from Otte et al., 1978).

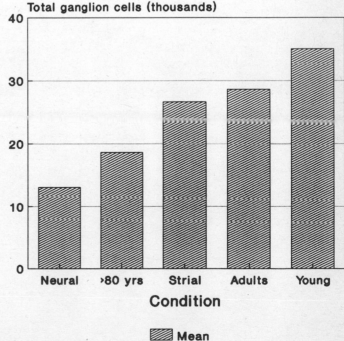

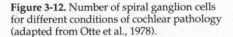

had, by far, the fewest ganglion cells (about 13 thousand), followed by individuals over 80 years of age regardless of otological diagnoses (18.6 thousand), and strial presbycusis (about 26.6 thousand). Young subjects (including children) had a mean of about 35 thousand ganglion cells.

The work of Otte et al. (1978) shows that ganglion cell losses of one third or more result in significant presbycusis. However, the relationship between ganglion cell loss and presbycusis is not a tight one. In the same study, Otte and colleagues counted ganglion cells in subjects having various degrees of hearing loss. As seen in Figure 3-13, elevations in pure tone average thresholds (PTAs) of 0 to 40 dB were associated with similar numbers of ganglion cells. The ranges indicate that fewer than 20 thousand ganglion cells remained in some of these subjects. Patients with threshold elevations of more than 40 dB had ganglion cell counts on the order of 20 thousand or less.

Apparently, good sensitivity to tones can be retained even when there is substantial reduction in the total number of ganglion cells. A striking demonstration of this point was made by Citron and colleagues (1963). A young patient with only about 20 percent of ganglion cells surviving had a normal pure tone audiogram. Schuknecht and Woellner (1953) obtained similar findings in the cat.

In summary, despite individual exceptions, by middle age most "normal-hearing" people are likely to have some loss of ganglion cells (Fig. 3-10). Although losses may occur throughout the cochlea, the basal turn is most vulnerable. (This is supported by high frequency audiometry; Chapter 8.) Importantly, the range of ganglion cell loss in subjects with good pure tone audiograms (Fig. 3-13) is rather broad. Individuals can endure losses on the order of one third yet still have good pure tone thresholds. More severe losses of ganglion cells are correlated with threshold elevations.

GANGLION CELL LOSS AND SPEECH RECOGNITION

In patients with poor speech recognition, 88 percent of whom were older than 60, Belal (1975) found ganglion cell loss to be severe. Eight cases had losses of 25 to 50 percent throughout the entire cochlea; 14 cases had 50 to 100 percent loss in the basal 9 mm; virtually all cases had significant ganglion cell loss extending at

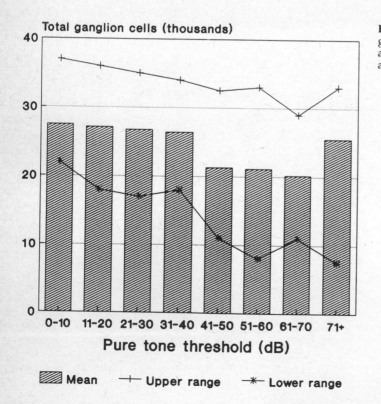

Figure 3-13. The number of spiral ganglion cells as a function of pure tone average threshold (adapted from Otte et al., 1978).

PTA for 500, 1000, 2000 Hz

Figure 3-14. The number of spiral ganglion cells as a function of speech recognition (adapted from Otte et al., 1978).

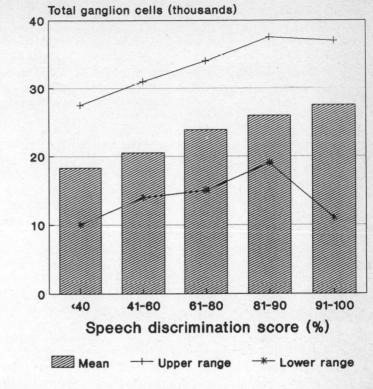

least half-way up the baso-apical coils. The correlation between ganglion cell counts and speech recognition was described in detail by Otte and colleagues (1978). As seen in Figure 3-14, a rather nice relationship between ganglion cells and speech recognition was found.

While a significant loss of ganglion cells may be associated with impaired speech recognition, the relationship is far from perfect. For instance, the ranges of recognition ability in the study of Otte et al. (Fig. 3-14) show that fairly good recognition (e.g., greater than 80 percent) can be achieved with substantially fewer than 20 thousand ganglion cells in some individuals. In fact, these researchers concluded that minimal speech recognition requires only 10 thousand neurons, with at least 3 thousand ganglion cells remaining in the apical 10 mm of the cochlea.

Deviations from the correlation between speech recognition ability and the degree of ganglion cell damage is also illustrated in Bredberg's important monograph of 1968. A case was reported in which patchy degeneration totaling about two-thirds loss

was accompanied by normal speech recognition in an 81-year-old subject.

Further information concerning ganglion cell loss and speech recognition was provided by Pauler, Schuknecht, and Thornton (1986). They selected temporal bones of patients aged 55 to 90 from the collection of the Massachusetts Eye and Ear Infirmary that met the following criteria: cochlear neuronal loss with a minimum of other cochlear pathologies; timely premortem tests of auditory function; technically satisfactory histological preparations. The ability to discriminate speech was highly correlated with the innervation density of the region of the cochlea 15-22 mm from the cochlear base. Pure tone thresholds from 1 kHz to 2 kHz, represented by this cochlear segment, were most strongly correlated with speech recognition (based on tests using phonemically balanced monosyllabic words at 40 dB SL)[2]. Despite the significant correlation, it was noted that the effect of neuronal losses on speech recognition varied greatly. For instance, three cochleas with 80 percent speech recognition performance had, respectively, 12 per-

[2] The studies by Otte et al. (1978) and Pauler et al. (1986), although from the same laboratories, identified different regions of the cochlea as being most critical to speech perception (the 22-32 mm and 15-22 mm segments, respectively). There are some differences in the two studies that might account for the different findings. The later study used subjects that were older (mean of 76.1 years compared to 61 years), used statistical correlations to draw conclusions, and chose cases with pathology primarily restricted to the ganglion cells. The study by Otte et al., used a sample of heterogeneous pathological types.

cent, 43 percent, and 60 percent loss of ganglion cells in the 15-22 mm segment. No significant correlation of the slope of the audiogram to speech recognition was evident.

To summarize, the correlation between ganglion cell loss and speech recognition tests is stronger than it is for pure tone thresholds (compare Figs. 3-12 and 3-13). Nevertheless, the range of ganglion cell counts for any recognition level is large. It must be concluded that the speech recognition performance is a limited predictor of the status of an individual's spiral ganglion.

AGE-RELATED HISTOPATHOLOGY OF THE STRIA VASCULARIS

BACKGROUND

The stria vascularis appears to be responsible for maintaining the ionic composition of the endolymph (e.g., secretion of potassium). This process is critical to the generation of the positive endocochlear electrical potential (Marcus, 1986) that is essential for normal cochlear function (e.g., Walsh and McGee, 1986). Thus, strial pathology would be expected to cause elevation of sensory thresholds.

There are three basic cell types in the stria vascularis. The marginal cells (or dark cells) form the surface boundary with the cochlear duct and are thought to be responsible for the production of endolymph (Marcus, 1986). The basal cells form a tight boundary between the stria and subjacent spiral ligament. The intermediate cells are found between the marginal and basal cells. All three cell types are contacted by capillaries.

HISTOPATHOLOGY

Virtually all older subjects in the group with high frequency-losses in the study by Crowe et al. (1934) had some strial pathology, as did 4 of the 15 non-elderly "control" subjects. The distribution of pathology varied considerably from case to case; whereas the left and right stria of some patients showed remarkably similar pathology, obvious differences in strial pathology between left and right ears also occurred. In most cases, pathology was not severe. Examples of strial presbycusis presented by Schuknecht and colleagues (Schuknecht, 1974; Schuknecht et al., 1974) indicate a good deal of variability in the extent of stria involved, ranging from almost the entire cochlea to circumscribed regions. The most common site of strial pathology is the apical region of the cochlea.

Johnsson and Hawkins (1972b) observed, in all patients beyond the fifth decade of life, some strial atrophy from the extreme basal region to the apical turn, with the least degeneration in the upper basal turn. Pigmentation increased, with clumps of pigment accumulating throughout the stria. With complete strial atrophy, the spiral ligament became covered with a flat epithelium with small roundish concretions often attached to the ligament.

Schuknecht and collaborators (1974) performed a detailed light- and electron-microscopic study of temporal bones in individuals for whom strial atrophy appeared to be the principal cause of deafness (six percent of the cases in their collection of temporal bones). Pathological changes consisted of degeneration of all three layers of the stria vascularis, being most severe in the marginal cells, followed by the intermediate cells and basal cells. Strial atrophy was most severe in the apical region of the cochlea. When the thickness of the stria was still normal, the following changes could be found: (a) intercellular edema in layers of the marginal and intermediate cells, (b) degenerative changes in the marginal cells with loss of mitochondria and other intracellular organelles, (c) the appearance of intracellular filaments, (d) an increase in the number of lysosomes, and (e) an increase in pigment granules, with fusion into large intracellular masses sometimes occurring. As atrophy progressed and the thickness of the stria began to decrease, marginal cells showed further changes, including a loss of many of their processes. They now constituted only 20 percent or less of the strial mass, compared to their normal 50 percent. When the stria became very thin, the luminal surface continued to be covered by atrophic marginal cells that were now abutted only by the basal cell layers. Ultimately, the marginal cells became disrupted and the underlying basal cells emerged to the fluid surface. During this progression, the intermediate and basal cells showed changes and accumulation of pigment, but tended to remain intact. Despite the changes, no instances were observed where communication between spiral ligament tissue, which contains perilymph, and the endolymph of the cochlear duct would be permitted.

Takahashi (1971) used electron microscopy to examine 14 post-mortem specimens that had been fixed within three hours of death; 8 of the 14 patients were aged 60 to 92 years. Degeneration was observed most frequently in the apical and lower basal cochlear turns. Within the same cochlea two types of atrophy could be observed: a localized type in which the stria had degenerated to a thin cell layer flanked by regions of normal or increased thickness, and a diffusely distributed pathology with normal thickness of the stria, but affecting all three types of strial cells. Takahashi also observed atrophy of the spiral prominence (a portion of the cochlear duct wall at the border of the stria vascularis), with no apparent relationship to strial pathology. The number of strial blood vessels decreased as degeneration increased. However, intact capillaries were sometimes seen in the atrophied regions, suggesting that diminished blood supply may not have

been responsible for strial degeneration. Pigment deposits were also more prominent in the stria vascularis of older patients. Belal (1975) also reported that strial lesions could be either localized to within 1 mm or generalized throughout most of the cochlea, but were most severe in the apical cochlea.

Age-related changes in strial vasculature are discussed below in the section on vascular histopathology. Table 3-3 summarizes studies showing age-related strial atrophy.

TABLE 3-3. STUDIES SHOWING AGE-RELATED ATROPHY AND/OR VASCULAR CHANGES IN THE STRIA VASCULARIS

Early reports (Jaehne, 1914; Manasse, 1906; Wittmach, 1916)[*]

Fabinyi (1931): occurred along with with sensory and neural degeneration

Crowe et al. (1934): observed in subjects with high tone hearing loss, but not prominent

von Fieandt and Saxen (1937): "angiosclerotic degeneration of the inner ear"

Saxen (1952): "Angiosclerotic degeneration of the inner ear" always involves strial pathology (with secondary organ of Corti atrophy); usually appears with spiral ganglion atrophy

Jorgensen (1961): hyalin-positive thickening of strial vessels

Schuknecht (1964, 1967, 1974, 1989): one of the four types of presbycusis

Krmpotic-Nemanic (1971): secondary to loss of blood supply to ossification

Takahashi (1971): ultrastructural strial pathology in apical and basal turns especially in patients older than 60

Johnsson and Hawkins (1972b): found in all subjects over 50

Schuknecht et al. (1974): principal cause of hearing loss in six percent of their cases

Suga and Lindsay (1976): often saw "diffuse senile atrophy" of the stria

Engstrom et al (1987): formation of lipofuscin with aging

---

*cited by Johnsson and Hawkins (1972b)

RELATIONSHIP OF HISTOPATHOLOGY TO HEARING IMPAIRMENT

About half of the "control" ears of Crowe et al. (1934) had a small degree of strial pathology throughout the lower cochlea. In "normal" hearing patients, Belal (1975) found vacuoles and cystic spaces in the intermediate cell layer, basophilic deposits beneath the basal layer, and thickening of capillaries in older subjects. Thus, a small degree of strial pathology may be of little consequence.

Cases presented by Schuknecht (1974) to illustrate strial presbycusis indicate the degree of histopathology associated with significant flat audiometric loss. Severe atrophy could be limited to fairly restricted regions of the cochlea (e.g., about 10 mm), yet hearing losses on the order of 50 dB or more resulted. Similar degrees of hearing loss occurred in other cases where strial degeneration was found in varying degrees throughout the cochlea. In Belal's (1975) sample, patients with flat audiometric losses of 40-50 dB had strial pathology ranging in extents from less than 1 mm to encompassing the entire cochlear duct. The severity of pathology ranged from "mild changes in cellular architecture" to complete atrophy. Figure 3-15 summarizes the audiogram and histopathology from a case of strial presbycusis presented by Nadol (1981).

The correlation between strial pathology (as indicated by strial cross-sectional area) and audiometric thresholds was computed by Pauler, Schuknecht, and White (1988) in patients with little nonstrial pathology. A strong negative correlation between strial thickness and threshold (500-4000 Hz PTA) was obtained, as seen in Figure 3-16. It can also be seen that speech recognition was not greatly affected by strial pathology, and that there was little relationship between strial pathology and the number of surviving ganglion cells.

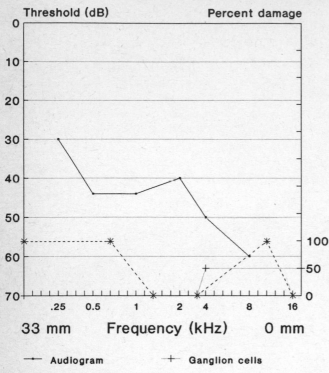

Figure 3-15. Strial presbycusis, audiogram and histopathology (adapted from Nadol, 1981). mm on abscissa refers to distance from cochlear base.

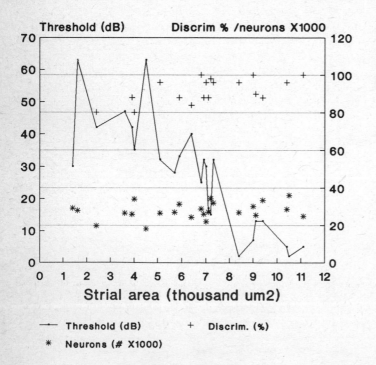

Figure 3-16. The relationship between thickness of the stria vascularis and absolute threshold (500-4000 Hz PTA), speech recognition, and the number of ganglion cells (adapted from Pauler et al., 1988).

AGE-RELATED SENSORINEURAL HISTOPATHOLOGY

BACKGROUND

Johnsson and Hawkins (1979), reviewing their own extensive histological observations of temporal bones, were unable to classify their material into distinct "sensory," "neural," or "strial" histopathological types as outlined by Schuknecht. The vast majority of their specimens "simply showed a sensorineural degeneration [pathology of both the organ of Corti and ganglion cells] that was most pronounced in the lower basal turn and usually was accompanied by vascular changes. ... All cases that had obvious strial atrophy also displayed hair cell loss" (p. 128). The fact that a significant number of elderly ears have combined pathology of various cochlear elements argues for a sensorineural type of histopathology distinguishable from either "pure" sensory, neural, or strial types. Presumably, regions of the cochlea in which both sensory and neural tissue have atrophied would be unable to participate in hearing.

HISTOPATHOLOGY

Because the survival of cells often depends on the integrity of neighboring tissue, three possibilities can be considered regarding the occurrence of combined sensorineural changes with aging. First, pathology of either hair cells or ganglion cells could be primary, with secondary degeneration of the other cell type following. Second, atrophy of both cell types could occur independently. Third, degeneration of one or both types could be secondary to changes in another type of cell (e.g., supporting cells), structure (e.g., stria vascularis), or system (e.g. cardiovascular).

Unfortunately, it is difficult to differentiate among these possibilities in post-mortem material because the changes have already occurred. Consequently, evidence of secondary degeneration is difficult to obtain. Nevertheless, insights to several questions can be gleaned from the literature.

DOES GANGLION CELL LOSS FOLLOW HAIR CELL LOSS AS A SECONDARY EVENT?

Johnsson and Hawkins (1972a) concluded that neural atrophy followed sensory cell loss because, in their

material, sensory cell loss (without apparent neural loss) was seen in infants, but adolescents and adults always had both sensory and neural loss. Bredberg (1968) concluded that neural degeneration was secondary to sensory cell loss; he identified a critical role of IHCs, but not OHCs in the survival of ganglion cells. A complete loss of inner and outer hair cells was invariably associated with an absence of nerve fibers in the osseous spiral lamina. A complete loss of OHCs alone was never associated with a noticeable loss of nerve fibers. Loss of IHCs with intact OHCs was highly correlated with loss or reduction of nerve fibers in the corresponding region of the cochlea. These findings, plus the work on animal models reviewed in Chapter 4, provide strong evidence that degeneration of IHCs, but not OHCs, is accompanied by a significant loss of ganglion cells.

The most direct evidence for the notion that IHC loss causes secondary neuronal degeneration comes from studies of experimentally induced cochlear damage in animal models. Johnsson (1974) and Johnsson and Hawkins (1972a) cited the experimental literature showing that secondary nerve degeneration follows destruction of the organ of Corti in animals. Spoendlin (1984) reviewed his research on retrograde degeneration of cochlear neurons in animals following experimental damage to the organ of Corti. Destruction of the organ of Corti by ototoxins or noise trauma was associated with an asymptotic curve for ganglion cell loss with about 10 percent of neurons surviving after 12 months. Because neural degeneration often occurred in the presence of normal supporting cells, Spoendlin concluded that the collapse or absence of supporting structures is not essential. Rather, with few exceptions, the critical event is damage to the peripheral afferent dendritic processes that occurs if IHCs are damaged.

Whereas it can be concluded that the destruction of IHCs by noise trauma or ototoxic drugs is followed by a secondary loss of nerve fibers, there are several reasons for skepticism in extrapolating the occurrence of this sequence to sensorineural damage associated with aging. First, the conclusion of Johnsson and Hawkins (1972a) might be questioned because it assumes that the same process is involved in hair cell loss of infants and in sensorineural loss in adults. It is feasible that the loss of hair cells in infants represents the late stages of a developmental process that has little to do with losses occurring with aging. Second, experimental destruction of hair cells and destruction associated with aging are likely to involve different physiological mechanisms; the fact that an ototoxic drug or noise traumatization results in secondary neural degeneration does not necessarily imply that the same will occur during aging. Third, species differences may exist in the interdependence of IHCs and ganglion cells. Altschuler, Miller, Zappia, Niparko, and Hawkins (1989) pointed out that, although the evidence for non-primates suggests that ganglion cell survival requires the presence of IHCs, this is not necessarily the case in primates. They reported a case study of a post-mortem human patient who had undergone a cochlear implant. An almost normal ganglion cell population was observed despite the loss of hair cells in much of the cochlea. In a patient who had profound deafness for 30 years, Nadol (1990) observed a substantial population of surviving ganglion cells despite total degeneration of the organ of Corti. Peripheral dendritic processes had degenerated, as well.

An even more cogent issue is how often primary IHC degeneration occurs during aging. Even if neural degeneration typically follows the loss of IHCs (when such loss occurs), the point is moot if IHC pathology rarely occurs as a primary age-related event. There have been observations of hair cell degeneration in aged ears without corresponding loss of radial fibers, suggesting that hair cell loss can precede atrophy of ganglion cells. In some cochleas of old patients, Johnsson (1974) found large portions of the organ of Corti to be devoid of hair cells while nerve fibers of the osseous spiral lamina appeared intact. Similarly, in a sample of 14 patients, Soucek, Michaels, and Frohlich (1987) observed instances in which hair cells were absent in a fairly extensive region of the cochlea, yet radial fibers survived. Furthermore, in cases of patchy degeneration of hair cells, atrophy of radial fibers was not always seen. It is *possible* in these cases that the loss of sensory cells would have been followed by degeneration of nerve fibers and ganglion cells, had the subjects survived for longer periods of time. However, the observations of ganglion cells persisting in humans with organ of Corti damage, cited above (Altschuler et al., 1989; Nadol, 1990), weakens this possibility.

Despite these observations of age-related atrophy of the organ of Corti without ganglion cell loss, the vast majority of histopathological cases indicate that when sensory cells degenerate with age, concomitant neural degeneration occurs (e.g., Crowe et al., 1934; Johnsson and Hawkins, 1979; Schuknecht, 1974). Furthermore, a good deal of human and animal research (reviewed in Chapter 4) has shown that when age-related inner ear degeneration is largely restricted to hair cells, the OHCs are more likely to be affected than IHCs (e.g., Figs. 3-3, 3-4). In short, there is little compelling evidence that aging results in primary IHC loss followed by secondary neural degeneration in humans. Rather, it may be the case that the correspondence of IHC and neural degeneration during aging is due to some factor(s) that directly affects both types of tissue.

DOES HAIR CELL DEGENERATION FOLLOW NEURAL DEGENERATION AS A SECONDARY EVENT?

The experimental literature shows that cutting eighth nerve axons results in transganglionic degeneration extending only as far as the habenula perforata, where fibers make their way to the hair cells (Johnsson and Hawkins, 1972a). Beyond this point, the unmyelinated portions of fibers, terminals, and organ of Corti can remain intact. While this suggests that primary degeneration of ganglion cell bodies would not necessarily result in degeneration of IHCs, it does not speak to the question of damage to the terminals that contact the IHCs. These terminals are very vulnerable to hypoxia or other insults. Thus, terminal degeneration could conceivably lead to secondary loss of IHCs, resulting in sensorineural pathology. However, the evidence for age-related neural pathology, reviewed earlier, indicates that loss of radial fibers often occurs without secondary sensory cell loss. At this time, there is not a strong case that less-than-total degeneration of neural tissue (terminals or ganglion cell bodies) causes secondary degeneration of IHCs during aging.

WHAT IS THE RELATIONSHIP BETWEEN SUPPORTING CELLS AND SURVIVAL OF SENSORY AND NEURAL CELLS?

The supporting cells may play a critical role in degeneration of sensory and/or neural cells. This possibility was recognized by Crowe et al. (1934). They observed that atrophy of supporting cells of Hensen and Claudius was always at least as extensive as that in the organ of Corti. In some cases, there was supporting cell atrophy with little other cochlear pathology. On the basis of these observations they felt that supporting cell atrophy precedes, and may contribute to, organ of Corti pathology.

Johnsson and Hawkins (1972a) stated that the presence of pillar and Deiters cells "seemed to determine" whether myelinated radial fibers survived. If these supporting cells remained, nerve fibers were also seen in corresponding areas of osseous spiral lamina. Conversely, if there were no supporting cells, no nerve fibers were seen. More recently, Johnsson and colleagues (1990) presented electron microscopic evidence that the survival of ganglion cell processes was correlated with the presence of supporting cells.

Schuknecht and colleagues also believed that the presence of Deiters and pillar supporting cells was very important for the survival of ganglion cells. In their studies, a loss of supporting cells was almost always associated with a severe loss of ganglion cells (Otte et al., 1978; Schuknecht, 1974).

The temporal bones of patients with sensorineural hearing loss were examined by Suzuka and Schuknecht (1988). Although none of these were presbycusis cases, the findings are instructive. The extent of neuronal degeneration was directly related to the extent of injury to inner pillar cells and inner phalangeal cells. A total loss of both IHCs and OHCs could occur without a concomitant loss of ganglion cells. The degeneration of inner pillar and phalangeal cells appeared to cause degeneration of terminals on the IHCs. When IHCs degenerated, the inner supporting cells also appeared to be responsible.

Zallone, Teti, Balle, and Iurato (1987) presented two cases prepared with the block surface technique in which there was complete loss of sensory cells in the basal organ of Corti. In one case, a 92-year-old man, innervation density in the osseous spiral lamina was normal, while the other case, a 72-year-old woman, had a clear reduction of radial fibers. The main difference between the two cases was that the pillar and Deiters cells were present in the former, but had been replaced by flat epithelial cells in the latter. These observations are consistent with the notion that supporting cells are important for the preservation of ganglion cell processes in the cochlea and that their destruction would cause sensorineural damage.

Spoendlin and Gacek (1963) concluded that the intimate relationship between supporting cells and afferent (but not efferent) terminals was critical for the terminals' survival: after cutting the eighth nerve in cats, afferent terminals survived despite degeneration of the spiral ganglion cells (from which the terminals emanate). It follows that experimental, and perhaps age-related, damage to supporting cells may have deleterious effects on afferent—but not necessarily efferent—fibers.

While an important role of supporting cells is indicated, supporting cell pathology is probably not a necessary element of age-related sensorineural pathology. Bredberg (1968) found that the correlation between sensory and supporting cell changes was not consistent. In some cases, even extensive loss of hair cells could be accompanied by no loss of pillar cells; in other cases comparable sensory cell loss was accompanied by collapse of Hensen cells and other supporting cells outside the tunnel of Corti. Bredberg also found cases where the organ of Corti was completely atrophied in a circumscribed region, but the Hensen cells appeared nearly normal. Complete loss of IHCs was invariably correlated with loss of ganglion cells. Johnsson (1974) also found that a good deal of nerve fiber degeneration may take place in older patients while supporting cells are still present.

As discussed previously, Spoendlin (1984) found that collapse or absence of supporting cells was not essential for retrograde degeneration of cochlear neu-rons of cats. Neural degeneration often occurred in the presence of normal supporting cells.

These negative findings do not mean that the loss of supporting cells does not cause sensorineural damage. They suggest that other causes exist. Johnsson and Hawkins (1972a) reasoned that, because pillar and Deiters cells often degenerate much later than hair cells and are involved in repair processes when hair cells do degenerate, they are probably not the primary site of cochlear pathology. Rather, the presence of pillar and Deiters cells can prevent or delay severe nerve degeneration, probably by providing protection and nutrition for unmyelinated nerve endings.

The role of supporting cells in age-related sensorineural pathology deserves further attention by researchers. It may be the case that subtle changes in certain types of supporting cells have not been detected by routine light microscopy, and that these changes could affect both hair cells and ganglion cells.

DOES PATHOLOGY OF THE STRIA VASCULARIS CAUSE SENSORINEURAL DAMAGE?

Age-related strial atrophy often occurs in combination with other types of pathology (Johnsson and Hawkins, 1979; Schuknecht et al., 1974), raising the question of the role of strial pathology in contributing to secondary changes in the organ of Corti and spiral ganglion. In the beginning of the century, German researchers (Jaehne, 1914; Manasse, 1906; Wittmaack, 1916) related atrophy of the spiral ligament and stria to degeneration of the organ of Corti (Johnsson and Hawkins, 1972b). The loss of sensory cells during aging was viewed by von Fieandt and Saxen (1937) as being secondary to vascular pathology in the stria. Support for this notion has been equivocal, however.

Johnsson and Hawkins (1972b,c) almost always found hair cell loss to accompany strial degeneration, and they felt that the severity and strial atrophy and hair cell loss were correlated and that strial pathology might be a "common denominator" in sensorineural pathology of various types. On the other hand, the spatial correlation between sensorineural degeneration and strial atrophy was not strong. There was always degeneration of both the stria and organ of Corti in the extreme basal and apical points; however, strial atrophy was generally greatest in the middle and apical turns, while organ of Corti degeneration was worst in the basal turn. With patchy sensorineural degeneration, sharply defined regions of strial atrophy were not seen.

Only one subject with neural atrophy and high-frequency losses in the study of Crowe et al. (1934) showed significant pathology of the stria vascularis. Similarly, Hansen (1973) found little evidence of strial pathology in his old patients and concluded, as have others (Saxen, 1952; Schuknecht, 1955; Jorgensen, 1961) that the degree of strial change does not parallel changes in the organ of Corti.

Schuknecht et al. (1974) described a number of cases in which strial atrophy appeared to have been the cause of hearing loss. They concluded that the other structures in the cochlea were typically normal, suggesting that strial pathology does not result in secondary sensorineural damage.

To summarize, the evidence that age-related strial pathology leads to secondary sensorineural degeneration is not compelling. However, it should be noted that this evidence is based on histopathological observations. The possible effects of age-related physiological changes in the stria have not been evaluated, and the issue remains an open one.

SUMMARY OF THE RELATIONSHIPS AMONG PATHOLOGY IN DIFFERENT TISSUES

Evidence was presented indicating that OHC loss can occur without the accompaniment of neural or other cochlear pathology. Likewise, pathology of the stria vascularis can occur without apparent effect on the organ of Corti or spiral ganglion. As discussed in the section on neural pathology, age-related loss of spiral ganglion cells can occur without the involvement of other cochlear tissues. A fourth type of pathology, sensorineural, appears to be caused by mechanism(s) that affect both spiral ganglion and organ of Corti tissue concomitantly.

RELATIONSHIP BETWEEN HISTOPATHOLOGY AND HEARING LOSS

Audiometric profiles of elderly patients with sensorineural damage are likely to include some loss of high frequency sensitivity because sensorineural pathology is usually most severe in the basal region of the cochlea (Johnsson and Hawkins, 1979). Presumably, a decline in speech recognition is also likely, as is the case with neural degeneration. However, stria vascularis pathology may often be present, as well (Johnsson and Hawkins, 1979), and this could lead to reduced sensitivity across a broad range of frequencies (see above). Because of the possible interaction of several types of histopathology, audiometric configurations associated with sensorineural atrophy are likely to vary considerably, with a common feature being high frequency loss.

AGE-RELATED HISTO-PATHOLOGY AFFECTING COCHLEAR MECHANICS

BACKGROUND

The basilar membrane is displaced by fluid motion within the cochlea and is, therefore, a critical element in cochlear mechanics. Age-related changes in its stiffness or other physical properties would be expected to affect sensory transduction. Also important in determining cochlear mechanics is the spiral ligament, situated between the bony labyrinth and cochlear duct, forming the outer wall of the membranous labyrinth. It is composed primarily of connective tissue cells (fibrocytes) and provides the external points of attachment for both the basilar membrane and Reissner's membrane. The spiral ligament was described by Henson and colleagues (1984) as containing an array of criss-crossing extracellular fibers connecting the bony wall of the cochlea with the outer margin of the basilar membrane (pars pectinata). Their observations suggested that this connection maintains radial tension on the spiral ligament-basilar membrane complex. Thus, alterations in the spiral ligament would be expected to affect the mechanical properties of the basilar membrane.

The presbycusis literature has typically not addressed the role of organ of Corti tissue with regard to age-related changes in cochlear mechanics. Loss of OHCs or other tissue might alter the properties of the mechanical system in a way that could affect the transduction process. For instance, Khanna and Leonard (1986) used laser inferometry to measure basilar membrane displacement as a function of sound frequency in cats subjected to cochlear trauma. A decline in the precision of basilar membrane frequency responses ("tuning" of the basilar membrane) was found to be correlated with the extent of OHC damage, particularly with regard to stereocilia and their relationship to the tectorial membrane. Furthermore, efferent activation of OHCs affects cochlear mechanics (Mountain, 1980; Siegel and Kim, 1982). Therefore, sensory and efferent neural atrophy has the potential for secondary effects on cochlear mechanics.

HISTOPATHOLOGY

SPIRAL LIGAMENT

Several researchers have observed age-related atrophy of the spiral ligament that might affect cochlear mechanics.

Johnsson and Hawkins (1972b) found that a loss of cell nuclei and cytoplasm, especially in the upper part of the spiral ligament, accompanied aging. When severe, only "scattered islands of pyknotic cells" remained on the vestibular surface of the spiral ligament. Nadol (1981) provided several examples of ligament atrophy in elderly patients.

The histopathology of the spiral ligament was evaluated by Wright and Schuknecht (1972) in their sample of temporal bones. Aging was associated with progressive changes in the spiral ligament, even in those patients having normal bone conduction audiograms. The distribution and shape of fibrocytes changed, acellular areas (which first appeared at a very young age) became more pronounced, and the density of cells decreased. In parts of the spiral ligament, clumps of cells became surrounded by acellular spaces. As the atrophy progressed, a zone of acellularity developed in the middle of the ligament and fibrocytes migrated toward the periphery. Ultimately, two distinct zones could develop: a larger, acellular, cystic, internal zone and a smaller zone with a matrix of scattered fibrocytes. A dense layer of closely packed fibrocytes could separate the two zones. Abnormalities were most pronounced in the middle and apical cochlear turns.

BASILAR MEMBRANE

Years ago, Mayer (1920) reported that, with aging, hyalinization, thickening, and calcification occurred in the basilar membrane. He felt that this could cause stiffening of the basilar membrane and proposed mechanical dysfunction as a cause of presbycusis. Calcareous deposits were observed by Crowe and coworkers (1934) in patients with normal hearing; however, such deposits were more common in older patients with high frequency losses.

Nomura (1970) found lipid deposits on the basilar membrane in almost half of the 71- to 95-year-old patients studied, and proposed that lipidosis of the basilar membrane should be considered as a cause of presbycusis. The deposits were observed on the filamentous structure of the pars pectinata (the outer segment of the basilar membrane) and were more numerous near the cochlear base. The organ of Corti was present in some cases and gone in others, suggesting that lipidosis was not a secondary response to organ of Corti pathology. The lipids were composed primarily of neutral fat and some cholesterol; however, the cholesterol content of the patient's serum was not correlated with the presence of lipid deposits. Nomura proposed that the lipidosis would affect basilar membrane impedance, contributing to presbycusis.

Nadol (1979) reported a case in which the basilar membrane, viewed with electron microscopy, showed

TABLE 3-4. STUDIES SHOWING AGE-RELATED CHANGES IN THE BASILAR MEMBRANE OR SPIRAL LIGAMENT

Mayer (1920):hyalinization and calcareous deposits of basilar membrane

Crowe et al. (1934): hearing normal despite moderate hyalinization and calcification of basilar membrane

Schuknecht (1964, 1967, 1974, 1989): one of the four types of presbycusis

Allam (1970): basilar membrane and spiral ligament pathology can be severe

Kraus (1970): age-related changes in basilar membrane

Nomura (1970): lipidosis of basilar membrane

Johnsson and Hawkins (1972b): observed devascularization in spiral ligament

Wright and Schuknecht (1972): loss of spiral ligament cells; correlation of width with descending audiograms

Nadol (1979): case study: thickening of basal basilar membrane

Nadol (1981): atrophy of spiral ligament

an increased number of fibrils in the basal turn. However, coincident loss of hair cells was probably sufficient to account for the patient's hearing loss.

Table 3-4 summarizes studies demonstrating spiral ligament and/or basilar membrane changes in the elderly.

RELATIONSHIP OF HISTOPATHOLOGY TO HEARING IMPAIRMENT

The occurrence of hyalinization or calcareous deposits on the basilar membrane was noted by Crowe et al. (1934) in their normal-hearing control group. It was concluded that such changes did not impair hearing when restricted to the basal 2 mm of the cochlea. Basilar membrane changes encompassing more than 3 mm were observed in several of the oldest subjects with high frequency losses; however, these subjects also had ganglion cell atrophy, so it was not possible to determine if the basilar membrane pathology contributed to hearing loss.

According to Belal (1975), an increase in the number of acellular areas in the spiral ligament appeared in older "normal" hearing patients. Wright and Schuknecht (1972) quantified the cell density and areas of acellularity in the spiral ligament by age for subjects with no known hearing deficits prior to death (Figure 3-17). Considerable age-related atrophy is observed in this population. Spiral ligament pathology,

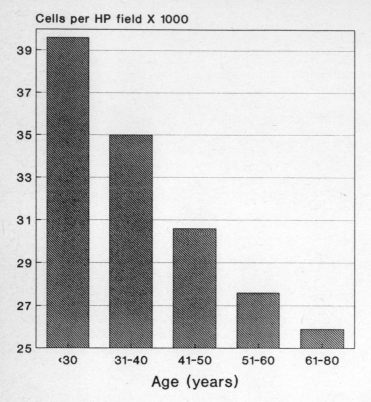

Figure 3-17. Density of spiral ligament cells (adapted from Wright and Schuknecht, 1972).

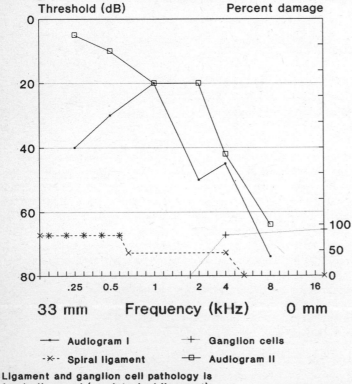

Figure 3-18. Mechanical presbycusis, audiogram and histopathology (adapted from Nadol, 1981). mm on abscissa refers to distance from cochlear base. Asterisks indicate detached spiral ligament.

in excess of what was observed by Wright and Schuknecht (1972) in normal hearing patients, was not observed in patients diagnosed as having Meniere's disease, primary pathology of the stria vascularis, or chronic otitis media.

The hallmark of Schuknecht's mechanical type of presbycusis is the descending audiometric pattern (Fig. 3-18). Some individuals who had descending audiometric curves in Belal's (1975) study exhibited "severe degenerative changes" of the spiral ligament. As shown in Figure 3-19, Wright and Schuknecht (1972) found that spiral ligament pathology was greater than normal for age in some cases of otosclerosis and in patients with descending audiometric curves. In all cases, spiral ligament atrophy was most severe near the apical turn. In 8 of the 15 cases, the basilar membrane had separated from the remnant of remaining spiral ligament, rupturing the cochlear duct. However, it was unclear if this was a fixation artifact or an actual phenomenon.

In unusual cases, basilar membrane/spiral ligament pathology can be severe (Allam, 1970). Schuknecht (1967) presented a case history of an 80-year-old man in whom the spiral ligament and basilar membrane were atrophied bilaterally, accompanied by progressive hearing loss. The greatly thinned basilar membrane ultimately ruptured, causing profound hearing loss.

AGE-RELATED CHANGES IN THE VASCULAR SUPPLY TO THE INNER EAR

BACKGROUND

Research on animal models has shown that cochlear responses to sound are associated with increased blood flow, presumably to meet metabolic demands. For instance, Ryan, Axelsson, Myers, and Woolf (1988) showed that blood flow/glucose metabolism in the eighth nerve, spiral ganglion, and organ of Corti of gerbils increased with exposure to moderately intense sounds. Similar increases were also observed in the stria vascularis of mice (Canlon and Schacht, 1983). In

Figure 3-19. Width of the spiral ligament of patients with otosclerosis or descending audiograms with respect to normal subjects (adapted from Wright and Schuknecht, 1972).

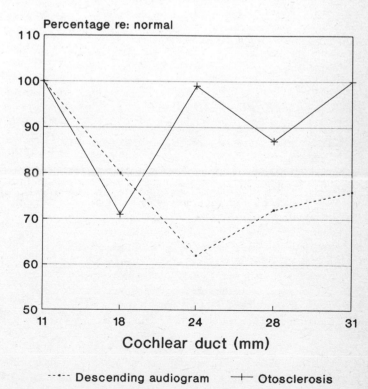

theory, if cochlear blood flow were impaired by aging, the increased metabolic demands could not be met and impaired hearing would result.

Arterial blood reaches the cochlea by successively traversing the vertebral, basal, and labyrinthine arteries. The latter gains access to the inner ear through the internal auditory meatus. The vasculature of the human cochlea was described in detail by Axelsson (1974). By this account, most of the cochlea is richly supplied with blood vessels, exceptions being Reissner's membrane, the tectorial membrane, and the peripheral portion of the basilar membrane. Blood is supplied by an artery running spirally around the modiolus with arterioles radiating out over the scala vestibuli and spiral lamina. Spiral capillary systems are found in the external wall of the cochlea (with the greatest density in the stria vascularis) and the spiral lamina. The vascular systems of the spiral lamina and external cochlear wall are drained by venules that empty into veins running spirally around the modiolus. Arteriovenous anastomoses are also found, especially in the basal turn, creating the potential for shunting blood past capillaries in segments of the cochlea. Additional capillary networks are found in the spiral ganglion, auditory nerve, modiolus wall, and extreme basal end of the cochlea. The vessels of the basilar membrane (i.e., spiral vessels) run under it from base to apex. However, the route from base to apex is not a continuous one. Rather, alternating radiating arterioles and venules provide an arrangement in which segments of the vessel can be occluded.

HISTOPATHOLOGY
INTRACOCHLEAR VASCULATURE

A number of investigators have observed age-related changes in cochlear vasculature, particularly in the stria vascularis (Table 3-3, 3-5). Von Fieandt and Saxen (1937) and Saxen (1952) identified "angiosclerotic degeneration of the inner ear" in elderly patients. They reported a thickening of strial and other cochlear vessels and loss of capillaries. In older patients, Jorgensen (1961) observed strial vessels that were thickened and stained positively for hyalin. Johnsson and Hawkins (1972b) often observed dilation of vessels and microaneurysms in the stria of older patients. Vascular changes within the stria have been found to occur throughout the length of the cochlea (Fabinyi, 1931; Crowe et al., 1934; Schuknecht, 1955; Jorgensen, 1961).

Johnsson and Hawkins (1972b) described the age-related changes in cochlear vasculature in detail. They noted that the cochlear vasculature was unusual in

TABLE 3-5. STUDIES SHOWING AGE-RELATED VAS-CULAR CHANGES IN THE INNER EAR OR INTERNAL AUDITORY MEATUS (OTHER THAN STRIAL)

Von Fieandt and Saxen (1937): "angiosclerotic degeneration"

Hansen and Reske-Nielsen (1965): thickening of vessels/ narrowing of lumen in internal meatus (more pronounced than in stria or modiolus)

Krmpotic-Nemanic (1971): ossification and cuffing of blood vessels

Fisch et al. (1972): progressive changes after first decade with thickening of vessels in internal auditory meatus

Johnsson and Hawkins (1972b; 1979): changes in blood vessels, especially in outer spiral vessels of basal cochlea

Suga and Lindsay (1976): vascular changes seen, but correlation with cochlear atrophy not demonstrated

Makishima (1978): internal auditory artery affected and related to other changes

that many vessels were surrounded by perivascular spaces. These were largest in the radiating arterioles, but also occurred in venules and capillaries (but not in the stria vascularis).

Gradual loss of capillaries with aging occurred in the spiral ligament and stria vascularis. Losses in the spiral ligament were more pronounced in the scala vestibuli than in the scala tympani. Capillaries were replaced by "intervascular strands" and "avascular channels" in the spiral ligament (Fig. 3-20). The strands were fibrous with occasional pyknotic nuclei, had a thickness of a few microns, and probably were the remnants of atrophied vessels. The channels appeared directly continuous with the perivascular spaces, often containing strands and elongated pyknotic cells, and apparently had been the perivascular spaces.

Less pronounced changes also occurred in the radiating arterioles of the spiral ligament and stria. They became narrower (with thicker walls), occluded, or atrophied and replaced by avascular channels.

By the end of the first decade there was already localized atrophy of the inner and outer spiral vessels. In old subjects a specific form of degeneration was seen in the outer spiral vessel of the hook region of the cochlea. This was characterized by thickening of the vessel wall, widening of the perivascular space, filling of the space by a hyaline substance, and "undulated" walls. The vessel's lumen was narrow or occluded.

EXTRACOCHLEAR VASCULATURE

Hansen (1973) examined temporal bones and found that circulatory pathways passing through the otic

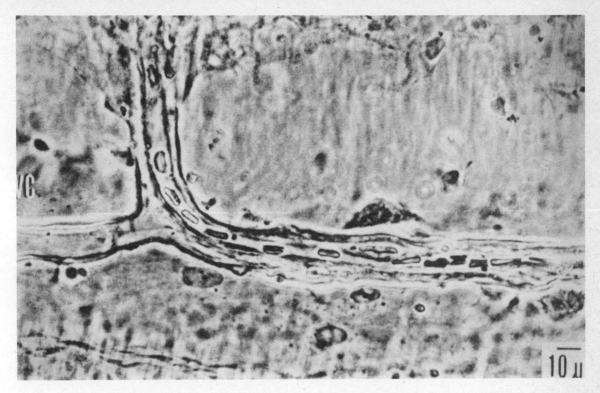

Figure 3-20. Outer spiral vessel with thickened wall and lumen almost occluded (in the most basal cochlea), from a 59-year-old male. Elongated red blood cells are seen in the narrow vessel to the right; the perivascular space appears to be filled with hyalinized substance; there is complete degeneration of the vessels to the left and only an avascular channel (AVC) remains; There is almost complete degeneration of nerve fibers in the osseous spiral lamina. From Johnsson, L.-G. and Hawkins, J.E., Jr. (1972b) Vascular changes in the human ear associated with aging. *Annals of Otology, Rhinology & Laryngology 81:* 364–376, with permission.

capsule to the cochlea appeared to remain viable in elderly patients. Hansen (1973) also measured the vascular density in the eighth nerve. Density in the peripheral (Schwann cell) portion of the nerve was uniform irrespective of age.

Fisch, Dobozi, and Greig (1972) observed degenerative changes in the wall of the arterial vessels of the internal auditory meatus beyond the first decade of life. The changes consisted of progressive thickening, particularly in the outermost layer, the tunica adventitia (Figs. 3-21; 3-22). This would affect the contractability and extensibility of the arteries. Ultimately, complete loss of cellular structure (hyalinization) resulted in some cases. The changes were seen in all sizes of vessels, but occurred earliest and with greatest severity in the smaller ones. They suggested that these changes could impair the blood supply to the inner ear. Fisch and colleagues noted similar findings by Pokotilenko (1965).

This limited evidence suggests that blood vessels serving the cochlea remain viable with age, but changes may occur that could diminish their functional capacity.

RELATIONSHIP OF HISTOPATHOLOGY TO HEARING IMPAIRMENT

While a good deal of evidence has been obtained for age-related histopathology in the vascular system of the cochlea, a link to hearing loss is yet to be established. We still await studies quantitatively relating the condition of cochlear vasculature to hearing loss in elderly listeners. Histopathological methods in postmortem tissue are rather limited in this regard, and research is needed to evaluate the cochlear vascula-

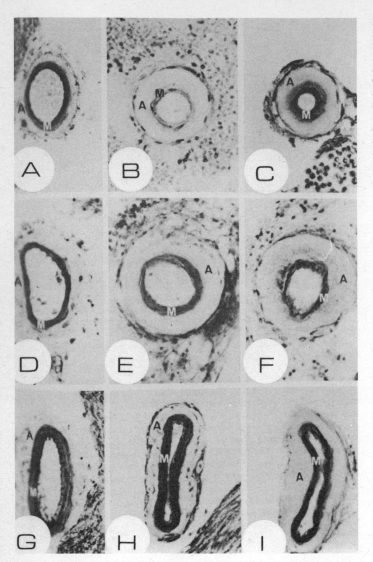

Figure 3-21. Histological pattern of change in the arteries of the internal auditory meatus. A,B,C: Vasa nervorum in the first, fourth, and seventh decade; D,E,F: Cochlear artery in the first, fifth, and seventh decade; G,H,I: labyrinthine artery in the first, fifth, and seventh decade. "A" = tunica adventitia; "M" = tunica media. From Fisch, U., Dobozi, M. & Greig, D. (1972) Degenerative changes of the arterial vessels of the internal auditory meatus during the process of aging. *Acta Otolaryngology 73:* 259–266, with permission.

ture and blood supply in living humans. Techniques such as laser Doppler blood flow measurements have great promise for animal and human research (e.g., Sillman et al., 1988), but the literature provides no indication of its use to study presbycusis. At the present time we must look to the literature on hypoxia and cochlear function to gain some insights into what *might* happen if the vascular supply to the cochlea were diminished in old individuals.

It is well established that hypoxia interferes with cochlear physiology. Cochlear potentials (endocochlear potential, compound action potential, cochlear microphonic) are reduced by hypoxia (Davis, 1957; Lawrence, Nuttall, and Burgio, 1975). Brown, Nuttall, Masta, and Lawrence (1983) measured frequency tuning curves from IHCs in guinea pigs whose respiration was transiently interrupted. They observed a decrease in sensitivity of tuning curve "tips" and a decrease in the

Figure 3-22. Thickness of the labyrinthine artery (adapted from Fisch et al., 1972).

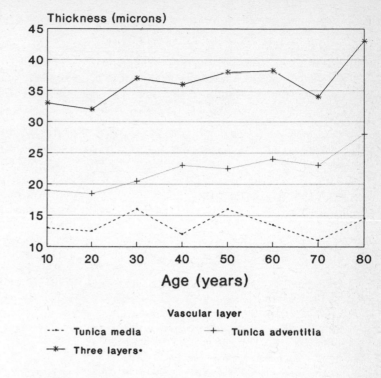

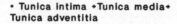

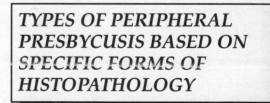

sharpness of tuning, suggesting that the frequency selectivity of IHCs was reduced. Sohmer, Freeman, and Schmuel (1989) experimentally produced hypoxia in cats and measured ABR thresholds. Hypoxia caused ABR thresholds to increase, with threshold being an inverse function of blood oxygen level. The authors interpreted threshold elevations to be due to depression of the endocochlear potential. In a study of humans Hotaling, Hillstrom, and Bazell (1989) reported that sickle-cell anemia crises were often accompanied by high frequency sensorineural hearing loss which can return to normal after the crisis. They suggested that cochlear ischemia was responsible.

When gradual anoxia is experimentally produced (e.g., by blocking of arteries or veins) the stria vascularis and OHCs are generally the most vulnerable tissues, and the basal cochlea is the most vulnerable region, followed by the apex, and finally, by mid-cochlear regions (Kimura, 1973).

Work of this type implies that a loss of hearing could result from age-related changes in the vascular system

if those changes reduced the supply of oxygen to the inner ear.

TYPES OF PERIPHERAL PRESBYCUSIS BASED ON SPECIFIC FORMS OF HISTOPATHOLOGY

This chapter has identified age-related histopathology in the organ of Corti, spiral ganglion cells and their processes, stria vascularis, tissue affecting cochlear mechanics including the spiral ligament, combined sensorineural tissue, and cochlear vasculature. With the exception of vascular pathology, each type has been shown to result in presbycusis if the severity of pathology surpasses a crucial level. We now address issues concerning the validity and utility of conceptual and/or diagnostic categories of presbycusis based on these various forms of pathology. These include the four types of presbycusis specified by Schuknecht, sensory, neural, strial, and mechanical, plus sensorineural presbycusis and vascular presbycusis.

The first issue to be examined is the validity of each type of presbycusis. The second issue concerns the usefulness of conceptualizing presbycusis according to distinct types of peripheral histopathology.

VALIDITY OF EACH TYPE OF PRESBYCUSIS

SENSORY PRESBYCUSIS

Schuknecht (1974) described sensory presbycusis as follows: the primary changes are in organ of Corti, with a loss of sensory and supporting cells, mostly at the base of the cochlea; the audiogram is characterized by a sharp loss of high frequency sensitivity (Fig. 3-6) but speech recognition remains well preserved.

An immediate reservation can be raised concerning Schuknecht's notion of sensory presbycusis because the occurrence of age-related atrophy of the organ of Corti is usually accompanied by ganglion cell damage. This was acknowledged by Schuknecht, and all of the cases presented by him (Gacek and Schuknecht, 1969; Schuknecht, 1964; 1974) indicate an extent of neural loss nearly comparable to that in the organ of Corti. Thus, on the basis of histopathology, these seem to be cases of sensorineural, rather than "pure" sensory presbycusis. The fact that speech recognition remains good in these cases does not rule out significant neural damage. As shown above, speech recognition can remain good despite significant loss of ganglion cells.

If the concept of "pure" sensory presbycusis is to be valid, a modification may be required, based on the involvement of OHCs and IHCs. Two compelling arguments can be made for modifying the concept of sensory presbycusis to focus on age-related atrophy of *OHCs*, rather than both OHCs and IHCs. Both arguments have been supported by the literature reviewed earlier. First, age-related loss of OHCs is typically more prominent than is the loss of IHCs. Second, age-related OHC degeneration can and often does occur

with minimum loss of spiral ganglion cells, whereas IHC degeneration is almost always complemented by ganglion cell loss. In other words, "pure" sensory presbycusis typically does not occur when IHC degeneration is involved, but can occur if the sensory damage is largely restricted to OHCs.

NEURAL PRESBYCUSIS

Schuknecht (1974) described neural presbycusis as characterized by a loss of spiral ganglion cells or their peripheral processes that is out of proportion to organ of Corti degeneration (Fig. 3-14 A,B).[3] The audiogram indicates high frequency losses (Fig. 3-14 A,B), but more importantly, speech recognition is depressed.

The histopathological literature reviewed earlier provides strong support for the validity of neural presbycusis as a distinct category of presbycusis. Some degree of ganglion cell loss—particularly near the base of the cochlea—is virtually inevitable in the elderly, and is often severe enough to cause clinically significant hearing loss (presbycusis). Furthermore, age-related cochlear neural pathology can occur without concomitant histopathological involvement of the organ of Corti. However, two issues are in need of further attention by researchers and clinicians.

THE RELIABILITY OF AUDIOMETRIC MEASURES

A hallmark of neural presbycusis, which distinguishes it from other diagnostic categories, is impaired speech recognition (Schuknecht, 1974). However, the literature reviewed above (e.g., Otte et al., 1978; Pauler et al., 1986) indicates that neither pure tone audiometric thresholds nor speech recognition tests are good predictors of the condition of the spiral ganglion. Consequently, these measures are not satisfactory diagnostic indices. This problem was underscored by a recent report on the Framingham Heart Study (Gates, Cooper, Kannel, and Miller, 1990). Less than one percent of (more than 1,000) elderly subjects exhibited speech recognition that was "disproportionally" poorer than pure tone thresholds would predict (based on norms established by Yellin, Jerger, and Fifer, 1989). Yet, based on histopathological studies reviewed earlier, it

---

[3] Degeneration of neurons in the central auditory system has been included in the neural presbycusis category (e.g., Schuknecht, 1974), but the present discussion restricts the use of the term to peripheral changes. Neural changes within the central auditory system, "central presbycusis," are discussed in Chapter 6.

would be expected that many of these subjects would have significant spiral ganglion pathology. Indeed, at this point, reliable audiometric measures of the condition of the spiral ganglion have not been developed.

THE EFFERENT NEURAL SYSTEM

The work on neural presbycusis by Schuknecht and others has focused on the afferent system (spiral ganglion cells and their radial dendrites). The role of pathology within the efferent neural system (fibers, synaptic terminals, parent cell bodies within the brain) is virtually unknown, and could be important.

STRIAL PRESBYCUSIS

Schuknecht et al. (1974) proposed that strial atrophy is a disease entity and a cause of hearing loss exhibiting specific clinical features: (a) symmetry of loss in both ears, (b) similar degree of threshold elevation across frequencies (Fig. 3-15), (c) good speech recognition ability, and (d) very slow progression. Schuknecht et al. (1974) had shown that atrophy of the stria vascularis can occur with minimal histopathological changes in the organ of Corti or spiral ganglion, as determined by light microscopy. Presumably pathology of the stria alters metabolic, chemical, and/or bioelectric properties throughout the cochlea. Schuknecht used the term "metabolic presbycusis" (Schuknecht, 1955; 1964; 1974) as well as "strial presbycusis" (Otte et al., 1978; Schuknecht, 1989) in referring to presbycusis associated with pathology of the stria vascularis. The latter terminology is used here, in keeping with the focus on histopathology.

There is no question that histopathology of the stria vascularis is associated with hearing loss, although a small amount of pathology can be tolerated. There is little apparent relationship between the baso-apical locus or extent of strial degeneration and the pattern of audiometric loss, which occurs across frequencies. However, the often-used term, "flat," may be a misnomer to describe the "strial" audiogram. As shown in Figure 3-23, audiograms associated with the diagnosis of strial presbycusis come in a variety of shapes.

Figure 3-23. Audiometric curves for examples of strial presbycusis (adapted from Schuknecht, 1974).

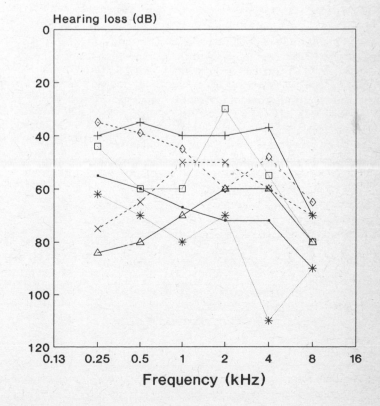

SENSORINEURAL PRESBYCUSIS

The term sensorineural presbycusis is used here to describe those cases of age-related hearing loss that are accompanied by a combination of organ of Corti damage plus a loss of ganglion cells or their processes, with possible strial involvement (as suggested by Johnsson and Hawkins, 1979).

Sensorineural pathology is undoubtedly a common cause of presbycusis—perhaps the most common of causes. As mentioned above, "pure" sensory presbycusis is not common, and organ of Corti degeneration is usually accompanied by neural damage. For instance, the data of Crowe et al. (1934) reveal no cases in which atrophy of the organ of Corti occurs without neural atrophy, and Johnsson and Hawkins (1979) found degeneration of both ganglion cells fibers and organ of Corti tissue to be typical of elderly inner ears.

The sensorineural classification of presbycusis does not contradict the notion of "pure" sensory, neural, or strial presbycusis. Rather, it indicates that pathological changes in cochlear tissues often go hand in hand. Indeed, it is possible that "pure" forms of presbycusis and sensorineural presbycusis have different etiologies (see Chapter 5).

MECHANICAL (COCHLEAR CONDUCTIVE) PRESBYCUSIS

Schuknecht (1974) described mechanical (also called cochlear conductive) presbycusis as follows. Significant pathology is not observed in the organ of Corti, spiral ganglion, or stria vascularis, yet there is a loss of sensitivity manifested by a "descending" audiometric curve (i.e., loss of sensitivity is directly related to frequency)(Fig. 3-18). Mechanical changes in the basilar membrane (e.g., altered stiffness), spiral ligament (e.g., diminished attachment of the basilar membrane), and/or other structures are presumed to be responsible for the loss of sensitivity. These putative changes could alter the motion mechanics of the cochlea (hence the alternative term, "cochlear conductive presbycusis"). Since patients with the characteristic descending curve typically have good speech recognition, Schuknecht (1964) felt that central involvement could be ruled out.

The rationale for associating the descending audiometric curve with mechanical change is based on two considerations. First, the basilar membrane has a physical gradient (progressively increasing width and decreasing thickness from base to apex) that is related to frequency representation: the frequency of sound is an important determinant of the locus of mechanical displacement of the basilar membrane. It is conceivable that physical changes (e.g., stiffness) in the basilar membrane could alter its displacement pattern in a manner that is directly related to the proximity to the cochlear base, producing the descending curve. Unfortunately, a convincing explanation for how this would produce a descending audiometric curve has never been provided. Second, the other types of age-related cochlear pathology have their own characteristic audiograms; cochlear conductive presbycusis emerges by the process of elimination (e.g., Ramadan and Schuknecht, 1989).

Glorig and Davis (1961) argued for the existence of cochlear conductive presbycusis on the basis of audiometric findings. They referred to a group of patients showing no loudness recruitment (a sign of hair cell dysfunction) in monaural loudness balancing tests, but having a descending audiometric curve. The explanation favored by Glorig and Davis was inner ear conductive impairment associated with physical changes in the cochlea. However, they did not provide a mechanism to account for the high frequency threshold elevations.

Lawrence (1979) questioned the validity of mechanical presbycusis as a diagnostic category, arguing that there was no evidence for its existence. To support this position, he cited Bekesy's (1960) classic cochlear model experiments. Lawrence inferred from this work that the types of changes resulting from spiral ligament or basilar membrane pathology would have little effect on basilar membrane motion. In addition, Bekesy performed experiments on temporal bones from human cadavers. When he mechanically manipulated the spiral ligament and basilar membrane, the amplitude and phase of the vibratory pattern of the basilar membrane appeared unaffected. While these experiments suggest robustness of the vibratory processes in the cochlea under certain experimental conditions, they provide little convincing evidence against the possibility of cochlear conductive hearing loss, given the types of histopathological changes that have been observed (see above).

To summarize, evidence of age-related changes in the basilar membrane that affect hearing is equivocal, and a clear link with mechanical presbycusis has not yet been established. However, the empirical evidence of spiral ligament pathology and its relationship to hearing loss, discussed earlier, provides tentative support for the validity of mechanical presbycusis.

VASCULAR PRESBYCUSIS

Johnsson and Hawkins (1979) concluded that vascular changes play an important role in presbycusis and suggested *vascular presbycusis* as a diagnostic category. Implicit in the inclusion of vascular presbycusis as a distinct category is the assumption that vascular insufficiency per se is a cause of impaired hearing (e.g., functional effects of hypoxia, etc.). It is conceivable that vascular deficiency could lead to degeneration of sensory, neural, or strial tissue, in which case it would be more appropriately viewed as a *cause* of other types of histopathology that result in presbycusis.

Because this research has been thwarted by technical limitations, a sound evaluation of vascular presbycusis in humans has not been forthcoming. Furthermore, a relationship between arteriosclerosis and hearing loss, which might provide indirect support for the validity of vascular presbycusis, is currently inconclusive, as discussed in Chapter 5. Work with animals (Chapter 4) does not present a consistent picture, either. Studies on guinea pigs (Axelsson, 1971) and rats (Hillerdal et al., 1987) provide no evidence of reduced cochlear blood flow in aged animals, whereas such evidence has been found in aging gerbils (Prazma, 1990).

At present, vascular presbycusis must be viewed as a compelling, yet hypothetical concept. It is compelling because blood supplied to the cochlea supports the metabolic requirements of the organ of Corti, spiral ganglion cells, and stria vascularis. It follows that age-related vascular pathology—which has been clearly demonstrated in humans—would likely result in an insufficiency of oxygen or other blood-borne metabolites supplied to the cochlea. The concept remains hypothetical because of a lack of evidence directly linking age-related vascular changes to hearing loss.

SUMMARY

Pathology of the organ of Corti in general, OHCs in particular, ganglion cells, stria vascularis, and spiral ligament are each correlated with presbycusis in humans. Cochlear vascular pathology occurs and is in theory sufficient to cause presbycusis. Sensorineural pathology, in which several types of tissue are involved, is also correlated with presbycusis. Thus, a good argument can be made for the validity of each of the six types of presbycusis based on histopathology—sensory (OHC), neural, strial, mechanical, sensorineural, and vascular.

THE USEFULNESS OF DISTINGUISHING SIX TYPES OF PERIPHERAL PRESBYCUSIS BASED ON HISTOPATHOLOGY

The evidence presented above indicates that each of the six types of cochlear histopathology can cause

presbycusis. Is it useful to distinguish six distinct types rather then viewing them as contributors to hearing loss under the rubric, "cochlear presbycusis?" To answer this question, three issues are relevant: the occurrence of the six types as distinct, independently manifested entities, the ability of audiometric tests to identify specific histopathologies, the ability of histopathological methods to assess the functional condition of the inner ear.

THE OCCURRENCE OF DISTINCT FORMS OF HISTOPATHOLOGY

Evidence from post-mortem histopathological studies, reviewed above, has shown that fairly specific sensory (OHC), neural, and strial forms of histopathology do indeed exist in some individuals, and the result is hearing loss. However, as noted by Schuknecht (1974) and Johnsson and Hawkins (1979), "pure" types of presbycusis are often not the case. This is especially true with respect to sensory presbycusis, which typically has concomitant neural involvement unless the hair cell injury is limited to the OHCs. With respect to mechanical presbycusis, it is unclear if damage to the spiral ligament has been observed in cochleas free of other pathology.

Undoubtedly, many cases of presbycusis do not fit neatly into any of the four categories of Schuknecht, limiting the utility of this classification scheme. This shortcoming is largely circumvented by inclusion of the sensorineural presbycusis category, which, by definition, encompasses cases without "pure" sensory or neural forms of pathology. The sensorineural classification is not merely a "catch-all" category. Evidence was presented earlier to indicate that age-related sensorineural pathology is not simply a secondary stage of either sensory, neural, or strial pathology, but is probably caused by factors different from those causing the "pure" forms (see also Chapter 5).

The existence of vascular presbycusis has not been verified, and the effects of age-related vascular pathology on various cochlear tissues, if any, are unknown. It is conceivable that vascular insufficiency could occur with or without concomitant pathology of other cochlear tissue. If secondary vascular effects on cochlear tissue were to occur in aging ears, the issue of the specificity of histopathology would be clouded.

In summary, with the inclusion of the sensorineural classification, the histopathological categories probably encompass and differentiate most cases of peripheral presbycusis. However, no matter what typology is adopted, many, if not most, cases appear to involve pathology of several types of cochlear tissue.

THE SPECIFICITY OF AUDIOMETRIC MEASURES AND THEIR RELATIONSHIP TO HISTOPATHOLOGY

There is little doubt that many patients have characteristic audiometric profiles appropriate for the histopathological classifications described by Schuknecht. However, it seems that caution is warranted in making inferences about cochlear histopathology from audiometric data. First, substantial audiometric variance exists within a given diagnostic category. Even when "textbook examples" of Schuknecht (1974) are plotted together, a degree of similarity among types as well as variance within types is evident (Figs. 3-23, 3-24). Second, when the histopathology involves more than one type of tissue (as is often the case), audiometric symptoms of one may mask another. For example, sensory cell loss in the base of the cochlea would alter the flat or descending audiograms that might otherwise be present due to strial and/or basilar membrane pathology. Thus, inferences of specific cochlear histopathology made on the basis of pure-tone audiometry may be suspect.

The addition of speech recognition tests to the audiometric battery accords only limited improvement in differentiating types of histopathology. The correlation between ganglion cell loss and speech recognition is not a tight one, as discussed earlier. Poor speech recognition can occur despite a relatively intact population of ganglion cells, and, conversely, substantial neural degeneration can occur without comparable losses in speech recognition.

Given these problems, it is not surprising that several studies have failed to show a close correspondence between audiometric data and cochlear pathology. In a sample of 17 aged patients, Suga and Lindsay (1976) found cases of gradually sloping audiometric curves, abrupt high tone hearing loss, and flat curves (i.e., the audiometric descriptors of Schuknecht's presbycusis categories). Cochleas of the patients demonstrated atrophy of the spiral ganglion, organ of Corti, and stria vascularis to varying degrees. However, no consistent correlation was found between the site of lesion and type of audiometric curve. The data of Crowe et al. (1934), which have been referred to repeatedly, show several histopathological subgroups all with hearing loss across high frequencies.

LIMITATIONS IN USING HISTOPATHOLOGICAL CRITERIA TO IDENTIFY THE CAUSES OF PRESBYCUSIS

Histopathological observations, especially at the light microscopic level, are most certainly limited in their ability to detect structural changes that may

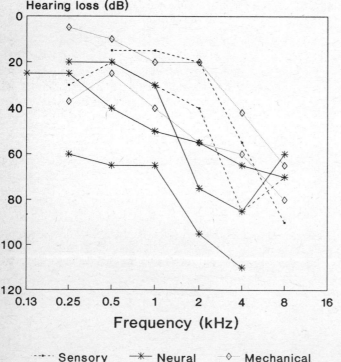

Figure 3-24. Audiometric curves for examples of sensory, neural, and mechanical presbycusis (adapted from Schuknecht, 1974).

produce physiological deficits that might cause hearing loss. "Normal looking" cochleas may not function at all normally if subtle physiological processes are disrupted. Thus, pathophysiological effects on hearing might be mistakenly attributed to presumed histopathological (e.g., degenerative) causes.

An example of how subtle cochlear changes might affect hearing is provided in a recent theoretical paper by Patuzzi, Yates, and Johnstone (1989). They present an account of OHC pathology that is based on current conceptions of cochlear physiology and may apply to presbycusis. They argue that much sensorineural hearing loss can be explained by disruption of the mechano-electrical transduction process of the OHCs.

Several assumptions are made. The IHCs are simple passive detectors of vibration that excite primary afferent neurons by chemical synapses. The OHC receptor current is related to transverse displacement of the organ of Corti in a nonlinear, frequency-invariant fashion. The OHCs apply a force to the organ of Corti that is dependent on the receptor current in a linear fashion. For near-characteristic frequency (CF) tones the vibration of the organ of Corti is determined by the pressure and frequency of the tone and by the active force generated by the OHCs; there is an active feedback loop linking organ of Corti vibration and OHC receptor current. For frequencies well below CF the active force of the OHCs is insignificant. The cochlear microphonic (CM) is used as an indicator of OHC currents; the compound action potential (CAP) is used as an indicator of organ of Corti vibration near CF.

The receptor current through the OHCs is intimately related to the mechanical sensitivity of the cochlea near CF. Even small disruptions of the currents are accompanied by a loss of sensitivity, presumably by interfering with the active OHC mechanism. Disruption of OHC current (particularly in the basal cochlea) is associated with temporary threshold shift, ototoxic drugs, asphyxia, anoxia, or non-linear processes. It is also likely that a loss of OHCs or their stereocilia, disruption of hair cell motility, or a change in the electrical impedance of OHCs would also affect the active process.

The differentiation between IHC and OHC systems also implies different forms of cochlear hearing loss associated with damage to each. Patuzzi and colleagues suggest that one type of pathological change would involve the OHC receptor currents and losses of mechanical sensitivity near CF; the other type would involve only the IHCs or synaptic processes and would produce approximately equal threshold elevation across the frequency threshold curve. Impairment of the OHC "motor" system would simultaneously produce reduced sensitivity, reduced frequency selectiv-

ity, and recruitment. Pathology involving the IHC system would also produce loss of sensitivity but would have smaller effects on frequency selectivity and compression of the intensity function.

If these events were to occur when cochlear changes are associated with aging, presbycusis would result. However the effects on hearing might not correspond well to any histopathological scheme, since the key dysfunctions may have no identifiable histopathological correlates.

CONCLUSIONS

The utility of the different histopathological classifications of presbycusis depends on one's perspective. From the practicing clinician's perspective, the usefulness of the histopathological classifications is limited. First, aging is typically associated with pathology in more than one type of inner ear tissue. Second, even when pathologies occur in relatively "pure" forms it is often difficult to distinguish them audiometrically. Third, presbycusis might result from physiological disturbances that have no detectable histological basis. For these reasons, audiometric measures could be irrelevant or misleading with regard to the underlying causes and treatments of presbycusis in many cases.

From the perspective of clinical and basic scientists, however, distinct categories of histopathology are useful because they can facilitate research on the mechanisms and etiology of presbycusis. With regard to the mechanisms underlying presbycusis, it is likely that damage to each type of tissue contributes to hearing impairment in a different manner. Therefore, in order to understand the underlying mechanism of presbycusis it is important to study the age-related changes in each type of tissue in detail. This can be done with animal models that exhibit the various types of histopathology found in humans (Chapter 4). For instance, research on an animal model such as the gerbil, which exhibits age-related strial pathology, can be used to gain insight into the changes in this particular type of tissue, whereas certain mouse strains can be used to investigate primary ganglion cell pathology. With regard to etiology, it is likely that pathology in different cochlear tissue is related to distinct causal factors. Different etiologies would imply different potential treatments or prophylaxis (Chapter 5).

CHAPTER 4

Aging and the Inner Ear of Animals

In this chapter research on aging and the inner ear of non-human animals is reviewed. The animal work complements the research on humans reviewed in Chapter 3. In some cases, techniques that are not possible to use on humans have been employed, providing details on age-related cochlear functioning that would otherwise be unavailable, and advancing our understanding of presbycusis in ways not possible with human work alone. In addition, by using such techniques, animals can be used as models to demonstrate what types of processes and events *can and do occur* in the aging mammalian ear. These may not be shared by humans, and one should never make a priori assumptions that they are. Nevertheless, the information obtained from animal research can be used to formulate credible, testable hypotheses about mechanisms underlying presbycusis or to suggest new clinical approaches to the human condition.

Some research methods can be used on both humans and animals (e.g., post-mortem histopathological studies). These methods provide data that speak to the ubiquity of certain age-related changes in the auditory system—their generality within the mammalian family. Such data can help sort out the roles of genetic and environmental variables in presbycusis.

The use of animals in research on presbycusis has been surprisingly sparse. This is exemplified by a 1975 "conference on animal models of aging in the auditory system" (Crowley, 1975) in which the majority of participants were not directly involved in animal research on presbycusis. Fortunately, the use of animal models of presbycusis has begun to accelerate.

RESEARCH CONSIDERATIONS

The use of animals in histopathological research lessens some of the problems associated with human post-mortem material discussed in Chapter 3. Excellent fixation of tissue can be obtained, and aged animals can be in good health at the time of euthanasia. In physiological, anatomical, or behavioral research, the effects of noise and other environmental insults can usually be accounted for and/or controlled.

However, research with animals is not without technical and practical limitations. The problems inherent in using carnivores or primates in aging research are apparent: they are expensive to maintain for long periods (preferably their entire life, to control for environmental influences on hearing), and they are long-lived. Nevertheless, when aged populations of larger laboratory animals are available, important findings can emerge, as shown below (e.g., Hawkins et al., 1985). Rodents, of course, are less expensive to maintain and shorter-lived; however, they have their own limitations as models for human presbycusis with regard to the frequency range of hearing, development of the neocortex, head size (re: spatial localization), etc.

THE ANIMAL MODELS

We shall review the animal models by species in order to obtain a sense of their advantages and shortcomings, as well as the extent and types of data available for each model.

GUINEA PIG

Guinea pigs are attractive for work on the peripheral auditory system because a considerable amount of work has been done on non-aged animals. Guinea pigs have a life span of more than seven years (Altman and Dittmer, 1972), which may present a practical difficulty for maintaining animals through old age. In fact, research on the auditory system of very old guinea pigs (older than five years) does not appear in the literature.

Thresholds of guinea pigs were measured by Dum and von Wedel (1983) using the auditory brainstem response (see also, Chapter 7). Thresholds were still near normal at 15 months, but were elevated by 30-40 dB at 24 months with little further change by 3 years. The threshold elevations were relatively "flat," being similar for frequencies of 500 to 15,000 Hz.

Covell and Rogers (1957) described the histological features of the guinea pig inner ear in animals ranging up to almost 5 years of age. Pathology of the stria vascularis was not consistent or striking, but did occur. Changes consisted of regional atrophy, "cystic degeneration," and increased pigmentation. The most prominent age-related change in the inner ear was a decrease in the number of ganglion cells near the cochlear apex and, to a lesser extent, in the basal end. The degeneration of ganglion cells, stained with hematoxylin and eosin, appeared as follows: eccentricity of the nucleus, chromatolysis, and loss of ground substance, followed by diminished stainability and swelling of the nucleus, loss of cytoplasm, cell membrane, and nucleus, and the appearance of macrophages.

The loss of peripheral dendritic processes of ganglion cells appeared to follow degeneration of the cell bodies. Degeneration of cell processes proceeded in each of the bipolar directions (into the eighth nerve and toward the organ of Corti), suggesting primacy of cell body degeneration. The efferent system was only "lacking a few fibers" in the basal turns of the oldest animals.

Degenerative changes in the organ of Corti were prominent only in the oldest guinea pigs, and only in the regions of ganglion cell loss. The changes consisted of a loss of supporting and sensory cells, collapse of the tunnel of Corti, and loss of mesothelial cells beneath the basilar membrane.

Other studies, counting hair cells of guinea pigs, were consistent with Covell and Rogers' work in finding minimal IHC losses in animals up to one year (Coleman, 1976a,b), two years (Dayal and Barek, 1975) (Fig. 4-1) and three years (Ulehlova, 1975). The Coleman (1976b) study showed some loss of OHCs (2.4-12.3 percent), with most damage occurring in the apical region.

Cochlear blood vessels of guinea pigs up to two to three years of age were evaluated by Axelsson (1971) by filling vessels with a contrast medium. No age-related changes were seen in the vessel of the basilar membrane, in the vessels in the basal region of the cochlea, or in vessels of the stria vascularis. Normalcy of cochlear blood vessels in older guinea pigs had also been described in the earlier study by Covell and Rogers (1957). They found no age-related changes in the walls of blood vessels in the modiolus; however, an increase in the amount of perivascular tissue was observed in older animals and was often associated with osteitis of the bony wall of the modiolus and new bone formation.

Pestalozza and co-workers (1957) measured cochlear microphonic and compound action potentials in guinea pigs similar to those used by Covell and Rogers (1957). They found age-related losses in the cochlear microphonic (believed to reflect OHC behavior) that seemed to be more severe than the reported cochlear pathology would warrant. There was also evidence of histological changes in the middle ear, suggesting to the authors that middle ear conductive hearing loss had occurred. The action potential data suggested losses even greater than the cochlear microphonics,

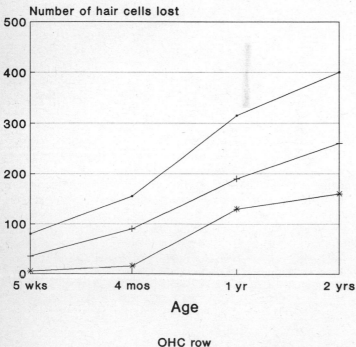

Figure 4-1. Guinea pig OHC loss (adapted from Dayal and Barek, 1975).

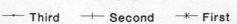

implicating a loss of spiral ganglion cells akin to that reported by Covell and Rogers. Thus, the aging guinea pigs appeared to demonstrate both middle ear conductive and peripheral neural impairment. However, the severity of impairment was rather mild.

A quantitative cytochemical study of the guinea pig basilar membrane was performed by Kraus (1970). The density of the basilar membrane decreased from 1.76 gm/cm³ in newborn animals to 1.33 gm/cm³ in adults; a small additional decrease to 1.29 gm/cm³ occurred in old animals. Kraus likened this pattern of change (decreased density with age) to that seen in the vitreous body of the eye, as contrasted with the increased density occurring in collagen. These findings suggest a basis for age-related changes in cochlear mechanics, although their actual functional significance is unknown.

RAT

Rats typically live up to three or four years, which is advantageous for life-span studies. A significant, if not extensive, literature on the rat auditory system exists. Importantly, rats have been used widely in (nonauditory) research on aging, behavior, and various aspects of biology, providing a rich background of gerontological data. The two most commonly used rat strains have been the Sprague-Dawley and Fischer 344.

SPRAGUE-DAWLEY RAT

Crowley and colleagues (1972a,b) assessed the utility of the albino Sprague-Dawley rat as a model of human presbycusis. Cochlear microphonics, masked and unmasked eighth-nerve compound action potentials (APs), and hair cell counts were obtained in rats as old as two years (i.e., moderately aged). The cochlear microphonic and AP indicated that maximum sensitivity for click stimuli was reached at 12 months and then declined by about 12 dB by 24 months. The derived AP amplitude (a method using masking to estimate the contributions of the different regions of the basilar membrane to the overall AP) indicated that the decline was greatest at high frequencies (Fig. 4-2). Cooper, Coleman, and Newton (1990) obtained brainstem-evoked response thresholds to tone bursts from 24- to 29-month-old Sprague-Dawley rats. Thresholds increased by about 18 dB at 3kHz, 14 dB at 8 kHz and 32 dB at 40 kHz.

Figure 4-2. Amplitudes of derived action potentials of Sprague-Dawley rats (adapted from Crowley et al., 1972).

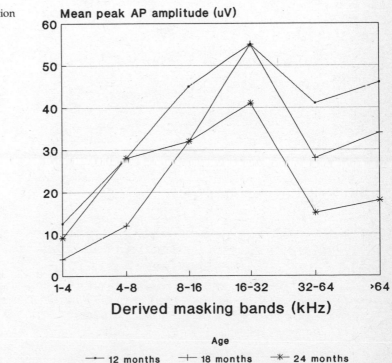

Mean peak AP amplitude (uV)

Derived masking bands (kHz)

Age

— 12 months —+— 18 months —*— 24 months

Age-related hearing loss in Sprague-Dawley rats has been measured behaviorally (Harrison, 1981; Harrison and Turnock, 1975; Turnock and Harrison, 1975). Thresholds were obtained for narrow noise bands with various center frequencies in a longitudinal study. Sensitivity remained unchanged through 14 months, showed a decline by 24 months and a further decline by 30-39 months. Animals over 30 months typically showed a hearing loss of 10-15 dB at frequencies above 32 kHz and below 1 kHz. The less pronounced age effect in this study, compared to that of Cooper et al. (1990) might be methodological. The ABR study used tone bursts whereas the behavioral work used filtered noise bands.

Crowley et al. (1972a,b) observed a small loss of OHCs (five percent) and an even smaller loss (one percent) of IHCs in two-year-old rats. Similarly, Keithley and Feldman (1982) found only small degrees of OHC degeneration beginning relatively early in the life span (e.g., by six months) but never progressing beyond ten percent (Fig. 4-3). IHC loss was minimal. They also noted the formation of phalangeal scars after degeneration of the hair cells and a loss of OHCs in clusters. The greatest losses of hair cells occurred at the cochlear base and apex.

Keithley and Feldman (1979) counted ganglion cells in Sprague-Dawley rats similar to those used for their hair cell counts. The median number of cells was significantly reduced by 23 months with little apparent further loss through 34 months. Although the losses occurred throughout the length of the cochlea, they were greatest near the base and apex. Keithley and Feldman also differentiated between Type I and II cells. Type I cells were lost throughout the spiral ganglion, whereas the loss of Type II cells occurred in the middle and apical regions, but not in the base. Loss of Type II cells appeared at a later age. The magnitude of loss of Type I and II cells was not highly correlated within individuals. On the basis of these differences in the pattern of cell loss, the authors proposed that the two types should be considered as different populations with respect to aging. An additional observation was the absence of new bone growth that might damage ganglion cell processes by occluding the openings through which they leave Rosenthal's canal.

In the Keithley and Feldman (1982) study, some cochleas were evaluated for the loss of both ganglion cells and hair cells. No correlation was observed between the degree of IHC loss and loss of Type I ganglion cells or between loss of OHCs and Type II

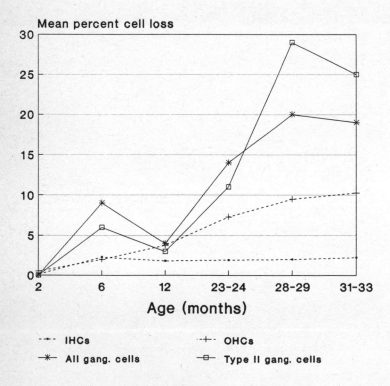

Figure 4-3. Mean hair cell and ganglion cell loss in Sprague-Dawley rats (computed from data in Keithley and Feldman, 1979; 1982).

Derived from data in Keithley & Feldman (1979; 1982)

ganglion cells. These observations are further supported by comparing the ganglion cell data from the 1979 study with the complete sample of hair cell data from the 1982 study, as shown in Figure 4-3. Ganglion cells were lost to a greater degree than IHCs. Thus, degeneration of Type I ganglion cells was not secondary to loss of the hair cells they innervated. Conversely, Keithley and Feldman observed a disappearance of OHCs at the cochlear base, but not Type II ganglion cells presumed to innervate them. This finding suggests that OHCs can atrophy without involving neural cells, a possible example of "pure" OHC sensory presbycusis.

Feldman (1990) recently described age-related changes in Reissner's membrane. A decrease in cellularity was seen in older rats, particularly those whose life spans had been extended to 41 to 48 months by dietary restriction. These animals showed cell density decreases of 29, 32, and 45 percent in the base, middle, and apex of the cochlea, respectively. Cells from aged cochleas often exhibited "blebs" or vacuolization, and focal areas of de-lamination between epithelial and perilymphatic cell layers were also evident. A good deal of variance in the baso-apical pattern of cell loss was observed, but the apical region was consistently affected in old animals. Since hair cell loss is greatest in the apex of Sprague-Dawley rats, Feldman suggested that the decreased cellularity of Reissner's membrane may impair its barrier function (protecting the organ of Corti from perilymph toxicity), thereby contributing to presbycusis.

The accumulation of pigment was studied in ganglion cell bodies of Sprague-Dawley rats aged 1 to 34 months by Feldman, Craig, and Keithley (1981). A greater accumulation of pigment was observed in type I cells than in type II cells. At age 23-29 months, 80 percent of type I cells had accumulated pigment, whereas the greatest percentage of OHCs with pigment was only 20 percent (at age 23 months). The distribution of pigment build-up was unrelated to the baso-apical location along the cochlea, suggesting it was independent of age-related ganglion cell loss. The functional significance of this finding is unclear at present.

The cochlear nerve of Sprague-Dawley rats was evaluated by Hoeffding and Feldman (1988). The median number of normal fibers was reduced by 21 percent at age 26.5 months and by 24 percent at 36 months. The number of degenerating myelin sheaths increased by 6 months, reached a peak at 26.5 months and declined at 36 months. The packing density of nerve fibers decreased across the life span. The cross sectional area of the cochlear nerve increased in older animals in conjunction with an increase in the thickness of myelin sheaths and in the area occupied by interneuronal elements. Removal of cellular debris by phagocytes continued across the life span, but the removal process appeared to be a slow one, perhaps requiring 6 months or more. The number of glial cells in the nerve was stable over the life span.

FISCHER 344 RAT

This strain shows a moderate loss of sensitivity with aging. An elevation in click thresholds of 20 dB occurs between 8 and 25 months of age (Simpson, Knight, and Brailowsky, Prospero-Garcia, and Scabini, 1985; see also Chapter 7). Cooper and colleagues (1986) measured ABR thresholds to tone pips (3, 8, and 40 kHz) in 12- and 25-month-old Fischer 344 rats. Thresholds increased by 30 dB or more at each frequency, with the greatest elevations occurring at 40 kHz.

A recent study by Hoffman, Jones-King, and Altschuler (1988) assayed putative efferent transmitters in the Fischer 344 rat cochlea. No differences were found in the levels of enkephalin, dynorphin, and acetylcholine for groups aged 3, 12, or 24 months. These data suggest that the efferent olivocochlear system (presuming it utilizes these transmitters) is robust in the face of aging (although 24 months is not extremely old for rats).

ALBINO WISTAR RATS

This strain was used by Hillerdal et al. (1987) in a study of cochlear blood flow. In rats that were either hypertensive or normotensive and had not been exposed to intense noise, blood flow measurements revealed no differences between young (3- to 6-month-old) and old (18- to 20-month-old) animals.

RATS WITH EXTENDED LIFE SPAN

Feldman (1984) examined the cochleas of Sprague-Dawley rats whose lives were extended to 45 to 48 months of age by dietary restriction. The cochleas of the extremely old rats exhibited degenerative changes more severe than those of normally aged rats. The excessive changes included complete atrophy of the organ of Corti in the basal cochlea, variable amounts of sensory cell atrophy throughout the cochlea, defective attachment of the tectorial membrane to the spiral limbus, cellular degeneration of the spiral limbus, very extensive loss of ganglion cells in the basal and apical cochlea, accumulation of lipofuscin in Type I ganglion cells (with Type II cells being less affected), changes in myelin, and changes in Schwann cells.

While the extended-life (restricted diet) animals showed substantially more severe pathology, there was no difference in severity between normal-reared and restricted-diet rats at age 26 months, the normal median life span of the strain. Therefore, the time spectrum of age-related change was not reshaped. Rather, the additional passage of time resulted in a continuation of degenerative changes that are normally terminated by the end of life in animals fed ad libitum. Feldman (1984) noted that the degree of pathology observed in the very old animals was similar to that seen in elderly humans.

CHINCHILLA

Chinchillas differ from other rodents in having a relatively long life span, on the order of 20 years, making this species a valuable model to assess the importance of variables that might act across an extended passage of time in contributing to presbycusis (Bohne, Gruner, and Harding; 1990).

Miller (1970) reported that one 14-year-old chinchilla had a 30 percent loss of ganglion cells, whereas another old one (12 years) showed no loss. Bhattacharyya and Dayal (1985) performed hair cell counts on surface preparations of chinchilla cochleas up to 4 years of age (not very old for chinchillas) and found a small (about 7 percent), but statistically significant, loss of OHCs. The loss of OHCs was much greater in the apical half of the cochlea. IHC loss was on the order of only 1 percent.

Bohne, Gruner, and Harding (1990) provided a detailed, quantitative description of the histopathology of the inner ear of chinchillas ranging in age from premature to 19.2 years. A total of 80 animals was examined.

A loss of sensory cells, albeit not severe, was found in all animals, as summarized in Figure 4-4. OHCs degenerated by about 1 percent per year compared to only 0.29 percent per year for IHCs. The outer row of OHCs was most often (but not always) the most severely affected. Many animals had circumscribed regions of hair cell loss, and these became more prevalent with age. The loss of OHCs was best described by a linear function, whereas IHC loss followed a power function. Morphological changes in hair cells, such as fused, missing, or disarrayed stereocilia, were not common but became more frequent with age. Inner and outer pillar cells degenerated, as well. A common age-related alteration in surviving pillar cells was a partial loss of cuticular-plate substance, particularly in the upper region of the cells, and a "moth-eaten" appearance. Lipofuscin accumulated in the subcuticular region of OHCs (more so than IHCs), inner and outer pillar cells, and the

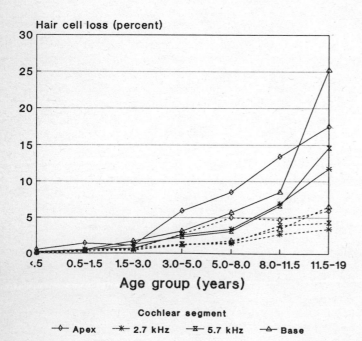

Figure 4-4. OHC and IHC loss in chinchillas (Bohne et al., 1990).

endolymphatic surfaces of many supporting cells. Total degeneration of regions of the organ of Corti was rare.

Five percent of the aging chinchillas demonstrated primary neural degeneration, manifested as a loss of dendritic processes of ganglion cells with minimal damage to the organ of Corti. The length of these neural lesions ranged from 0.27 mm to 10.12 mm, with a mean of 3.46 mm. They were found in the apical end of the cochlea.

Combined sensorineural lesions occurred in 24 percent of the animals. These were most typically located in the basal half of the cochlea: 14 percent of organ of Corti lesions in the apical half of the cochlea were associated with degeneration of ganglion cell processes, whereas 36 percent of organ of Corti lesions in the basal half had concomitant neural loss. Combined sensorineural pathology occurred, almost exclusively, when IHCs were involved. Sensory degeneration that was restricted to OHCs rarely involved neural pathology.

Strial degeneration occurred in 13.6 percent of the chinchillas over three years of age. Degeneration involved all three types of strial cells and capillaries.

Vascular changes other than degeneration of strial capillaries were not detected by Bohne and colleagues, as indicated by the dimensions of vessels below the basilar membrane and other observations. Intravascular strands and avascular channels (as noted in Johnsson and Hawkins's 1972 study of humans; Chapter 3) were not found.

GERBIL

Gerbils feature a relatively short life span (about three years), a range of hearing similar to that of humans, and an excellent research data base (Mills, Schmiedt, and Kulish, 1990). This small rodent has received growing attention in recent years as a model of presbycusis. For instance, Mills, Schmiedt, Adams, and colleagues at the Medical University of South Carolina have performed a comprehensive examination of the aging gerbil ear (Adams, Tarnowski, Heaple, Hellstrom, and Schmiedt, 1989; Hellstrom and Schmiedt, 1989, 1990, 1991; Mills and Schmiedt, 1989; Mills, Schmiedt, and Kulish, 1990; Schmiedt, Hellstrom, and Lee, 1990; Schmiedt, Mills, and Adams, 1989, 1990; Schulte and Adams, 1989).

Electrophysiological measures indicate a "flat" loss of sensitivity by two years of age (Henry, McGinn, and Chole, 1980; Fig. 4-5). A somewhat greater loss of

Figure 4-5. Eighth nerve AP thresholds of gerbils (adapted from Henry et al., 1980).

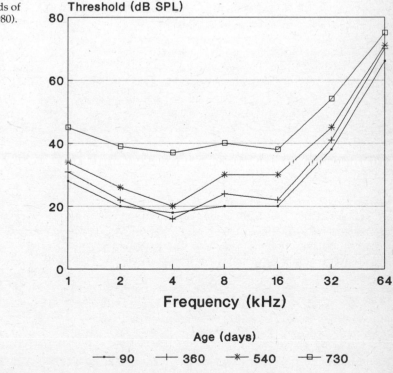

sensitivity (22 dB versus 10 dB) has been found with high frequencies (32 kHz) by Woolf, Ryan, Silva, Keithley, and Schwartz (1987). Schmiedt, Mills, and Adams (1987, 1990) obtained AP recordings from gerbils reared in a quiet environment. They showed elevations of threshold: by two years, threshold elevations of about 10 dB occurred at all test frequencies; by three years elevations at the lower frequencies (1-4 kHz) were about 20 dB while those at higher frequencies (8, 16 kHz) were about 30 dB. No significant gender effects occurred, but some marked individual differences were observed despite homogeneity in the environmental history and genotype of the aged animals. In summary, the loss of sensitivity in aging gerbils extends across the entire frequency range and is, in the absence of evidence for conductive loss, suggestive of strial pathology. The slightly greater severity of losses at high frequencies observed by Woolf, Mills, and coworkers may only appear at ages beyond two years.

Keithley, Ryan, and Woolf (1988) examined the gerbil cochlea and found a loss of ganglion cells, appearing first at 24 to 30 months of age. In the oldest animals (36 to 42 months) a 15 to 25 percent loss occurred. Degeneration of the stria vascularis was also observed in the apical turn of the oldest animals, as was some degeneration of the organ of Corti. The development of vacuoles, a peculiar age-related development in the central auditory system of gerbils, was seen in the auditory nerve, but only central to the Schwann-glial border. Because no vacuoles were seen in the ganglion cells and their proximal axonal portions, it was concluded that the vacuoles were associated with glial cells of the central nervous system.

Scanning electron microscope material obtained by McGinn and Chole (cited in McGinn and Faddis, 1987) revealed little loss of hair cells or other cochlear pathology in gerbils as old as 30 months that were free of middle ear disorders. Schmiedt et al. (1990) likewise found minimal OHC loss and virtually no loss of IHCs in old gerbils reared in quiet.

Cochlear histopathology was evaluated and correlated with the degree of hearing loss at 36 months by Adams et al. (1989). Animals with minimal hearing loss had few histopathological changes. Animals with moderate hearing loss had a moderate loss of hair cells; however, the losses were most pronounced in the apical cochlear turn, whereas threshold elevations were greatest at high frequencies (to which the basal cochlea responds best). In gerbils with severe hearing impairment, hair cell loss was more widespread, but there was little loss of IHCs or radial fibers or disruption of stereocilia. Strial atrophy was evident (Schulte and Adams, 1989). Aging animals showed complete

atrophy of strial marginal cells in the apical turn, extending into the second turn in very old animals. Strial pathology was observed in the basal and first cochlear turn of old gerbils, as well. Pathology of stromal cells in regions of the spiral ligament was seen when strial pathology was severe. The endocochlear potential, presumably generated by the stria, was also reduced in older gerbils (Schmiedt et al., 1990).

A consistent finding was age-related loss of epithelial cells in Reissner's membrane (Adams et al., 1989). Changes in Reissner's membrane could affect the ionic barrier that is necessary to maintain the ionic composition of the scala media. The possibility was offered that alterations in Reissner's membrane could contribute to—or cause—strial dysfunction and/or histopathology.

Prazma and colleagues (1990) measured regional cochlear blood flow with surface dissection and microspheres. They morphometrically quantified capillary density in the stria vascularis of old and young gerbils. Blood flow in the cochlea was decreased in the old gerbils, particularly in the stria. The decrease of blood flow in older animals was clearly not related to a loss of strial capillaries. Rather, they concluded, decreased blood flow must arise from either decreased perfusion pressure or from increased vascular resistance.

MOUSE

Several inbred mouse strains have been used to study the relationship between aging and hearing because their age-related patterns of cochlear pathology occur reliably. The most commonly used strains have been the C57BL/6J (C57) and CBA/J (CBA). In the author's colony, these strains have a median life span of about 2 years, with many animals surviving to 30 months or older (particularly C57 mice).

HEARING IN C57 AND CBA MICE

Peripheral function in C57 mice develops in an apparently normal fashion, being optimum between one and two months of age (the typical age for maturation of the auditory system in mice). Sometime during the following few months, however, high-frequency sensitivity begins to decline (Fig. 4-6). By 6 months of age loss of high-frequency sensitivity (e.g., greater than 20 kHz) is significant; by 1 year, losses are severe and have begun to encompass lower frequencies; after about 15 months of age, thresholds for all frequencies are typically in excess of 80 dB SPL (Henry, 1983; Hunter and Willott, 1987; Willott, 1986).

Figure 4-6. Electrophysiologically obtained thresholds of C57 mice (adapted from Mikaelian, 1979).

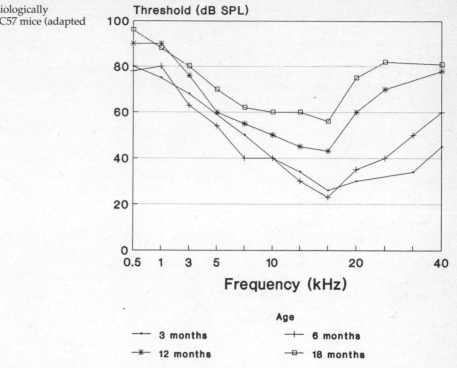

Unlike C57 mice, the CBA strain retains good sensitivity to sound for most of its 2-year life, with moderate losses across frequencies occurring at relatively old ages (Henry, 1983; Hunter and Willott, 1987; Wenngren and Anniko, 1988a; Willott, 1986).

HISTOPATHOLOGY IN C57 AND CBA MICE

The age-related elevation of hearing thresholds in CBA and C57 mice is correlated with cochlear histopathology. Comparison of these strains provides a striking contrast in the range of age-related peripheral changes that can be found in mice. The C57 cochlea has been studied by several researchers (Henry and Chole, 1980; Mikaelian, 1979; Willott et al., 1987; Willott and Mortenson, 1991; unpublished work by Willott and Pujol) and a consistent pattern has emerged. Prior to 2 to 3 months of age, little cochlear pathology is evident in C57 mice. Between 6 and 12 months, degenerative changes of the organ of Corti (e.g., distortion, clumping, and loss of OHCs) are observed, being most pronounced in the basal turn. The outer pillar cells also show degenerative changes at this time. The loss of OHCs is more severe than, and precedes, the loss of IHCs, as seen in Figure 4-7. In fact, relatively little IHC loss is evident in many C57 mice,

even at 2 years of age, except in the extreme basal cochlea (Henry and Chole, 1980; Willott and Mortenson, 1991). By 2 years of age the basal region of the C57 organ of Corti is virtually devoid of recognizable structures (Fig. 4-8). By comparison, CBA mice show virtually no loss of hair cells at 16 months of age; at 2 years of age a few IHCs have been lost, and there is a small loss of OHCs with a total loss only at the cochlear base (Henry and Chole, 1980).

Age-related loss of spiral ganglion cells also differs dramatically between the C57 and CBA strains. As shown in Figure 4-9, a pronounced loss of ganglion cells occurs in aging C57 mice, with nearly complete loss in the basal cochlea during the second year of life. The sparsely populated Rosenthal's canal of a 2-year-old C57 mouse is shown in Figure 4-10. A few ganglion cell bodies and myelinated fibers remain; debris and "homeless Schwann cells" (Cohen and Bullers, 1990) are present, as well. In contrast, there is little loss of ganglion cells during the first year of life of CBA mice, and only a minimal decrease throughout the cochlea by 2 years (Fig. 4-9). Only at an extreme old age is there a significant loss of ganglion cells.

The degeneration of ganglion cells in C57 mice follows several stages (Cohen and Grasso, 1987; Cohen, Park, and Grasso, 1990): (a) incipient demyelination, with loosening and unraveling of myelin sheaths,

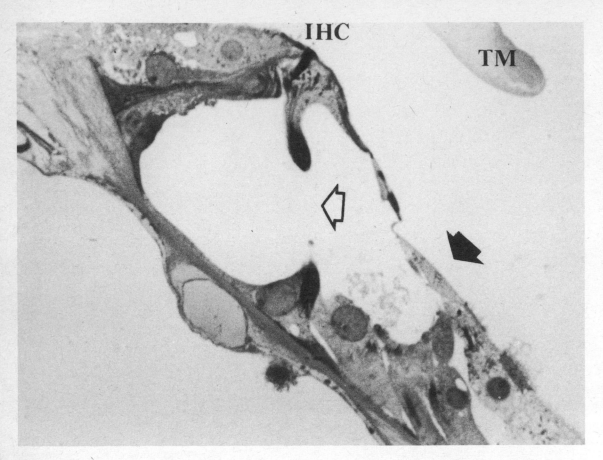

Figure 4-7. Semithin (2um) section of organ of Corti from 7-month-old C57 mice (toluidine blue stain; original magnification 1000X). The section was taken from the basal cochlea, where complete loss of OHCs (filled arrow) and a degenerated pillar cell (open arrow) are evident.

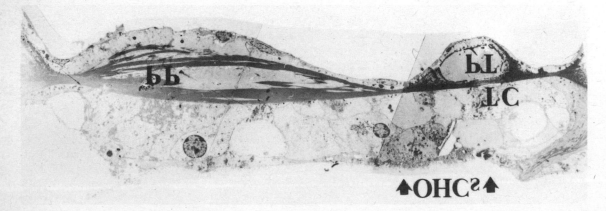

Figure 4-8. Low-power electron micrograph of organ of Corti in the basal cochlea of a 2-year-old C57 mouse. PP = pars pectinata of basilar membrane; PT = pars tecta of basilar membrane; TC = tunnel of Corti; arrows indicate former location of OHCs. The organ of Corti is completely degenerated and the tunnel of Corti is filled. Microvilli are visible at the organ of Corti surface at former location of OHCs. Original magnification 2400X; scale: the length of the specimen is about 130 um (obtained in collaboration with R. Pujol).

Figure 4-9. Relative density of spiral ganglion cells in C57 and CBA mice as a function of age and cochlear region (adapted from Willott and Mortenson, 1991).

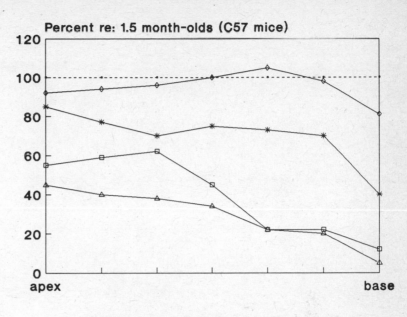

Percent re: 1.5 month-olds (C57 mice)

Segments of Rosenthal's canal

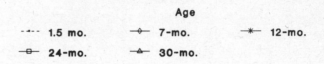

Age
- - - 1.5 mo.   ◇ 7-mo.   ✳ 12-mo.
—□— 24-mo.   —△— 30-mo.

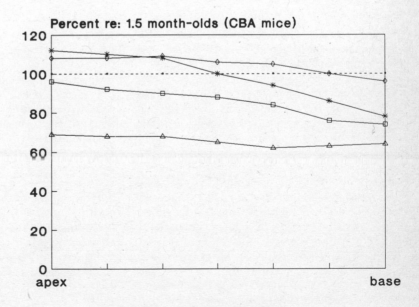

Percent re: 1.5 month-olds (CBA mice)

Segments of Rosenthal's canal

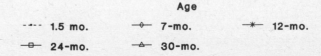

Age
- - - 1.5 mo.   ◇ 7-mo.   ✳ 12-mo.
—□— 24-mo.   —△— 30-mo.

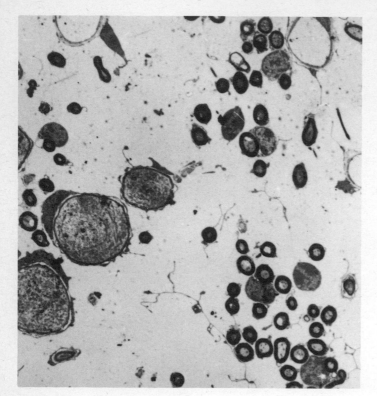

Figure 4-10. Low-power electron micrograph of Rosenthal's canal of a 2-year-old C57 mouse, basal region. Note ganglion cell bodies, cross sections of myelinated fibers, and glial processes. Original magnification 2400X; scale: diameter of ganglion cells is about 10 um (obtained in collaboration with R. Pujol)

(b) contact and fusion of partially demyelinated cells, (c) clumping of naked perikarya, which become surrounded by cytoplasmic processes, and (d) resorption. During the second stage, the basal lamina disappears at the sites of contact between myelinated neuronal cell bodies, and the myelin sheaths become disheveled. During stages two and three, Schwann cells encircle the clumping ganglion cell bodies (Cohen and Bullers, 1990). Plasma membranes of clumping ganglion cells remain intact (i.e., multinucleated syncytia are not formed). The neuronal clumps show characteristic degenerative changes, including pronounced mitochondrial death. After the fourth stage, the empty spaces, formerly occupied by ganglion cells, are not filled by formation of new tissue.

Some biochemical correlates of the early stages of ganglion cell degeneration in C57 mice have been provided by Cohen and colleagues. Cohen and Lawrence (1989) measured acid phosphatase (a lysosomal enzyme closely associated with intracellular digestion) in ganglion cells of C57 mice up to eight months of age and found reaction products associated with age pigments. They also stained for carbonic anhydrase (the zinc-dependent enzyme that catalyzes carbon dioxide to and from carbonic acid) and found

that degenerating ganglion cells stained less darkly for this enzyme. Cohen and Bullers (1989) stained the C57 cochlea for neuron specific enolase (an enzyme involved in glycolysis). In 8-month-olds, ganglion cells in the cochlear apex stained lighter than their counterparts in young animals. Degenerating cells in the cochlear base stained less darkly than apical cells.

The fate of efferent fibers has not yet been evaluated in aged C57 mice. However, injection of horseradish peroxidase (see Chapter 6) into the cochlea of an old C57 mouse results in retrograde labeling of numerous cell bodies in the superior olivary complex (a source of efferent fibers), indicating that many viable efferent fibers remained (Fig. 4-11). The labeled SOC neurons were on the side ipsilateral to the cochlear injection and were primarily located within the lateral superior olivary nucleus (LSO), the origin of the lateral efferent system that projects to the IHCs (Warr, Guinan, and White, 1986). However, some labeled cells were also found outside of the LSO. Even in a totally degenerated organ of Corti of a 30-month-old C57 mouse, an efferent terminal can be seen (Fig. 4-12). These preliminary observations suggest that the efferent system may be rather robust despite sensorineural presbycusis (see also Chapter 3).

Figure 4-11. Superior olivary complex neurons labeled with horseradish peroxidase transported from the cochlea of a 2-year-old C57 mouse. The labeled cells are on the side ipsilateral to the cochlear injection are found mostly, but not exclusively, within the LSO. Original magnification 100X.

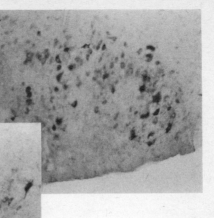

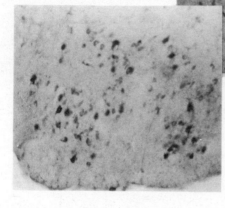

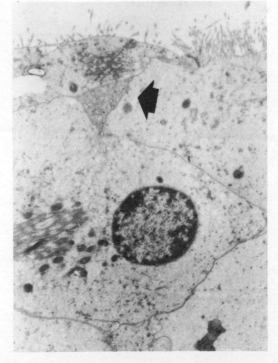

Figure 4-12. Electron micrograph of basal organ of Corti in an old C57 mouse (original magnification 15,000X). Arrow points to an efferent terminal (obtained in collaboration with R. Pujol).

Mikaelian (1979) observed some atrophy of the stria vascularis of aging C57 mice. However, a striking correlate of aging in the C57 stria vascularis that is evident in the histological specimens of the author's laboratory is an increase in pigment. At the electron microscopic level, pigment (presumably melanin) and inclusions can be seen throughout the stria (Fig. 4-13). We have not observed increases in pigment of this magnitude in CBA mice.

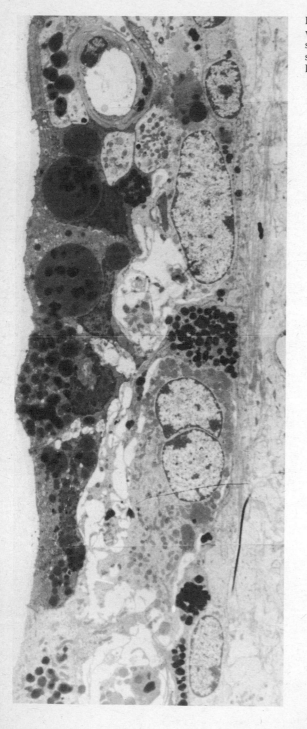

Figure 4-13. Low-power electron micrograph of the stria vascularis of an old C57 mouse showing pigment inclusions. Original magnification 2,400X; scale: length of the specimen is about 80 um (obtained in collaboration with R. Pujol).

SEQUENCE OF HISTOPATHOLOGICAL CHANGES IN C57 MICE

A comparison of Henry and Chole's (1980) hair cell counts with the ganglion cell counts shown in Figure 4-9 suggests that ganglion cells degenerate independently of IHCs. In the apical half of the aged cochlea IHC counts were near normal at 2 years of age, whereas ganglion cell counts were reduced drastically. Recent work (Willott and Mortenson, 1991) found that IHCs generally persisted in aging C57 mice unless there was a near-total the loss of ganglion cell processes innervating them.

It is more difficult to assess the relationship between atrophy of OHCs and ganglion cells in C57 mice because both begin relatively early in the extreme basal cochlea. The evidence suggests that OHC loss occurs first because cochlear microphonic recordings indicate a small elevation in high-frequency thresholds as early as 2 months of age (Henry, 1984; Saunders and Hirsch, 1976), and changes in ganglion cells have yet to be observed at this age.

Because few spiral ganglion cells innervate OHCs, and pathology and loss of ganglion cells precedes a significant loss of IHCs, the neuronal pathology is not secondary to hair cell loss. To the contrary, IHC loss appears to occur only when denervation is severe.

At least three possibilities can be considered regarding the relationship between the pathology of OHCs and ganglion cells. First, it may be that the same mechanism(s) is responsible for pathology of both OHCs and spiral ganglion cells, but OHCs are more vulnerable. This would explain why OHC pathology appears to precede spiral ganglion cell pathology. Second, OHC loss may be secondary to spiral ganglion cell pathology (as seems to be the case with IHCs), but the early ganglion cell pathology is too subtle to be detected by routine light microscopy. Third, pathology of OHCs and spiral ganglion cells could be caused by specific, independent genetic mechanisms.

OTHER TYPES OF MOUSE

Other inbred strains exhibit various time courses, severity, and frequency patterns of presbycusis. The "BDF1" strain, presumably derived from one C57 parent, demonstrates age-related loss that progresses through 18 months (Church and Shucard, 1986); however, threshold elevations are probably not as severe as those found in C57 mice during the first year of life. Threshold elevations between 50 days and 240 days in other strains are shown in Figure 4-14. The variance among strains is obvious. Sensorineural pa-

Figure 4-14. Electrophysiologically determined thresholds for 8 mouse strains: difference between 240-day-olds and 50-day-olds (adapted from Henry, 1983).

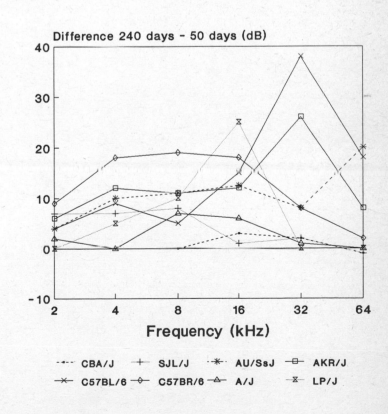

Difference 240 days - 50 days (dB)

Frequency (kHz)

--·-- CBA/J —+— SJL/J —*— AU/SsJ —□— AKR/J
—×— C57BL/6 —◇— C57BR/6 —△— A/J --×-- LP/J

thology has been demonstrated in most of these mouse strains, although the relationship of peripheral histopathology to hearing loss is not always clear (Chole and Henry, 1983). Age-related losses more drastic than any of these are seen in the DBA/2J strain, which has severe sensorineural loss before 2 months of age (Willott, 1981).

Examples of cytocochleograms from two inbred strains are shown in Figures 4-15 (LP/J) and 4-16 (A/J). IHC loss is quite limited in the LP/J strain, while OHC loss is more severe but confined to the basal cochlea. Both IHC and OHC loss are much more severe in the A/J strain and occur throughout the cochlea.

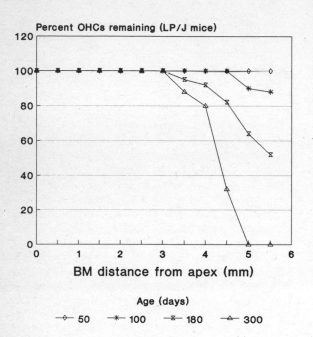

Figure 4-15. Cytocochleograms from LP/J mice (adapted from Chole and Henry, 1983).

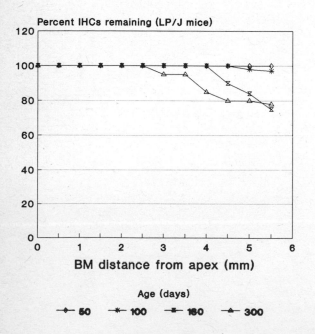

Mice with single gene mutations often have severe congenital or early onset ear pathology (Steel et al., 1983). However, some of these mutants may be useful in aging research. For instance, the Dancer mutant succumbs to progressive hearing loss during adulthood (Wenngren and Anniko, 1988b), making it a potential model to study the genetics of presbycusis.

An outbred strain, the NMRI mouse, was tested behaviorally for thresholds across a range of ages (Ehret, 1974). Thresholds were progressively elevated through 18 months of age, but the losses were less than 20 dB except at the highest frequency tested (80 kHz), where the increase was about 40 dB.

Figure 4-16. Cytocochleograms from A/J mice (adapted from Chole and Henry, 1983).

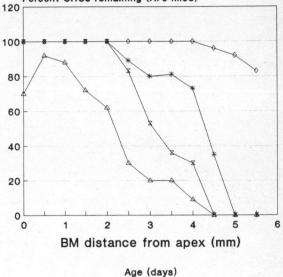

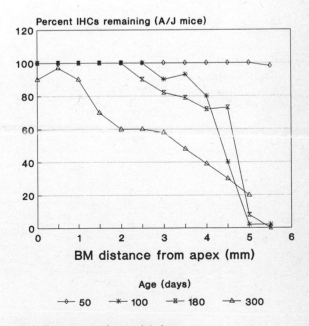

Note: there was nearly complete loss of IHCs and OHCs in 500-day-olds

OTHER SPECIES

RABBIT

Bhattacharyya and Dayal (1989) evaluated surface preparations of cochleas from rabbits as old as 4 years. While this is not an extremely old age for rabbits, which may live to 13 years (Altman and Dittmer, 1972), damage to the organ of Corti was observed in both base and apex. By 4 years of age, a 7 percent loss of OHCs and less than a 2 percent loss of IHCs had occurred. This difference, while small, was statistically significant. No differences were seen in the magnitude of loss between the three OHC rows.

CAT

Auditory thresholds become elevated in aging cats. Harrison and Buchwald (1982) used the brainstem-evoked response to measure click thresholds. The mean threshold for clicks presented in the free field was 34 dB SPL in young cats. Cats aged 12 to 23 years had a mean threshold of 75 dB, which was significantly

different from the young group. All of the old cats had high thresholds (range 57-91 dB).

Schuknecht (1955) presented histological findings on the cochleas of four adult cats of unspecified age. In each cat, atrophic changes in the organ of Corti and loss of efferent and afferent nerve fibers, especially nearer the cochlear base, were observed. No changes in blood vessels were evident. Despite the similarity in the types of pathology, the degree of pathology varied substantially. The state of the tectorial membrane ranged from normal to absent in the base; the condition of the efferent nerve bundle ranged from normal to missing along some distance; the stria vascularis and spiral ligament showed varying regions of degeneration or normalcy throughout; the spiral limbus showed some acellularity in three cases, but was normal in one case. Thus, the histopathological profiles were actually rather variable within the general framework of sensorineural atrophy. Behavioral audiograms differed substantially as well (Fig. 4-17). "Pure" neural presbycusis was apparently not seen in any of the available cats.

Spoendlin (1970) presented electron micrographs obtained from a 13-year-old cat "which apparently did not hear well." Large lysosomal bodies, filled with

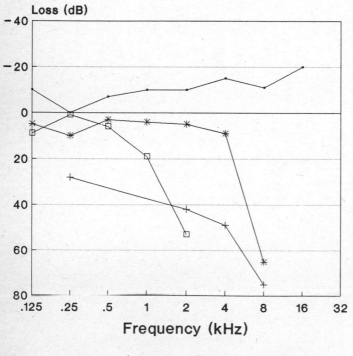

Figure 4-17. Behavioral audiograms from four cats (adapted from Schuknecht, 1955). Thresholds are plotted with respect to average normal levels for cats. Cat 1 had sensorineural pathology in the basal 2-3 mm of the cochlea; Cat 2 had sensorineural pathology in the basal 10 mm of the cochlea; Cat 3 had sensorineural pathology in the basal 6 mm of the cochlea; Cat 4 had sensorineural pathology in the basal and middle regions of the cochlea. In all cases, damage occurred in ganglion cells, hair cells, and supporting cells to similar degrees.

dense inclusions, were seen in the OHCs but were rare in IHCs. Spoendlin's EM material also showed a marked decrease in the number of internal spiral fibers, an important part of the efferent innervation of the organ of Corti.

An age-related increase in stria vascularis pigment has been reported in old cats (Conlee, Parks, Schwartz, and Creel, 1989).

DOG

Johnsson and Hawkins (1972c; 1979) indicated that the inner ear of several dogs they examined histologically had changes similar to those found in aged humans, including strial atrophy, sensorineural degeneration, and vascular disturbances. They suggested that the carnivorous diet of dogs might contribute to the changes (as it would in humans), making the canine an attractive model. Recently, Knowles and colleagues (1989) examined the middle and inner ears of dogs aged 1.5 to 17 years. No histological abnormalities were detected in the middle ear ossicles. The density of spiral ganglion cells was reduced, primarily in the basal turns of the cochlea, and the degree of loss was correlated with severity of hearing loss (deter-

mined from ABRs). In their "hearing impaired" group, the density of ganglion cells was reduced to 40 percent in the lower basal region (compared to the normal-hearing dogs). In the "deaf" group the lower basal turn density was reduced to 15 percent, and the upper basal turn to 44 percent.

RHESUS MONKEY

Hawkins and collaborators (1985) presented histopathological data on 15 rhesus monkeys, aged 4 to 31 years (the upper limit of the life span). Scattered phalangeal scars replacing missing hair cells (particularly in the extreme the cochlear base and apex) were seen in all cases, becoming more pronounced with age. Their three 31-year-olds had a complete loss of inner and outer hair cells and nerve fibers in the first 2-5 mm of the basal turn. A representative cytocochleogram is presented in Figure 4-18. Loss of nerve fibers was seen in the same regions as hair cell loss (i.e., sensorineural damage). A partial loss of spiral ganglion cells in the basal turn was characteristic of older animals. Few changes were seen in the stria vascularis, aside from some scattered vacuoles in two older monkeys. The spiral ligament showed changes

Figure 4-18. Cytocochleogram from a 31-year-old rhesus monkey (adapted from Hawkins et al., 1985).

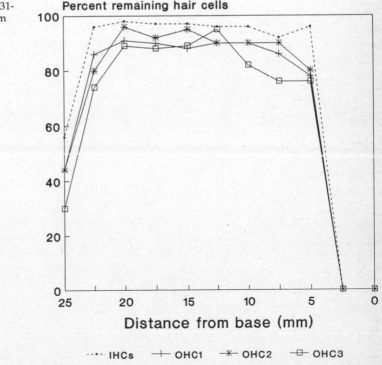

in one 24-year-old only. Reissner's membrane showed no age-related differences except for an increased number of lipofuscin granules in the oldest group. Taken together, the authors saw the changes as similar, albeit of lesser magnitude, to those typical of sensorineural presbycusis in humans (i.e., organ of Corti atrophy with concomitant nerve loss). Some evidence was seen for ganglion cell degeneration independent of hair cell loss in at least one animal, suggesting a parallel to "pure" neural presbycusis. However, little evidence was found for strial, vascular, or mechanical types of presbycusis. The formation of new bone was observed in the areas through which nerve fibers pass, possibly putting ganglion cell axons at risk (see Chapter 5).

SQUIRREL MONKEY

Dayal and Bhattacharyya (1986) examined surface preparations of the organ of Corti of this New World monkey. They observed a small degree of hair cell loss beginning at the apex, with virtually no losses in the basal half of the cochlea through 6 years, the oldest age studied (Fig. 4-19). As the authors pointed out, squirrel

monkeys may live 15 to 20 years under favorable conditions, so their animals were hardly "old." Nevertheless, the data do indicate that hair cell loss begins in the cochlear apex.

CHIMPANZEE

Johnsson and Hawkins (1972c) examined the temporal bone of a 39-year-old chimp. The animal exhibited relatively mild OHC loss, mainly in the basal turn, and diffuse strial atrophy throughout the cochlea.

QUAIL

Ryals and Westbrook (1988) counted hair cells and ganglion cells in young adult (3-month-old) and old (3- to 6-year-old) quail. Age-related hair cell loss was minimal, amounting to less than 10 percent in the oldest birds. However, 20 to 60 percent losses of ganglion cells were found in the old group, with the greatest losses occurring in the middle section of the papilla. Accumulation of lipofuscin was also seen in aged ganglion cells. The authors point out that these

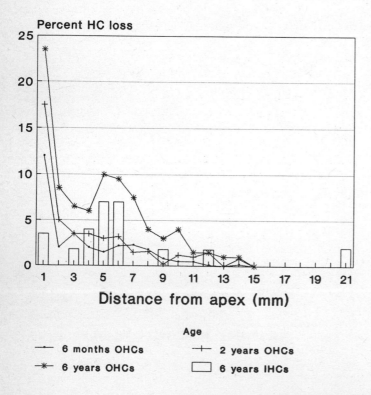

Figure 4-19. Hair cell loss in squirrel monkeys (adapted from Dayal and Bhattacharyya, 1986).

findings indicate generality of the primary age-related loss of ganglion cells reported in mammals by many authors.

SUMMARY

Aging animals exhibit the various types of peripheral histopathological changes observed in humans, described in Chapter 3. Indeed, the occurrence of some sort of cochlear pathology appears to be a ubiquitous concomitant of aging across species. As summarized in Table 4-1, age-related degeneration of OHCs, spiral ganglion cells and their processes, the stria vascularis, and/or sensorineural tissue have been observed in most of the animal species that have been evaluated. Evidence of changes in the spiral ligament or basilar membrane ("mechanical" changes) and vascular insufficiency (vascular presbycusis) is less widespread, but has been obtained. Also in common with humans, the cochlear base and (in some species) the apex are particularly vulnerable to age-related sensorineural pathology, and OHCs (particularly those in the outermost row) are more vulnerable to age effects than IHCs.

PHYSIOLOGICAL STUDIES OF THE EIGHTH NERVE

The ability to obtain physiological data from individual auditory nerve fibers has not yet been exploited in aging animal models, with the exception of work on gerbils by the group in South Carolina.

RECORDINGS FROM AGING GERBILS

Recordings from individual eighth-nerve fibers of gerbils maintained in quiet conditions (Schmiedt et al., 1989; 1990) revealed threshold elevations of about 10-40 dB around the fibers' characteristic frequency (CF). Because sensorineural pathology was minimal in these

TABLE 4-1. SUMMARY OF AGE-RELATED HISTOPATHOLOGY IN ANIMAL MODELS

Species	OHC	Neural	Strial	Mechanical	Sensorineural	Vascular
Guinea pig	+	+	+	+	+	
Rat	+	+		+	+	
Chinchilla	+	+	+		+	
Gerbil		+	+			+
Rabbit	+					
Mouse	+	+	+		+	
Cat	+		+	+	+	
Dog			+		+	+
Rhesus monkey		+			+	
Squirrel monkey	+					
Chimpanzee	+		+			
Quail		+				

+ = evidence for the existence of pathology has been reported.
Note that a lack of current evidence does not preclude the existence of histopathology for species that have not been thoroughly studied.

animals, the authors felt the threshold elevations were likely due to strial dysfunction. The shapes of tuning curves and tuning curve "tails" (the thresholds for frequencies below the CF) were normal. However, measures of the "sharpness" of tuning curves (Hellstrom and Schmiedt, 1991) indicated that old fibers with CFs above 4-5 kHz tended to be less frequency-selective (although there was overlap in the data from old and young animals). Two-tone suppression (the reduction in the vigor of responses to one stimulus by the presentation of a second stimulus with a different frequency) was often robust. Two-tone suppression was present both above and below CF even with CF threshold shifts of up to 40 dB.

A diminution in AP amplitudes and in the steepness of amplitude-intensity functions was found in older gerbils, whereas the rate-level functions (evoked discharges as a function of SPL) were fairly normal for single fibers (Hellstrom and Schmiedt, 1990). The difference in intensity functions between compound AP and single-fiber recordings suggests that the reduction in AP amplitude may be caused by a smaller number of (relatively normal) nerve fibers whose summed responses influence the AP. A reduction in the synchrony of firing of the single fibers could likewise lead to reduced AP amplitudes.

In quiet-aged gerbils, the proportion of auditory nerve fibers with high rates of spontaneous activity increased for fibers with CFs greater than 6 kHz (high frequencies) (Schmiedt and Mills, 1991).

Data were also obtained from gerbils allowed to age in the presence of continuous noise (85 dBA for 700 days). Threshold shifts around fiber CF were typically greater in these animals compared to their quiet-reared counterparts, with tuning curve tails being about normal. The most notable correlate of noise rearing involved two-tone suppression: it was often absent or only occurred with higher level tones. Also, in contrast to quiet-reared animals, the proportion of fibers with high spontaneous rates decreased (Schmiedt and Mills, 1991).

summarized in Table 4-2. Loss of OHCs alone or OHCs and IHCs in combination is associated with alterations in the tuning curves. These changes are not simple upward shifts in thresholds but may involve a variety of changes in tuning curve shape, including a shift of the CF, sensitization of the tuning curve tail, or selective elevation of the tuning curve tip. Damage to stereocilia (which may accompany aging; Chapter 3) appears to be sufficient to produce significant changes. The spontaneous firing (i.e., in the absence of intended acoustic stimuli) of auditory nerve fibers is altered. Changes may occur in the temporal pattern of discharges as revealed by post-stimulus time histograms of discharges, and the ability of fibers to phase-lock to tones may diminish. Abnormal responses of nerve fibers associated with combinations of tones (two-tone inhibition and distortion products) have been observed. Intensity functions for discharges of nerve fibers are altered.

The primary correlates of damage to the OHCs appear to be threshold elevations and reduced sharpness of tuning curve tips. The effects of IHC damage are difficult to assess because they are less vulnerable to noise or ototoxic drugs. Cochlear pathology is also associated with changes in response properties of auditory nerve fibers relevant to frequency, intensity, and temporal parameters of sound.

SUMMARY

Sensorineural pathology resulting from aging plus noise exposure (gerbils) or from ototraumatic agents applied to young adult animals (Table 4-2) can result in a number of alterations in response properties of auditory nerve fibers in addition to elevated thresholds. Aged gerbils reared in quiet tended to have minimal sensorineural damage, with the primary dysfunction appearing to be strial. These animals also exhibited abnormal responses but they differed somewhat from their noise-exposed counterparts.

RECORDINGS FROM EIGHTH NERVE FIBERS AFTER SENSORINEURAL DAMAGE

In the absence of an extensive literature on the effects of aging on auditory nerve fiber responses, we may look to studies of the effects of noise-, drug-, or trauma-induced pathology. Because the damage done to the cochlea by these experimental means has a number of similarities with age-related pathology, these studies provide insights into the types of changes that might be expected. These are briefly

IMPLICATIONS OF THE ANIMAL MODELS WITH RESPECT TO HUMAN PRESBYCUSIS

The similarities in the forms of pathology in humans and other species bodes well for the use of animal models to further enhance our understanding of the nature of age-related change in humans. In this regard,

TABLE 4-2. PHYSIOLOGICAL RESPONSES OF AUDITORY NERVE FIBERS (SINGLE-UNITS) WITH COCHLEAR PATHOLOGY.

Study	Experimental Manipulation	Result of Manipulation
Kiang et al. '70	kanamycin (cats)	fibers no longer responding to low intensities responded to high intensities; abnormal tuning curves
Dallos & Harris '78	kanamycin (chinchillas)	abnormal tuning curves in and near region of OHC damage; with no OHCs: broad tuning, normal tuning curve tail with elevated CF threshold, *or* undetermined CF; latency, spontaneous rate, and PSTH unaffected
Liberman & Kiang '78	noise exposure (cats)	altered tuning curves; hypersensitivity of "tails"; some changes in spontaneous activity; OHC loss associated with elevation of tuning curve tips
Liberman & Beil '79	acoustic trauma (cats)	some threshold elevations not correlated with HC loss; orderliness of stereocilia was most closely correlated with threshold shifts
Robertson & Johnstone '79	kanamycin guinea pigs	outer hair cell loss associated with change in tonotopic map
Cody & Robertson '80	mechanical trauma (guinea pigs); N1 response	spatial extent of damage was more important than number of HCs lost; lesions only damaging OHCs also produced threshold elevations
Salvi et al. '79	noise exposure (chinchillas)	fewer peaks in PSTHs in response to clicks
Salvi et al. '80	noise exposure (chinchillas)	more "damping" of neural response to clicks; no change in latency re: SPL, but latency shorter re: SL; broad tuning curves
Schmiedt et al. '80	acoustic trauma or kanamycin (gerbils)	effects of midcochlear and basal OHC damage differed; basal damage: elevated CF thresholds correlated with OHC loss; no two-tone inhibition above CF; altered tuning curves
Schmiedt & Zwislocki '80	acoustic trauma or kanamycin (gerbils)	two-tone responses often showed no inhibition; changes in slopes of intensity functions; "two-tone summation" often seen
Woolf et al. '81	kanamycin (chinchillas)	loss of OHCs associated with threshold elevations; fibers whose CF corresponded to area of OHC damage exhibited a reduction in frequency range for which phase locking occurred
Evans & Klinke '82	furosemide (cats)	tuning curve tip elevated, but tail not affected
Santi et al. '82	kanamycin & bumetanide (chinchillas)	behavioral audiograms were not closely correlated with innervation density as long as a few IHCs were present; OHC damage correlated with threshold elevations
Siegel et al. '82	noise exposure (chinchillas)	amplitude of two-tone stimulus distortion products reduced
Patuzzi & Sellick '83	acoustic trauma (guinea pigs)	reversal of neural response re: direction of BM displacement
Liberman '84	acoustic trauma (cats)	CF shifts down as threshold rises
Liberman & Dodds '84a	acoustic trauma (cats)	decrease in spontaneous rates associated with loss of tallest row of OHC stereocilia
Liberman & Dodds '84b	acoustic trauma (cats)	elevation of tuning curve tips & hypersensitivity of tails, associated with OHC stereocilia damage; OHC + IHC damage causes elevation of tuning curve tail & tip
Liberman & Kiang '84	acoustic trauma (cats)	abnormal intensity functions, especially for low intensity component; associated with IHC stereocilia damage

the fact that some species are particularly well suited as models for certain types of pathology supports the view that it is valuable, for research purposes, to maintain specific histopathological categories in conceptualizing presbycusis.

Since animals reared in institutional or commercial animal facilities are not usually exposed to consequential noise or ototoxic drugs, presbycusis appears to occur despite minimal "contamination" by exogenous environmental factors. Nevertheless, the magnitude of age-related pathology is typically less severe in animals than in humans. This may be due to a number of factors including the effects of environmental insults, diet, and genotype. For instance, aged gerbils maintained in noise exhibit a greater degree of hearing loss than quiet-reared gerbils; the severe sensorineural pathology in dogs might be related to their carnivorous diet, as suggested by Johnsson and Hawkins (1979); and the differences among inbred mouse strains implicates genetic factors. While the involvement of these factors is far from being fully understood, research on experimental animals, with its ability to systematically control genetic and environmental variables, provides our best hope of future progress in elucidating their relevance to presbycusis.

The animal data also speak to the issue of the relevance of the passage of time per se (e.g., the number of years the organism has lived) versus the percentage of the species life span achieved (irrespective of the absolute passage of time). Bohne et al. (1990) speculated about the possibility that the generally more severe pathology in aged humans, compared to other species, might be due to the greater number of years the human ear has for aging to occur. This would certainly be an important factor with respect to the accumulation of exogenous influences such as exposures to noise. However, the comparative data indicate that the life span is a critical variable with respect to presbycusis. Significant presbycusis is observed in rats and mice by 3 years of age and in dogs and cats by 13 to 15 years. In human terms, 3 to 15 years of age is obviously nowhere near old age. It is clear that presbycusis is an aspect of each species' aging process, and is not simply due to the passage of time outside of this context.

The ability to control the genetics and environment of laboratory rodents provides an opportunity to investigate the variability of presbycusis that can occur despite invariance of these factors. Indeed, variance of age-related hearing loss can be considerable, even with animals maintained under controlled conditions. Mills, Kulish, and Adkins (1989) maintained gerbils in an 85 dBA noise environment or in quiet for most of their life span (Mills, Kulish, and Adkins, 1989). The

median threshold data indicated a significant contribution from the noise. However, the variance among quiet-reared individuals was substantial; some had higher thresholds than some noise-exposed animals. In another study, Sjostrom and Anniko (1990) obtained ABR thresholds from CBA mice that were heterozygous for the jerker gene (homozygous jerker mice, *je/je* mice appear to be congenitally deaf; CBA mice without the jerker gene, +/+, retain good hearing through most of their life). Compared to normal CBA mice, by 9 months of age the *je/+* mice began to show hearing loss, which progressed thereafter. Despite the fact that all of the aging *je/+* mice were genetically identical and were reared under the same conditions, the variance in the magnitude of age-related hearing loss was considerable by 12 months of age (e.g., threshold ranges on the order of 40 dB at frequencies of 8-20 kHz). These findings suggest that individual differences in presbycusis in a population of humans or other species are not a simple function of genetic and environmental variance.

The neurophysiological recordings from auditory nerve fibers in aged gerbils reared in noise and other species with sensorineural damage suggests that the "message" received by the central auditory system is likely to be *distorted* when sensorineural pathology occurs (e.g., impaired two-tone suppression; decreased spontaneously active fibers). Presumably, whenever sensorineural damage accompanies aging, some sort of distortion of the cochlea's neural messages would likewise result. However, if aging occurs in the absence of significant sensorineural pathology (quiet-reared gerbils), the consequences on the quality of the neural message may be less severe (e.g., normal two-tone suppression) or different (e.g., an increase in spontaneously active fibers).

CHAPTER 5

The Etiology of Inner Ear Pathology in Presbycusis

This chapter examines the factors that may cause the age-related changes in the inner ear that are associated with presbycusis. The boundaries between different etiological factors are somewhat arbitrary because many of them are probably interrelated. For example, biological aging of cochlear tissue is likely to be influenced or controlled by genes. Genetics also may be important in determining the impact of other variables involved in the etiology of presbycusis such as alterations in bone, arteriosclerosis, and exogenous ototraumatic agents.

PRESBYCUSIS AND BIOLOGICAL AGING

Perhaps the most fundamental cause of age-related cochlear pathology is the biological aging of the cells of the inner ear. In the early literature, the decrease of ganglion cells with age was explained on the basis of theories that nerve substance is "consumed" over time, resulting in their degeneration (Wittmaack, 1916; Steurer, 1926, cited in Jorgensen, 1961). More modern views of the causes of cellular aging have implicated diminished immune system responses and auto-immune damage, neuroendocrine failure that alters cellular homeostasis, cellular malfunction due to molecular cross-linking, waste-product accumulation within cells, somatic mutations, DNA replication and repair, damage caused by free radicals, and other mechanisms.

It is generally assumed that virtually all tissues in the body undergo some sort of change as aging ensues, and as Schuknecht (1974) noted, the cells of the ear are presumably subject to biological aging, as well. However, this is not an a priori certainty; some cells, such as certain neurons in the brain, are relatively resistant to age-related change (Chapter 6; Duara, London, and Rapoport, 1985). In fact, at this time we know virtually nothing about how (or if) the inner ear is affected by somatic mutations, waste-product accumulation, or any of the other putative mechanisms of biological aging to an extent sufficient to cause the histopathological abnormalities observed in elderly ears, such as cell loss, tissue degeneration, and alterations in structure (e.g., fusion of stereocilia).

In the ensuing discussion, three basic possibilities are offered to suggest how biological aging might affect the inner ear to cause presbycusis. Because of the paucity of research on this topic, this discussion is meant to provide a conceptual framework, rather than a review of empirical evidence.

SLOWLY ACTING ENDOGENOUS OTOTOXIC FACTORS

One way to conceptualize the means by which biological aging could affect the inner ear is in terms of the presence of slowly acting "endogenous ototoxic factors." The notion here is that these factors are produced by the body and are present well before old age, or even at birth, and accumulate over time (e.g., waste-product accumulation; somatic mutations, free radical damage). They would cause slow, chronic degeneration of auditory tissue that progresses to clinically significant degrees during adulthood or old age. An ototoxic factor could be a generic "cause of aging" that affects the body's tissues in general, or it could have an affinity for inner ear tissue in particular.

The existence of endogenous ototoxic factors is at present a heuristic construct. However, a well-established agent of cell damage, free radicals associated with cellular metabolism, illustrates the concept. Free radicals are atoms and molecules with unpaired electrons that are ubiquitous in cellular metabolism but cause cellular damage because of their biochemical reactivity. It has been proposed that free radical damage is the most fundamental cause of biological aging (Harman, 1986), but we shall view the phenomenon with respect to inner ear damage. Because the production of free radicals is related to the level of metabolic activity in cells (Harman, 1972), it would be predicted that portions of the inner ear that are particularly active metabolically would be susceptible. The stria vascularis is metabolically active and, as we have seen, exhibits age-related pathology, as well as a build-up of melanin (a possible correlate of free radical damage). The implication is that free radicals may act as endogenous ototoxic agents whose relentless assault on strial and other metabolically active tissue would cause presbycusis.

To continue with the hypothetical example, if free radicals were an endogenous ototoxin, vulnerability to presbycusis might then be determined by the ability of inner ear tissue to be protected from oxidative processes (associated with free radicals) by anti-oxidants such as glutathione. Glutathione acts as a "scavenger" for potentially damaging free radicals. It is found in the inner ear, as well as in liver, kidney, and other tissue. Some preliminary experiments by the author, in collaboration with Dr. Douglas Hoffman, suggest possible involvement of the glutathione system in presbycusis in the C57 mouse. Assays of the oxidized form of glutathione (GSH) revealed that, irrespective of age, GSH levels differed between C57 mice (a strain with progressive age-related hearing loss) and CBA mice (a strain that retains normal hearing with age). GSH levels in the liver were lower in C57 mice, but higher in the kidney and inner ear. At this point the data cannot be interpreted (e.g., perhaps the elevated GSH levels in the inner ear and kidney are compensatory responses to lower levels in the liver; perhaps they reflect the body's attempts to prevent the destruction of especially vulnerable tissue in these organs). Nevertheless, the findings are interesting in that they suggest that systems fighting destructive oxidative processes differ in the inner ear and other tissue of certain mouse strains with and without progressive presbycusis.

An intriguing aspect of the endogenous ototoxic factors hypothesis, from a clinical perspective, is the possibility of assessing an individual's risk and developing clinical methods to attenuate their effects. For example, if a defective anti-free radical system (glutathione) were responsible for presbycusis in certain individuals, and the defect could be detected at early age, treatment or prevention strategies (e.g., with antioxidants) might then be developed.

LATE-EMERGING DAMAGING FACTORS

Whereas endogenous ototoxins are presumably deleterious to inner ear tissue throughout life, it is also possible that other harmful factors emerge only later in life. Such factors could involve the termination of essential processes and/or the alteration of processes that are normally benign so that they come to have damaging effects. For example, failures of the immune system and the appearance of auto-immune disorders often occur in the elderly (Hausman and Weksler, 1985), and auto-immune diseases are known to affect hearing (Yoo, 1985).

Another possible illustration of the concept of late-emerging factors is provided by the *glutamate hypothesis* of Pujol and colleagues (e.g., Pujol et al. 1990). Glutamate is an excitatory amino acid that is likely to be a neurotransmitter at the synapse between the IHCs and radial fiber afferent terminals of spiral ganglion cells. It is therefore, essential to the functioning of the inner ear. Hypoxia and other physiological insults cause swelling of these terminals, presumably due to an excess release of glutamate and entry of water into the terminals, and may lead to the destruction of radial afferent terminals. With respect to presbycusis, it is conceivable that glutamate toxicity at the IHCs might be triggered during old age by (a) hypoxia due to vascular insufficiency, (b) deficits in the inhibitory effects of efferents on the terminals, or (c) other changes at the synapse or in the ganglion cells that might cause excess release of glutamate or influx of water. While these possibilities are worthy of consideration, it should be noted that there is presently no evidence for or against a role of glutamate toxicity in presbycusis.

PRESBYCUSIS RESULTING FROM AGE-RELATED ABNORMALITIES IN METABOLISM

The third theoretical means by which biological aging might affect hearing is via metabolic deficits that develop with age and are deleterious to hearing.

A variety of clinical syndromes associated with metabolic disorders are known to affect hearing (Meyerhoff and Liston, 1980). These involve impaired glucose metabolism (diabetes mellitus), adrenocortical insufficiency, metabolism of certain proteins and lipids (e.g., hyperlipoproteinemia), deficiencies in thyroid hormone, and alterations in fluid and electrolyte metabolism caused by kidney disorders (e.g., Alport's syndrome). Kidney transplants or dialysis are also often associated with hearing impairment (Bergstrom et al., 1980).

While these conditions are not aspects of "normal aging," changes in metabolism often do occur in the general elderly population. For instance, as reviewed by Minaker, Meneilly, and Rowe (1985), it is not uncommon to have age-related changes in glucose metabolism, thyroid hormone, and adrenal function. Protein metabolism may be slowed in the elderly (Reff, 1985), and kidney function typically declines (Vestal and Dawson, 1985).

A possible role of altered calcium metabolism in presbycusis has received recent interest. Jastreboff (1990) noted the existence of evidence that calcium metabolism can be altered with age (e.g., Liang et al., 1989). He also reviewed literature indicating that alterations in calcium metabolism may affect the cochlea in a variety of ways including alteration of the tectorial membrane with decoupling of OHC stereocilia and changes in OHC membrane permeability. Jastreboff hypothesized that such calcium-related changes in cochlear physiology would result in auditory dysfunction, including tinnitus. It follows that age-related changes in calcium metabolism could contribute to hearing problems in the elderly. Shapiro and colleagues (1990) also suggested that alterations in calcium metabolism might play a role in presbycusis. They measured ABRs in young and old monkeys (older than 22 years) in response to calcitonin-induced hypocalcemia. Hypocalcemia was associated with elevated thresholds in all animals, but the effects were more pronounced and longer lasting in the old monkeys. The findings were interpreted as suggesting a role of calcium regulation in hearing loss.

In short, alterations in metabolism can cause hearing loss, and metabolic changes occur during aging. It is conceivable that declines in certain types of metabolism might be sufficient to cause, or contribute to, hearing impairment in the elderly.

CONCLUSIONS

Biological aging has the potential to cause damage to the inner ear in various ways—slowly acting endogenous ototoxicity, late-emerging damaging factors, and changes in metabolic processes critical to inner ear physiology. It is imperative that researchers begin to evaluate these possibilities if we are to understand the nature of presbycusis.

GENETIC FACTORS IN PRESBYCUSIS

It is often assumed that at least certain types of presbycusis have a strong genetic component. Schuknecht and colleagues (1974) have suggested that strial presbycusis is likely to have a genetic etiology because of clinical impressions that the disorder is prevalent in certain families. They further note that strial presbycusis does not appear to be secondary to vascular pathology because there is a lack of association with generalized vascular disease (see below). Furthermore, its onset often occurs at an early age, and there is little histological evidence for antecedent vascular disease in the strial capillary system.

While such arguments are compelling, they do not provide direct evidence for genetic causes of presbycusis. In fact, little is known about the genetics of presbycusis, and we are again relegated to a theoretical, conceptual discussion. Conceptually, three fundamental variants of genetic determinants of presbycusis can be suggested: those affecting biological aging in general, those affecting the inner ear in particular, and those determining various non-auditory traits that affect hearing indirectly.

GENETIC INFLUENCES ON BIOLOGICAL AGING IN GENERAL

The degree and type of biological changes that accompany aging can be strongly influenced by genes (e.g., Kirkwood, 1985). Thus, any of the hypothesized mechanisms of presbycusis outlined above—endogenous ototoxic factors, late-emerging damaging factors, age-related metabolic disorders—could theoretically be influenced by genetic mechanisms that affect aging of the body's tissues in general. In these cases, it might be expected that relatively early or late cochlear pathology would be correlated with age-related change in other, non-auditory tissue, as well.

A study by Buchanan (1990) may be relevant to this issue. Thresholds were obtained from subjects with Down syndrome (age range: 5.4 years to 59.1 years) and compared to those obtained from other mentally retarded subjects and normal individuals. Down syndrome subjects had an earlier onset of age-related hearing loss than either of the other groups, being evident by at least the second decade of life. The data were interpreted as a manifestation of precocious aging that is a general characteristic of Down syndrome (Tice and Setlow, 1985). Research evaluating correlations between presbycusis and other signs of aging in the general population would be welcome.

GENETIC MECHANISMS WITH PARTICULAR EFFECTS ON THE AGING AUDITORY SYSTEM

There is no doubt that certain types of progressive cochlear pathology occurring during adulthood in both human and non-human animals are genetically determined. In these instances, the age-related loss of hearing does not appear to be correlated with a general acceleration of aging.

NON-HUMAN ANIMALS

A number of inbred mouse strains exhibit genetically determined, progressive, age-related hearing loss fitting the criteria outlined in Chapter 1 to be classified as presbycusis. Several of these, including the C57BL/6J strain, were described in detail in Chapter 4. A basic experiment performed in the author's laboratory in collaboration with Dr. Lawrence Erway serves to demonstrate the genetic nature of hearing loss in the C57 mouse. When crossbred to the CBA/J strain, which retains good hearing during aging, F1 hybrids do not exhibit the severe losses by middle age, characteristic of their C57 parents. Since all of the F1 hybrids have one allelic gene from the CBA/J parent and one from the C57, the data indicate that the gene(s) causing presbycusis in the C57 mouse are recessive or co-dominant. When the F1 hybrids are bred with one another to produce F2 hybrids, a proportion of these mice (presumably the ones that have inherited the appropriate C57 genes in matched pairs) exhibit presbycusis. Because the mice of different strains are raised under standard dietary and environmental conditions it is quite certain that the occurrence of presbycusis is under the control of genes in these animals.

HUMANS

Of the more than 1,000 genetic syndromes known to affect man, many are associated with sensorineural hearing loss, with onset during adulthood and with the most significant pathology occurring in old age (Konigsmark, 1972; Proctor, 1977). This group of syndromes includes several in which hearing loss occurs without non-auditory anomalies. These conditions may be symptomatically indistinguishable from sensorineural presbycusis. Proctor (1977) described two basic types. *Dominant hereditary sensorineural hearing loss without associated defects* may occur as late as age 40 and usually slows after age 50, reaching losses of 60-70 dB, especially for high frequencies. It occurs in approximately one in 40,000 people. *Recessive sensorineural hearing loss without associated defects* slowly progresses from early childhood, becoming severe in old age. The incidence is approximately one in 4,000.

A potential type of inherited presbycusis, *lipofuscinosis of the cochlea*, was proposed by Engstrom and collaborators (1987). They suggested that the formation of lipofuscin may represent one cause of presbycusis. They pointed out that hereditary lipofuscinosis is associated with deterioration of sensory organs and dementia. Lipofuscin is deposited in cells of the organ of Corti, spiral ganglion, and probably in stria vascularis[1] (Engstrom et al., 1987; Ishii et al., 1967b; Schuknecht, 1974). At this time, however, it has not been established that lipofuscin deposits of this type cause hearing loss.

GENETICALLY DETERMINED NON-AUDITORY TRAITS THAT COULD AFFECT HEARING IN THE ELDERLY

It is conceivable that any number of genetically determined traits might be associated with increased susceptibility to presbycusis. These could be global traits such as race and gender, or constitutional traits, such as the normalcy of metabolism and physiology.

RACE

In reviewing the literature on presbycusis, Kryter (1983; 1985) concluded that there was little evidence to indicate that race was an important variable. There are, however, indications that pigmentation, a major correlate of race, may be a relevant factor in presbycusis.

Some evidence suggests that pigmentation may affect susceptibility to presbycusis or ototoxic drugs, but the evidence is contradictory. Some researchers have found pigmented guinea pigs to have a greater degree of age-related cochlear hearing loss than albinos (Conlee, et al., 1988; Dum, 1983; Dum, Schmidt, and von Wedel, 1980). On the other hand, pigmented animals may be more resistant than albinos to certain ototoxic drugs (Conlee et al., 1988; 1989). In contrast to these findings, Keithley and Feldman (1991) evaluated the spiral ganglion and stria vascularis in four rat strains, albino and pigmented, and found no evidence that degeneration in old animals (27-36 months) differed as a function of pigmentation. In light of the research on animals, it would seem that the effects of pigment in hearing loss may depend on factors such as species or the type of cochlear histopathology involved. In any event, further research on pigmentation and presbycusis seems warranted to clarify their relationship to one another.

GENDER

In most surveys of hearing on industrialized populations presbycusis is less pronounced in women than in men (Chapters 1 and 8). Of course, numerous exogenous ototraumatic variables are likely to differ between the sexes, such as military and industrial

---

[1]Because cells in the stria vascularis accumulate melanin pigment with age, it is difficult to determine if some reports of pigment have identified lipofuscin or, in fact, melanin.

noise exposure. In reviewing the epidemiological literature, Kryter (1985) concluded that such factors were indeed responsible for gender differences in populations, and there was no evidence for an intrinsic gender difference in vulnerability to age-related hearing loss.

One way of determining if intrinsic, biological differences between sexes contribute to the severity of presbycusis is to control or minimize the exogenous ototraumatic factors. This has been done with human subjects by studying the hearing of non-industrialized populations. No gender differences in the degree of presbycusis were found in the Mabaans of the Sudan (Rosen et al., 1962) or the natives of Easter Island (Goycoolea et al. 1986), both of whom lived in non-noisy environments.

Another way of controlling exogenous factors is by using animal models. Hunter and Willott (1987) obtained ABR thresholds from male and female C57BL/6J and CBA/J mice and found no significant gender differences in any age group. Likewise, gender effects were not observed in AP thresholds of aged gerbils (Schmiedt et al., 1990).

In summary, at this time there is no indication of an intrinsic, biologically determined gender difference in the susceptibility to presbycusis.

CONSTITUTIONAL TRAITS

Inherited abnormalities in physiology or metabolism sometimes are associated with the manifestation of hearing loss during adulthood (Konigsmark, 1971; Proctor, 1977). One example is diabetes mellitus, mentioned earlier. Another is an inherited disturbance in lipid metabolism, *familial hyperlipoproteinemias*, which can be accompanied by sensorineural hearing loss. The existence of inherited syndromes like these supports the feasibility that other, less apparent genetic influences might also contribute to the risk of presbycusis. For example, a familial history of atherosclerosis (arteriosclerosis) increases one's risk for acquiring this cardiovascular disorder (Bierman, 1985). In turn, arteriosclerosis may contribute to presbycusis (see below).

CONCLUSIONS

In many cases, genetic mechanisms can and do determine the severity of age-related hearing loss and/or changes in the inner ear. Some genetic syndromes are symptomatically indistinguishable from presbycusis. It is conceivable that the genotype of each individual predetermines the risk or inevitability of presbycusis. Perhaps the only thing that differentiates the known genetic syndromes from sensorineural, strial, or other types of presbycusis is the fact that we have not yet identified the genes that cause, or contribute to these types of presbycusis.

AGE-RELATED CHANGES IN THE TEMPORAL BONE AND OTIC CAPSULE THAT MAY CAUSE PRESBYCUSIS

OSTEOSIS IN TEMPORAL BONE

A group of researchers in Yugoslavia proposed as a major cause of presbycusis the process of progressive osteosis of the channels through which nerves and vessels pass to penetrate the bony regions of the cochlea (Sercer and Krmpotic 1958; Krmpotic-Nemanic, 1969, 1971; and Krmpotic-Nemanic, Nemanic, and Kostovic, 1972). They observed progressive formation of osteoid and bone tissue to occur in the bottom of the internal auditory meatus. Progressive osteosis would result in stricture of the holes through which auditory nerve fibers pass, compressing the nerve fibers and the arteries passing through the spiral tract (the pathway from the internal auditory meatus to the cochlea), to cause atrophy of nerve fibers and ultimately ganglion cells. In a similar manner, compression of arteries by osteosis could lead to a reduction of blood supply to the organ of Corti, stria vascularis, and spiral ligament.

According to Krmpotic-Nemanic and colleagues, osteosis occurs in several stages. During the first decade of life spiral ganglion cells form a compact mass. Slight but constant apposition of the dense fibrous tissue in the basal region of the spiral tract separates the nerve bundles passing through. Some fibers and ganglion cells atrophy and disappear, leaving groups of nerve fibers and cells. In the next stage the osteoid and bony tissue become localized at the entrances of the nerve bundles, compressing them first in the periphery of the bundle. By 80 to 90 years of age, the channels for nerve bundles become almost closed. At this age bony cuffs may also form around the arteries in the basal cochlea, compressing them as well.

Krmpotic-Nemanic (1971) felt that this process could explain most forms of presbycusis described by Schuknecht and others. The loss of ganglion cells could lead to primary neural degeneration; the loss of sensory cells could be secondary to neural atrophy or loss of blood supply; degenerative changes in the stria vascularis and spiral limbus could be secondary to lost blood supply.

While this hypothesis is of great interest, osteotic changes have not been reported by most researchers. For instance, Suga and Lindsay (1976) described primary loss of ganglion cells but found no evidence in their temporal bone material to support the ossification hypothesis. In animals, osteotic changes have been reported in guinea pigs (Covell and Rogers, 1957) and rhesus monkeys (Hawkins et al., 1985), but corroboration by other studies of animals is lacking (Chapter 4).

One explanation for the scarcity of supporting evidence is that osteosis occurs only under certain conditions (e.g., secondary to vascular insufficiency as suggested by Belal, 1980) or in certain subpopulations of the elderly (e.g. living in Yugoslavia). However, it is also likely that many histopathological studies have not adequately evaluated the spiral tract, having focused on cochlear tissue. In any event, this hypothesis is deserving of further assessment.

CONTRIBUTIONS OF OTOSCLEROSIS TO COCHLEAR PATHOLOGY IN THE ELDERLY

As mentioned in Chapter 2, otosclerosis is a disease affecting the bone of the otic capsule, often producing sensorineural deficits, particularly in the elderly. Whereas otosclerosis can cause sensorineural impairment without conductive loss (Balle and Linthicum, 1984), a progression from conductive to sensorineural impairment is more typical. Otosclerosis is not usually included as a type of presbycusis, and we shall not do so here. Nevertheless, hearing loss associated with otosclerosis fits reasonably well within the definition of presbycusis given in Chapter 1: its severity and occurrence are correlated with aging; it is not caused by exogenous ototraumatic agents. The fact that it is often manifested in young adults does not distinguish it from the other forms of presbycusis, all of which can begin to develop prior to old age. Furthermore, its impact on the elderly listener is presumably no different from other types of presbycusis with similar symptoms; we simply know more about the genetic and histopathological properties of this disorder. Despite its kinship to presbycusis, we shall avoid nosological controversy and view otosclerosis as a special type of sensorineural hearing impairment affecting a significant number of older adults. As such, it is appropriate to discuss otosclerosis in the context of the etiology of age-related sensorineural hearing loss.

Several mechanisms have been proposed that would account for sensorineural hearing loss with otosclerosis. Vascular shunts between intra- and extra-labyrinthine structures have been found (Hansen, 1967; Ruedi, 1965) that could provide routes for the infiltration of otosclerotic foci, inflammatory products, or toxins into the cochlea. Ruedi and Spoendlin (1966) hypothesized that the vascular shunts result in congestion of cochlear veins; the congestion leads to sensorineural pathology. Alternatively, the encroaching lesion may directly affect the cochlea, with the spiral ligament being particularly vulnerable. In a study of spiral ligament histopathology, Wright and Schuknecht (1972) found that about half of their sample of otosclerotic temporal bones showed involvement of the external cochlear wall. When the focus of otosclerosis had reached the cochlear endosteum (the tissue lining the inner boundary of the bone), flattening of the bony cochlear contour and narrowing of the spiral ligament were observed. The external layer of the spiral ligament was replaced by dense, homogeneous tissue. Finally, changes in the dimensions of the cochlear duct could contribute to hearing loss (Linthicum et al., 1975; Ruedi and Spoendlin, 1966). The scala tympani can become filled with bone in severe cases (Nager and Fraser, 1938).

Despite the variety of insults that otosclerotic lesions can render, there has been some disagreement regarding the significance of otosclerosis in sensorineural hearing loss. Audiometric evidence suggests that otosclerosis is a significant cause of sensorineural hearing loss. Sataloff et al. (1964) compared air- and bone-conduction thresholds in patients with unilateral otosclerosis and concluded that sensorineural loss occurred at high frequencies. Carhart (1966), evaluating audiometric data, suggested that there was sufficient parallel between groups of patients with cochlear otosclerosis and a large sample of patients with sensorineural hearing loss of unknown etiology to support the hypothesis that cochlear otosclerosis was probably a common etiology in the latter group.

Several studies have provided histological support for the audiometric data. Freeman (1979) evaluated 100 cases of progressive sensorineural hearing loss of uncertain pathogenesis using polytomography. Fifty-three of the patients were diagnosed as having cochlear otosclerosis/otospongiosis (a condition associated with otosclerosis); 40 of these patients were aged 50 years or more. Linthicum, Filipo, and Brody (1975) examined 100 pairs of temporal bones from adults with premortem evidence of otospongiosis and repeated audiometric testing during their lifetime. In 36 patients with otospongiosis involving the cochlear endosteum, sensorineural hearing loss was far greater than would be expected in the general population of the same age group. In all but 3 cases, the ear with the greater involvement of the cochlear endosteum had the greater sensorineural loss. In examining the histopathology of three elderly patients with sensorineural hearing loss and otosclerosis, Altmann (1966) felt that the lesion was sufficient to contribute to the hearing loss in at least two of the cases. From an examination of temporal bones, Hinojosa and Marion (1987) concluded that the pattern of sensorineural degeneration associated with otosclerosis was often similar to that observed in presbycusis.

In contrast to these authors, Guild (1944), in a histological study, concluded that sensorineural atrophy in patients with otosclerosis was no more severe than in like-aged non-otosclerotic patients. Further negative evidence was provided by Schuknecht and Gross (1966) and Gross (1969), who also concluded that otosclerosis did not cause sensorineural hearing loss in a significant number of cases. In a collection of temporal bones from patients at the Massachusetts Eye and Ear Infirmary, a few specimens from old patients had histological evidence of otosclerosis. Examination of cochleas in these cases led the authors to believe that the otosclerosis was not the cause of sensorineural pathology.

Three factors may be responsible for the disagreements in the literature. First, the relationship between the light-microscopic histological condition of the cochlea and hearing loss may be equivocal. The conclusion by Schuknecht and Gross (1966) that histological evidence did not support sensorineural involvement was made despite their observation of changes in the spiral ligament of the otosclerotic patients. They dismissed these observations because there was no apparent correspondence between the baso-apical location of the histopathological change and the frequency of hearing loss. However, the spiral ligament, like the stria vascularis, may influence cochlear chemistry (Takahashi and Kimura (1970); histopathology of the spiral ligament can be associated with changes in the stria vascularis (Altman Kornfeld, and Shea, 1966); and subtle changes in the spiral ligament might change the tension of the basilar membrane, altering cochlear mechanics (Henson, Henson, and Jenkins, 1984). Thus, conclusions that an otosclerotic histopathology is *not* responsible for hearing loss must be made with caution.

Second, the severity of the otosclerotic lesion is likely to play an important role in determining the degree of hearing loss. Lindsay and Beal (1966) found evidence of a sensorineural component in their collection, but mainly in those cases with the most extensive or multiple foci. Linthicum (1966) determined that there was a relationship between the amount of cochlear endosteum involved by the otosclerotic lesion (especially when the spiral ligament was involved) and the degree of sensorineural loss. In severe cases the cochlear duct may rupture (e.g. about 10 percent of the cases of Schuknecht and Gross, 1966), causing pronounced hearing loss. Nager (1966) reexamined the temporal bone collection used by Guild and found it to be largely comprised of small lesions, a sample not typical of cases seen by clinicians. This, of course, could be the reason for Guild's conclusion that cochlear otosclerosis is not a significant factor in sensorineural hearing loss.

Third, it may be the case that sensorineural symptoms of otosclerosis are more likely to occur in older patients. Glorig and Gallo (1962) performed an audiological comparison of like-aged otosclerotic and normal subjects in several age groups. Sensorineural hearing loss was *not* greater in young otosclerotic patients, but it *was* significantly more severe in subjects over 60 years of age. These data suggest an interaction between the sensorineural effects of otosclerosis and aging.

In conclusion, otosclerosis appears to be a significant cause of sensorineural hearing loss in the older population.

AGE-RELATED CHANGES IN THE CONDITION OF BONE

Several workers have examined the general condition of temporal bone in the elderly (Covell, 1952). A study by Nager (1947) found osteoporosis of the temporal bone of older patients. The most extensive changes occurred in the periosteal layer, with involvement of endochondrial bone occurring as well. Earlier work described by Mayer (1930) and Guild (1936) indicated that aging temporal bone may become increasingly brittle and subject to fracture. Whether weakening of the temporal bone might affect cochlear blood supply or otherwise contribute to presbycusis is not clear, and little attention has been given to this topic in recent years.

Temporal bone appears to remain metabolically active during aging. Gussen (1968) found that bone construction and decomposition (e.g., remodeling) were occurring in the otic capsule throughout life. Zechner and Altmann (1969) used a variety of stains to assess enzymatic activity in the bone of the otic capsule. The bone was found to be metabolically active, and this activity persisted "throughout life" (although the ages of their temporal bones are unclear). Hansen (1973) found the bone tissue of old people to be well provided with vessels, with high rates of metabolism indicated by histological stains. These findings indicate that blood supply to the bone of the otic capsule remains good.

To summarize, little evidence has been generated to indicate that alterations in the temporal bone or otic capsule associated with "normal aging" are a significant etiological factor in presbycusis.

RELATIONSHIPS AMONG CARDIOVASCULAR DISEASE, INNER EAR PATHOLOGY, AND HEARING LOSS

Cardiovascular and other circulatory disorders are the most prevalent causes of death and disability in elderly, industrialized populations (Brody and Brock, 1985). Even healthy older people tend to have reduced cardiovascular function, particularly in response to stress or if a high level of physical activity is not maintained (Lakatta, 1985). Since diminished or impaired cardiovascular function is so widespread in the elderly, it warrants consideration as a potential cause of presbycusis (Chapter 1).

Arteriosclerosis[2], the thickening and hardening of arterial walls, and cardiovascular disorders in general, have long been suspected to be a contributor to, if not a major cause of, presbycusis. Arteriosclerosis has certain epidemiological parallels with presbycusis: it can develop progressively over the years, can have a strong genetic component, and tends to be more severe in men than in women; it is very common in industrialized societies and has been taken to be a widespread biological concomitant of aging (Bierman, 1985).

It is assumed that cardiovascular insufficiency can result in reduced blood supply to the cochlea, having either of two general effects. On the one hand, diminution of oxygen and other blood-borne metabolites could result in physiological changes associated with vascular presbycusis as discussed in Chapter 3. On the other hand, secondary damage to tissue essential for hearing (sensory cells, etc.) could result from hypoxia causing one or more of the "types" of presbycusis discussed in Chapter 3. For example, Shirane and Harrison (1987) observed changes in the stereocilia

and cytoplasmic protrusions from the cuticular plate of IHCs of chinchillas made hypoxic. Such changes would be expected to interfere with the sensory transduction processes of the IHCs and could contribute to or cause sensorineural presbycusis.

At this time, the research supporting either potential effect of cardiovascular disorders is controversial.

Some investigators have been unable to discern a clear relationship between arteriosclerosis and intracochlear vascular changes in older subjects. Saxen (1952) concluded from his material that sclerosis in vessels of the inner ear and those of the internal auditory meatus were not well correlated. Crowe et al. (1934) found arteriosclerosis to be characteristic of many older patients with high-frequency losses. However, there was little sclerosis of the labyrinthine artery or its branches, suggesting that a general condition of arteriosclerosis did not necessarily extend to the inner ear.

Others have concluded that there may be a relationship between arteriosclerosis and intracochlear vascular changes, but that these do not necessarily lead to cochlear pathology or hearing loss. Jorgensen (1961) felt that thickening of capillary walls in the stria vascularis was most pronounced in arteriosclerotic patients. However, the severity of vascular pathology did not appear to be correlated with the severity cochlear pathology. Ishii (1967; cited by Hansen, 1973) was unable to establish a correlation between changes in the arteries of the internal auditory meatus and lesions of the inner ear. It was maintained by von Fieandt and Saxen (1937) that a correlation existed between vascular pathology of the kidney and inner ear pathology, but they found little correlation between arteriosclerosis and cochlear pathology. Johnsson and Hawkins (1972b), who studied the vasculature of the aging ear in detail, felt that the relationship between systemic vascular disease and presbycusis is unclear. They did not see characteristic arteriosclerosis but did not exclude it, since they did not study modiolar vessels or the internal auditory artery. Arteriosclerosis was observed by Suga and Lindsay (1976) in the internal auditory meatus of many of their cases. However, a consistent relationship between arteriosclerosis and the degree of strial atrophy or the degree of sensorineural degeneration was not found. Furthermore, sensorineural pathology often occurred without changes in the vessels serving the inner ear.

Gussen (1968; 1969) provided histological evidence that arteriosclerosis, vascular insufficiency, and changes in the bone tissue of the otic capsule are

---

[2] Some of the work cited uses the term "atherosclerosis," an age-related type of arteriosclerosis affecting the larger arteries (Bierman, 1985). Because it is sometimes impossible to determine which form(s) of arteriosclerosis have been included in certain studies, we shall employ the more general term, "arteriosclerosis."

related. In patients with arteriosclerosis, plugging of vascular canals and other changes in bone tissue—manifestations of aging of bone—were observed. Gussen suggested that these would lead to vascular insufficiency, which in turn would contribute to further breakdown of cochlear bone. However, an effect on hearing was not demonstrated.

Fabinyi (1931) concluded that the relationship between arteriosclerosis and cochlear pathology was unclear in post-mortem tissue from patients aged 47 to 78 years. Eleven of 15 patients in which arteriosclerosis was seen in vessels of the internal auditory meatus had a greater than average loss of hearing. However, even those patients in which inner ear pathology was not observed (mostly patients younger than 60 years) had sclerosis of the meatal and cerebral vessels.

A recent study conducted in Germany by Bohme (1989) failed to find evidence for a relationship between the extent of hearing loss and degree of carotid artery occlusion in a group of patients whose average age was 65 years.

Other workers have concluded that arteriosclerosis is correlated with hearing loss. Rosen and colleagues (Rosen, 1966; Rosen and Olin, 1965; Rosen et al., 1970) have argued for a relationship between coronary heart disease/arteriosclerosis and hearing loss on the basis of epidemiological grounds. In populations where arteriosclerosis (associated with high fat diets) is prevalent, hearing loss tends to be greater than normal. For example, people living in Moscow were found to have higher levels of arteriosclerosis, coronary heart disease, and blood cholesterol levels than those living in Soviet Georgia. Hearing levels of young Georgians and Muscovites did not differ, but middle-aged clerical workers living in Georgia had better hearing at 4 kHz than their counterparts living in Moscow (Rosen et al., 1970).

Bochenek and Jachowska (1969) obtained a statistically significant relationship between the diagnosis of arteriosclerosis and what they termed "accelerated presbycusis" (i.e., apparently, more severe hearing loss than their "pure" presbycusis group), and suggested that arteriosclerosis plays a causal role in presbycusis.

A comprehensive study of the vasculature and temporal bones of 40 patients over 50 years of age (with audiometric and blood pressure histories) was performed by Makishima (1978). The degree of lumen narrowing of the internal auditory arteries was quantified and correlated with severity of audiometric threshold elevations and inner ear histopathology. Narrowing of the internal auditory artery lumen was correlated with both atrophy of the spiral ganglion (the most prominent histopathological change seen) and severity of hearing loss. A positive correlation between the degree of arteriosclerotic changes in the internal auditory artery and that in the renal artery was also noted.[3]

Rubinstein and colleagues (1977) compared the hearing of elderly patients suffering from chronic cardiovascular disturbances with the hearing of healthy subjects. The cardiovascular patients had poorer pure tone audiograms (but comparable performance on suprathreshold tests). Shapiro, Purn, and Raskin (1981) observed moderate, bilateral high-frequency hearing loss in patients who had undergone cardiopulmonary bypass surgery. Most of the patients were males older than 50 years. Based on the fact that most patients showing such losses were atherosclerotic and had prolonged periods of blood pumping during surgery, Shapiro and colleagues concluded that reduced blood supply to the ear was responsible for the hearing loss.

A relationship between ischemic heart disease and hearing loss was detected by Susmano and Rosenbush (1988) using regression analysis. The probability of patients with hearing loss of unknown cause was much greater if they suffered from ischemic heart disease than if they were in normal health. Hearing loss always preceded the clinical signs of ischemic heart disease, leading the authors to conclude that it was particularly sensitive to vascular or generalized arteriosclerotic conditions.

To summarize, the evidence linking arteriosclerosis and other cardiovascular disorders to hearing loss is conflicting. A body of evidence exists to imply a relationship between arteriosclerosis and hearing loss, at least in some older individuals. However, if hearing loss can be caused by arteriosclerosis, it is apparently not inevitable, since several studies have found that patients with arteriosclerosis do not have especially severe hearing loss.

The formation of solid conclusions from correlative research is hampered because both cardiovascular disease and presbycusis typically accompany aging and could be causally unrelated. Furthermore, when hearing loss has been found to be correlated with arteriosclerosis, there is little evidence of enhanced cochlear pathology, suggesting that vascular insufficiency may be responsible (vascular presbycusis?). As discussed in Chapter 3, the efficacy of the cochlear vasculature and the physiological effects of vascular insufficiency are difficult to measure, especially in humans. Future work on the auditory system of animal models in which arteriosclerosis can be manipu-

---

[3] Makishima also divided the patient population into normotensive and hypertensive (systolic pressure greater than 160 mm Hg; diastolic pressure greater than 90 mm Hg) groups. Normal hearing individuals were not found in the hypertensive group.

lated is warranted to clear up this issue. In the meantime, a tentative, but conservative conclusion is that hearing loss is likely to result from arteriosclerosis and other cardiovascular disorders in some individuals.

THE ROLE OF NOISE EXPOSURE IN THE ETIOLOGY OF PRESBYCUSIS

As mentioned in Chapter 1, the accumulation of the effects of exposure to noise of everyday life (sociocusis) is thought by some to contribute to audiometric threshold elevations over the years. Exposure to intense (e.g., industrial) noise most certainly can cause permanent hearing loss. A detailed review of the histopathological consequences of traumatic and chronic low-level noise exposure is beyond the scope of the present discussion. It is important, however, to illustrate how noise exposure might contribute to or mimic the histopathology associated with presbycusis, described in Chapters 3 and 4. This can be done by briefly reviewing some research on the effects of exposure of animals or humans to intense noise.

HISTOPATHOLOGICAL EFFECTS OF EXPOSURE TO INTENSE NOISE

It has been known for more than a century that exposure to intense noise can cause the destruction of hair cells, especially OHCs, and collapse of the organ of Corti (Engstrom, 1983). The patterns of histopathology can be quite varied from patient to patient (Ward and Duvall, 1971). Johnsson and Hawkins (1972a) identified two patterns of histopathology associated with exposure to intense noise. The first is a localized, well defined lesion involving the sensory and neural cells of the cochlea in the middle of the lower basal turn—producing the 4kHz "dip" in the audiogram. This appears to be distinct from the patterns of atrophy accompanying aging in nonexposed persons. The second pattern consists of varying degrees of severe sensorineural pathology in the lower basal turn, associated with high-frequency loss.

Sensorineural changes associated with noise exposure are reminiscent of those described in Chapters 3 and 4 for some types of presbycusis. Wright (1976) observed noise-induced damage of the organ of Corti and myelinated nerve fibers of guinea pigs. The neural loss was accompanied by hair cell loss in some cases and independent of hair cell loss in other cases. Replacement of degenerated hair cells by phalangeal scars, similar to what is seen in presbycusis was reported by Bohne and Rabbitt (1983). Engstrom (1983) described the more subtle effects of noise on hair cell stereocilia. Stereocilia of rabbits, particularly those on the IHCs, were particularly susceptible to noise damage, and "giant cilia" could result. Noise-induced swelling of dendrites below the IHCs was reported by Spoendlin (1971) and Robertson (1983). The stria vascularis is also affected by noise. Duvall, Ward, and Lauhala (1974) exposed chinchillas to noise and saw changes in the stria vascularis, including alterations of the intermediate cells and the internal membrane system.

Research on the effect of noise exposure on cochlear blood flow has been somewhat controversial, but a number of studies have indicated noise-induced impairment of cochlear circulation (Bohne, 1976). For instance, a recent study on hypertensive rats exposed to noise for 6 months found the microcirculation of the cochlea to be diminished (Sidman, Prazma, Pulver, and Pillsbury, 1988), and Vertes et al. (1982) found some vascular change in guinea pigs exposed to moderately intense tones.

In conclusion, some of the effects of intense noise (e.g., the localized damage in the 4 kHz region) are not typical of presbycusis. However, obvious similarities also exist, with sensorineural damage to the basal cochlea, giant stereocilia, and impairment of cochlear blood flow being examples. Thus, exposure to intense noise prior to old age can affect the cochlea in ways that mimic presbycusis.

THE INTERACTION OF PRESBYCUSIS AND NOISE-INDUCED HEARING LOSS

There is no question that exposure to intense noise for a sufficient period of time, prior to old age, can cause permanent damage to the ear. However, the manner in which damage from noise combines with that associated with aging is not a simple one.

As reviewed by Humes (1984), several studies have concluded that the effects of noise trauma and presbycusis are additive (Macrae, 1971; Mollica, 1969; Welleschik and Raber, 1978). These conclusions are based on audiometric data from noise-exposed young and old subjects showing that aging plus noise exposure results in greater threshold elevations than aging minus noise exposure. Corso (1976) pointed out that the data of the American Standards Association (1954) also indicated additivity of noise exposure and presbycusis. The presence of presbycusis did not protect the ear from further, noise-induced damage, nor did presbycusis make the ear more sensitive to noise-induced damage.

On the other hand, Novotny (1979a,b) found similar degrees of hearing loss in young and old subjects with comparable degrees of noise exposure; there were no additional effects of age on noise-induced losses. Schmidt (1969) argued against additivity on the basis of a study by Gallo and Glorig (1964). For high frequencies, hearing loss was approximately a linear function of the time of exposure to noise. However, most of the hearing loss was manifested during the first 15 years of exposure with little further increase thereafter. In nonexposed subjects thresholds continued to rise into old age (see Chapter 8).

It stands to reason that if a portion of the cochlea has been virtually destroyed by noise in middle age, little additional damage can be induced by presbycusis and the "effects of aging" will not be additive. A ceiling effect would be operative. Similarly, if the 4 kHz region of the cochlea has been minimally affected by presbycusis through middle age the "opportunity" for noise-induced loss will be provided, and additivity may result. In other words, the potential for additivity will depend in part on the differences in histopathology due to aging and noise exposure (Corso, 1976). Since there is a great range in age-related histopathology, a general additivity rule is probably not valid, and it is not surprising that contradictions have arisen in the literature.

Several age-related changes in the auditory system might be expected to influence the vulnerability of the ear to noise and the additivity of effects. First, it is possible that age differences in biochemical, metabolic, or mechanical properties of the cochlea could affect the ear's response to intense noise. Such changes could conceivably render the cochlea more or less susceptible. For instance, if the ability to recover from metabolic stress were reduced in aging cochlear cells, they might be more vulnerable to noise trauma; conversely, reduced physiological responses might actually protect cells from over-stimulation.

A second possibility is that age-related changes in the outer or middle ear (Chapter 2) might influence the vulnerability of the cochlea to noise. On one hand, a reduction in the conductive transmission of sound to the cochlea might afford some protection. On the other hand, reduced effectiveness of the middle ear reflex or elevated reflex thresholds to noise that often occur with aging (Chapter 7) might put the cochlea at greater risk. While it is plausible that these factors could have some effect on age-related vulnerability to noise exposure, they are probably not of major importance since the outer and middle ear seems to provide little protection from noise exposure over extended periods of time (Tonndorf, 1976).

A third possibility is that noise-induced cochlear damage can interact with central processing of auditory information (Chapter 6) or cognitive hearing skills (Chapter 10). It will be shown in later chapters that degradation of the peripheral neural message may have an exaggerated impact on central processing of information in older listeners. Thus, from the broad perspective that presbycusis encompasses central processes (Chapter 1), sensorineural hearing loss induced by noise or other agents may have a disproportionately severe effect on older persons.

While the relationship between aging and vulnerability to acoustic trauma is an important issue, it has generated little interest by researchers. Two studies have addressed the question using mouse models. Henry (1983a) measured noise-induced threshold elevations in CBA mice and found evidence of decreased susceptibility shortly after maturation of the auditory system; no threshold elevations were induced for low and middle frequencies in mice aged 4 months or older, and threshold elevations for high frequencies were less pronounced with respect to those observed in young mice. Shone et al. (1991) exposed 6-month-old and 21-month-old CBA mice to intense noise and observed no significant differences in threshold elevations. Both studies indicate that, once middle age is reached in CBA mice, susceptibility to noise-induced threshold shifts does not change with further aging. Since CBA mice retain good hearing through old age, these findings suggest that aging (in the absence of significant presbycusis) does not result in a change in susceptibility to noise-induced hearing loss. Shone et al. (1991) also compared middle-aged C57 and CBA mice and found a greater degree of threshold shift in the C57 mice. They suggested that presbycusis in C57 mice may render the ear more vulnerable to noise trauma. However, to support the latter conclusion it must be shown that young CBA and C57 mice do not differ in vulnerability to noise exposure. If young C57 mice were more susceptible than young CBA mice, a genetically determined factor other than hearing loss would be suggested as the cause of the differences between strains at middle age.

THE CONTRIBUTION OF EXPOSURE TO "EVERYDAY NOISE" (SOCIOCUSIS)

Whereas exposure to *intense* noise can damage the cochlea, the effects of exposure to everyday noise is difficult to assess and not well understood. Kryter (1983; 1985) reviewed the literature and concluded that most surveys of presbycusic hearing loss in industrialized societies reflect the effects of age-related hearing loss plus sociocusis, especially in men. This conclusion is based in part on the well-known work of Rosen and colleagues on the Mabaan tribe of the Sudan (Rosen et al., 1962; 1964; 1966). When surveys from industrialized societies are compared to audiometric data from the Mabaans, it appears that presbycusis is less severe and differences between males and females are less pronounced in the Mabaans. A study of Bantu and Bushmen also suggested decreased severity of presbycusis in these tribes as well (Dickson (1968).

While the inference of sociocusis from cross-cultural comparisons may very well be valid, several cautionary points must be raised. Bergman (1966) pointed out that the comparison group in the 1962 study of Rosen and colleagues was from the 1954 World's Fair data, in which thresholds are unusually high (see Chapter 8). When other U.S. surveys that have excluded subjects exposed to excessive noise are used for comparison, the thresholds are more similar. The accuracy of reported ages could also influence the comparisons. For instance, the tenth percentile values (worst 10 percent) of 40- to 49-year-old American males are similar to those of of 50- to 59-year-old Mabaans (Fig. 5-1). Questions can also be raised regarding the possibility of genetic differences in vulnerability to age-related changes in the Mabaans versus the heterogeneous populations of industrialized societies, differences in dietary or ototoxic variables, and differences in audiometer calibration in the field. Thus, it is difficult to extrapolate these types of comparative findings to determine the contribution of sociocusis to presbycusic hearing loss in industrialized societies. Cross-cultural comparisons could easily lead to overestimations of the contribution of sociocusis to presbycusis.

Another factor that could influence the validity of the comparison between Mabaans and industrialized people is the population variance. The variance is low in the homogeneous Mabaan population and high in the heterogeneous U.S. population. In 50- to 59-year-olds, the poorest hearing U.S. subjects had worse thresholds than the poorest Mabaan subjects (e.g., about 20 dB difference in the tenth percentiles), as shown in Figure 5-1. However, there was little difference in the ninetieth percentiles of the two cultures (Fig. 5-1) and less than 10 dB difference for the medians (not shown). Thus, the majority of Americans have a degree of presbycusis similar to the Mabaans. Relatively few older Americans have more severe presbycusis than the Mabaans, and their losses may reflect the variance due to atypical noise exposure or numerous other factors that might affect performance on hearing tests.

Another method of estimating sociocusis is to compare males and females in industrialized societies (Kryter, 1985). Because males tend to have more age-related hearing loss than females, it is concluded that this is due to the presumed greater exposure of males to everyday noise that causes sociocusis. However, gender comparisons may be confounded by smoking habits, life expectancy, susceptibility to cardiovascular disease, hormonal status, and numerous other variables that could affect hearing. Consequently, this means of determining sociocusis is not without difficulties.

There is also the question of whether hearing loss would be expected to result from moderate noise exposure. The relationship between exposure to moderate levels of noise and hearing loss is difficult to assess. However, data indicate that minimal permanent threshold shifts result from exposure to 85 dBA noise for 8 hours per day for 10 years (Ward, 1976). After 40 years of 8-hour exposures, the risk increases for 4 kHz sensitivity but is still rather small for the lower frequencies. Presumably, even less severe effects would result when exposure is intermittent (i.e., non-occupational). Thus, the contribution of sociocusis is not necessarily significant for many individuals.

Finally, the physiological mechanisms by which moderate levels of noise would damage the cochlea are not clear. There is neither compelling experimental evidence nor theoretical reason to believe that such should be the case.

While the role of sociocusis is difficult to assess, a recent study by Goycoolea et al. (1986) presents evidence that it can be a significant factor, but not a necessary one. They measured the hearing of natives of Easter Island. These people were genetically homogeneous, having descended from 111 persons and had no evidence of genetic sensorineural deafness in the lineage. Goycoolea and colleagues compared hearing in natives that had spent their whole life in the unusually quiet environment of Easter Island with those who had left and returned after spending 3 to 5 years or more than 5 years off the island in industrialized settings. The natives remaining on the island demonstrated progressively worse hearing with age (Fig. 5-2), indicating that significant sociocusis is not necessary for presbycusis to occur. However, the degree of hearing loss was worse for those who had spent 3 to 5 years, and more so for those away from the island for more than 5 years (Fig. 5-3). Unfortunately, it is impossible to differentiate the influence of industrial noise exposure from nonindustrial levels because almost half of the subjects who had left the island and returned were employed in military or industrial professions.

In summary, there may very well be a significant contribution of sociocusis to age-related hearing loss in industrialized societies. However, the magnitude and ubiquity of this effect and the noise levels required are difficult to determine.

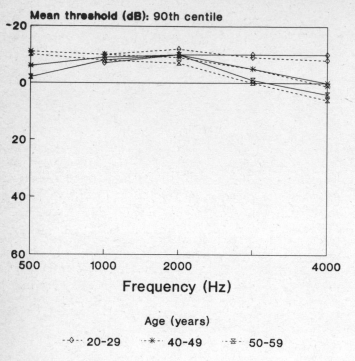

Figure 5-1. The 90th and 10th centiles of thresholds in the Mabaans and a U.S. survey (adapted from Bergman, 1966).

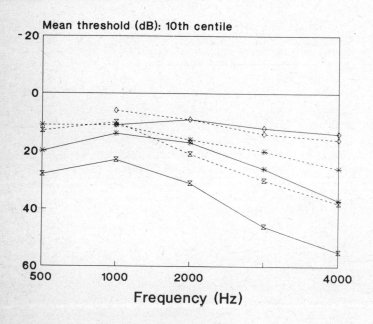

Figure 5-2. Thresholds of Easter Island natives who have never left the island (adapted from Goycoolea et al., 1986).

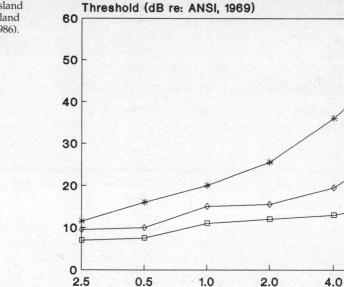

Figure 5-3. Thresholds of Easter Island natives who have never left the island or left and returned after 3 to 5 years or more than 5 years on the mainland (adapted from Goycoolea et al., 1986).

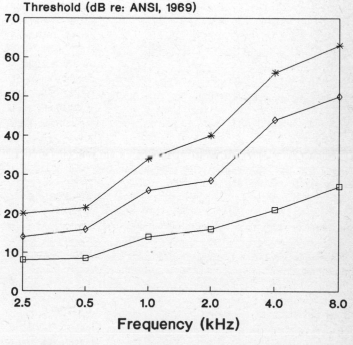

CONTRIBUTIONS OF OTHER EXOGENOUS FACTORS TO PRESBYCUSIS

As discussed in Chapter 1, variables that are prevalent in the environment (in addition to noise) have the potential to contribute to presbycusis. Many such variables have been suggested including anoxia due to spasms, sludging of blood cells, emotional strain, various toxins, infections (Fowler, 1959), smoking, head trauma, zinc deficiency (Shambaugh, 1989), to name but a few.

While it seems likely that various life experiences may contribute to age-related hearing loss, much work remains to be done in determining which factors are relevant and under what conditions they are significant. There is disagreement in the literature regarding the role of general health problems and hearing loss in the elderly. A longitudinal study conducted in China (Wang, 1990) compared the annual loss of hearing in elderly subjects over a ten-year period. Individuals with various health problems (which included arteriosclerosis, hyperlipidemia, hypertension, and diabetes) had a greater annual decline in hearing than did healthy people. In contrast, Soucek, Michaels, and Mason (1988) compared hearing of elderly people with and without various medical conditions and found no relationship between hearing level and general medical condition. The same researchers also compared hearing of elderly subjects in hospitals (many with coronary disease) with other elderly subjects. Hospitalized patients had less severe loss of hearing than other elderly people (Soucek and Michaels, 1991).

OTOTOXIC DRUGS

Various therapeutic drugs have side effects that include inner ear pathology (see reviews by Hawkins, 1976; Rybak, 1986). Aminoglycoside antibiotics, such as kanamycin, destroy OHCs in the basal cochlea at minimal ototoxic levels; at higher doses, damage to IHCs and afferent terminals also occurs. Complete regional degeneration of the organ of Corti results in phalangeal scarring. Damage to the stria vascularis (atrophy, thinning) may result from aminoglycosides, as well. Loop diuretics, such as ethacrynic acid and furosemide, have their primary effect on the stria vascularis (e.g., reversible edema), but may have more widespread sensorineural effects when administered in conjunction with other drugs. Salicylates (e.g., aspirin) cause hearing loss and tinnitus, usually of a transient nature but potentially permanent in some cases (Kisiel and Bobbin, 1981).

Similarities between the effects of the known ototoxic drugs and the peripheral correlates of aging suggest that exposure to various ototoxic substances could contribute to presbycusis in some cases. It is also conceivable that other ototoxic substances, whose effects may be less pronounced and unappreciated, could play a larger role in presbycusis than is currently realized.

Another issue regarding aging and ototoxicity is the relative susceptibility of elderly individuals. Little is known about this topic. On the one hand, it is theoretically possible that older individuals could be less sensitive: inner ear melanin appears to have an ameliorative effect on some ototoxic drugs (Conlee et al., 1989), and melanin may increase in the inner ear with age (Chapters 3 and 4). On the other hand, a study by Henry et al. (1981) indicated that older CBA mice were more sensitive than young adults to kanamycin ototoxicity. Grigor, Spitz, and Furst (1987) showed that elderly people are more susceptible to the toxic effects (e.g., tinnitus) of salicylates. It may be the case that the interaction of age and/or presbycusis with ototoxic drugs is a complex process that depends on several variables, as is the case with noise exposure (see above).

THE ROLE OF DIET

Dietary fat is known to contribute to arteriosclerosis (Bierman, 1985). As discussed earlier, however, it is not yet clear if arteriosclerosis is a significant factor in presbycusis. If arteriosclerosis is proven to contribute to presbycusis, a corollary cause would be dietary habits.

Rosen and colleagues (e.g., Rosen, 1965; 1966) provided evidence indicating that the superior hearing of elderly Mabaans may be due to their low-fat diet and low-stress lifestyle which are conducive to cardiovascular health. When Mabaans moved to the city, changing diet and lifestyle, they often developed cardiovascular disorders. This suggests that the lesser severity of presbycusis in rural Mabaans may have been in part related to their low-fat diet. However, the effects of lifestyle and urban noise cannot be differentiated from dietary effects, and the study is inconclusive vis a vis the effects of diet. More convincing is Rosen's work (discussed in Chapter 2) on Finnish patients. Those patients who were put on a low-fat diet had better hearing than those eating the normal, high-fat Finnish diet. The high-fat group also had a greater prevalence of heart disease and, presumably, arteriosclerosis. The difference between the groups was seen for bone conduction thresholds, indicating an inner ear disorder. However, the air-bone gap at 4000 Hz was also enhanced in the high-fat group, indicating a conductive disorder as well.

A link between hearing loss (not necessarily in the elderly) and diet was made by Spencer (1973). He showed that 42 percent of patients with hearing loss (not necessarily presbycusis) also had hyperlipoproteinemia. He suggested that dietary control would greatly benefit hearing in these patients. Elevated levels of cholesterol in the blood was found by Pyykko et al. (1988) and by Hesse and Hesch (1986) to be a major risk factor in contributing to the development of sensorineural hearing loss in adults.

In conclusion, the potential contribution of diet (particularly high fat levels) to presbycusis may be significant. However, the evidence is inconclusive at present.

The effects of *dietary restriction* on presbycusis in rodents are receiving attention. Henry (1986) and Sweet, Price and Henry (1988) evaluated the effects of dietary restriction on presbycusis in mice. The effects of dietary restriction on presbycusis appeared to depend on genotype and the period during which diet is restricted. CBA mice restricted for their entire life and those restricted for the latter half of life had less pronounced loss of sensitivity at an old age than mice fed ad libitum. Life span was not affected. Restriction until mid-life had no effect on hearing. Dietary restriction in AKR mice had no effect on presbycusis or life span while in AU/Ss mice, presbycusis was reduced and life span was increased (Henry, 1986).

Park, Cook, and Verde (1990) examined the temporal bones of C57BL/6NNia mice (a variant of the C57BL/6J) that had been maintained on either ad libitum or restricted diets. In 18-month-olds, the number of spiral ganglion cells in the restricted group was about 4000, whereas the ad libitum group had only about 3000 cells. The data of Park and colleagues indicate that the age-related loss of ganglion cells can be slowed by dietary restriction. In contrast, in a study of rats maintained on restricted diets to extend their lives, Feldman (1984) found that the restricted diets did not ameliorate age-related cochlear pathology.

These studies suggest that reduced caloric intake may have the effect of diminishing the severity of presbycusis, but genetic factors play a key role. Thus, certain strains of mice benefit, whereas some strains of mouse and rat do not. The the possibility that genotype determines the effects of diet on presbycusis indicates that no simple relationship will be found in humans. Rather, individual differences, determined genetically, may be critical. This promising area of research deserves further attention.

THE PRESENCE OF OTHER TYPES OF SENSORINEURAL PATHOLOGY

Nadol, Young, and Glynn (1989) counted the number of spiral ganglion cells in patients who had suffered from various types of sensorineural pathology (e.g., postnatal viral or bacterial labyrinthitis, congenital, ototoxic). Cell counts were lowest in patients who were old at the time of death or had a long duration of deafness. However, multiple regression analysis indicated that the contribution of age and duration of impairment was minimal; the cause of the deafness was the main determinant of ganglion cell survival. Three patients (mean age at death, 63 years) diagnosed as having presbycusis and/or otosclerosis had a mean of 18,885 ganglion cells. This number of cells was greater than all other types of pathology except aminoglycoside ototoxicity and sudden idiopathic deafness (about 21,000 cells). Normal hearing patients had a mean count of 28,418. Thus it would appear that aging does not necessarily add to the severity of other types of sensorineural pathology.

ETIOLOGY OF THE DIFFERENT TYPES OF HISTOPATHOLOGICAL CHANGES IN THE COCHLEA

An adequate account of the etiology of peripheral presbycusis must deal with the specific properties of histopathology that accompany aging, in particular, the occurrence of six different types of peripheral pathology and the vulnerability of the base and apex of the cochlea.

ETIOLOGY OF DIFFERENT FORMS OF COCHLEAR PATHOLOGY

Evidence was presented in Chapters 3 and 4 that pathology of OHCs, spiral ganglion cells, the organ of Corti and ganglion cells in combination, and the stria vascularis can sometimes occur as independent age-related events. This suggests that specific histopathological outcomes may have different etiologies. This is an important issue because different etiologies imply different strategies for treatment or prevention of the disorders. Although little is known about the etiology of specific age-related tissue damage, findings reviewed in this and earlier chapters provide evidence that the different tissues of the cochlea are indeed differentially vulnerable to various insults. The following findings lend credence to the notion of specific etiologies.

(a) OHCs are particularly vulnerable to noise trauma and aminoglycoside antibiotics, suggesting that they are more sensitive to certain deleterious factors than other cochlear tissue. In addition, the OHCs are among the first cells to degenerate in certain inbred strains, such as the C57BL/6J, suggesting that genetic mechanisms may selectively affect OHCs during aging.

(b) The afferent terminals synapsing with IHCs are vulnerable to hypoxia, perhaps due to glutamate toxicity. Hypoxia or other age-related changes that affect glutamate synapses would have the potential to damage both IHCs and the terminals of dendritic processes of ganglion cells. OHC synapses would not be affected because they do not use glutamate as a neurotransmitter.

(c) There is a good deal of evidence that primary pathology of ganglion cells often occurs in aging humans, and these cells seem to be particularly affected by some genetically determined mechanisms of presbycusis in mice. Furthermore, if there were age-related pathology of neurons in the cochlear nucleus of the central auditory system, the efferent targets of auditory nerve fibers (Chapter 6), ganglion cells might be affected by retrograde degeneration. Finally, the axons of ganglion cells could be damaged by the formation of bony cuffs at the openings through which they leave Rosenthal's canal.

(d) It is possible that the high level of metabolic activity of the stria vascularis renders it susceptible to destructive oxidative processes, and its high degree of vascularity would be especially affected by impaired circulation. The stria vascularis is the primary site of loop diuretic ototoxicity, indicating the sensitivity of this tissue to certain ototoxic factors that have little effect on other cochlear tissue.

(e) Vascular insufficiency in the cochlea might be caused by arteriosclerosis or changes in the circulatory system. It is conceivable that moderate decreases in cochlear blood supply would have minimal histopathological consequences on other tissue but produce hearing loss by disturbing cochlear physiology.

The relevance of observations like these with regard to the etiology of different forms of age-related cochlear pathology remains to be determined by future research. Nevertheless, they underscore the feasibility that various etiological factors can cause damage to specific types of cochlear tissue.

VULNERABILITY OF THE BASAL AND APICAL COCHLEA

The basal region of the cochlea is usually the region most seriously implicated in sensorineural presbycusis.

The apex also exhibits a significant loss of hair cells and is often the site of strial atrophy. The middle of the cochlea is generally the least seriously affected in elderly individuals.

The reason(s) for this differential baso-apical vulnerability to age-related damage is unknown, but potential clues are suggested by the literature. The cochlea is not uniform from base to apex in several respects, providing possible substrates. For instance, the way energy is metabolized in the base and apex of the cochlea differs (Krzanowski and Matschinsky, 1971; Thalmann et al., 1972), and the thickness of the metabolically active stria vascularis varies. Furthermore, there are differences in the vascular organization in the base and apex of the cochlea leading Johnsson and Hawkins (1972b) to suggest that the the basal cochlea might be at risk from circulatory insufficiency. In this regard, Billett, Thorne, and Gavin (1989) have recently shown that cells of the basal cochlea, irrespective of type, are most vulnerable to ischemia in the guinea pig. The effects of ototoxic aminoglycoside antibiotics and noise exposure tend to be greatest in the basal organ of Corti as well, suggesting that this region is fragile in general. Taken together, these observations suggest that age-related hypoxia, alterations in energy metabolism, or other stressors that accompany aging might impact the basal cochlea most severely. Why the apical cochlea is susceptible to strial and other pathology is not clear.

CONCLUSIONS

Major gaps exist in our understanding of the causes of age-related inner ear pathology. This chapter has presented a great deal of speculation, but little empirical evidence. A preliminary conceptual framework has been provided here to help deal with what are likely to be multiple, often interactive etiological factors.

An understanding of the causes of the various types of cochlear pathology associated with aging is extremely important from both applied and theoretical perspectives. From the applied, clinical perspective, identification of causes of presbycusis may lead to prevention or effective treatment. From the theoretical perspective, etiological factors are fundamental pieces in the puzzle of presbycusis. This must certainly be a major emphasis of future, interdisciplinary research.

CHAPTER 6

Aging and the Anatomy and Physiology of the Central Auditory System

Stach, Jerger, and Fleming (1985) evaluated the hearing of a man several times between the age of 75 and 79 years. As seen in Figure 6-1, the patient's audiometric pure tone average (PTA) and scores on the maximum phonetically balanced word (PB max) test changed little during this period. By comparison, his synthetic sentence identification (SSI) score (which requires the identification of words in competing babble), dropped precipitously. Since performance on the SSI decreased, whereas the other measures did not, dysfunction of the central auditory system is suggested. This longitudinal case study provides an example of how clinical measures are used to infer the decline of central auditory processing with age.

Despite well-documented cases like this and the long-held assumption that "central presbycusis" occurs, few researchers have attempted to examine neurobiological aspects of the aging central auditory system (CAS). The paucity of CAS research is unfortunate because the brain is the "organ" of hearing and perception, with CAS neurons providing the infrastructure. For a full understanding of the perceptual deficits   that accompany aging, it is imperative that the fate of the central auditory system be known. In this chapter we review much of what is currently known about the anatomy and physiology of the aging CAS. The involvement of the CAS in psychophysical and other measures of auditory performance are discussed in Chapters 7 to 10.

The central auditory system is threatened by two concomitants of aging: changes in the structure or function of central auditory neurons due to biological aging and the removal or attenuation of neural input from the ear caused by peripheral pathology. The concept of "central" presbycusis has typically been associated with the former—age-related pathology of central auditory neurons. This condition can presumably cause auditory perceptual problems irrespective of peripheral hearing loss. However, an otherwise "healthy" central auditory system may be secondarily affected by the elimination of portions of the peripheral input from an impaired ear. As a result of the loss of some cochlear neurons (e.g., from neural presbycusis) or disruption of the relative contributions of cochlear components (e.g., from various types of pathology), some neurons in the cochlear nucleus (the first CAS station) may be completely relieved of their auditory input (e.g., high-frequency neurons), others may be partially relieved (e.g., neurons receiving both high- and low-frequency input), whereas some neurons may retain their input if it arises from healthy regions of the cochlea. Removal or attenuation of synaptic input to the CAS would disrupt the information received by the neurons and, in addition, could alter the physiological properties of post-synaptic neurons. Because the affected neurons provide input to other neurons, the effects could spread throughout the CAS. Central neural circuitry would be disrupted or altered because various circuit components (neurons) have become abnormal or nonfunctional to a greater or lesser extent.

Because both aging and peripheral impairment may affect the CAS, it is useful to differentiate two theoretical age-related effects that could result in central presbycusis. The deleterious effects of histopathology and/or pathophysiology of neurons and neural circuits within the central auditory system that are associated with biological aging[1] (irrespective of peripheral impairment) will be described by the term "central effects of biological aging" (CEBA); the deleterious effects of the age-related removal or alteration of cochlear neural input to the CAS (associated with peripheral presbycusis) will be described by the term "central effects of peripheral pathology" (CEPP).

The concepts of CEBA and CEPP are heuristics that provide a framework for examining research on the age-related anatomical and physiological changes that occur in the CAS. Presumably, central presbycusis can be caused by CEBA, CEPP, or a combination of the two.

STRUCTURE-FUNCTION CONSIDERATIONS

All ongoing auditory information is encoded by brief electrical impulses (action potentials) that travel along the 30,000 or so nerve fibers that leave the human cochlea (if the individual is young and normal hearing) and enter the CAS. These impulses have virtually no phenomenological similarity to speech and other sounds, yet the CAS somehow manages to transform them into the perceptual experiences of speech, music, and all of the sounds we hear. While we are far from understanding this feat, several aspects of CAS organization seem to be important, and each is potentially vulnerable to the aging process.

---

[1] As discussed in Chapter 5, the notion of "biological aging" encompasses a variety of events that can affect cells of the brain directly or indirectly via changes in metabolism, blood supply, etc.

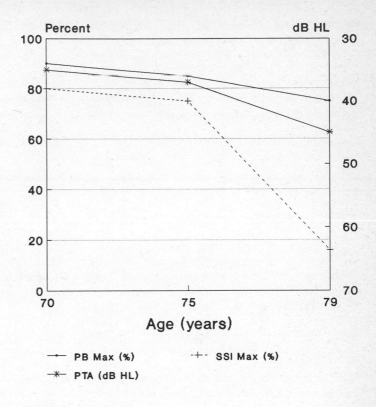

Figure 6-1. An example of clinical indications of central presbycusis. Maximum score on phonemically balanced words (PB Max), maximum score on Synthetic Sentence Identification test (SSI), and pure tone average (PTA). Depressed performance on the SSI relative to the other tests is thought to indicate central processing disorder. Only the SSI declines in this longitudinal study (adapted from Stach et al., 1985).

THE GENERAL ORGANIZATION OF THE CAS

The central auditory system is composed of many component parts. The "short list" of parts that often must suffice for clinical applications includes the cochlear nucleus (CN) and superior olivary complex (SOC) in the lower brainstem, the inferior colliculus (IC) in the midbrain, the medial geniculate body (MGB) in the thalamus, and the auditory regions of the neocortex. However, these terms have little meaning from an anatomical standpoint because each of these "nuclei" is in reality a collection of "subnuclei" or subdivisions. For instance, the cochlear nucleus may be subdivided into the anteroventral (AVCN), posteroventral (PVCN), and dorsal (DCN) subdivisions. As if this were not enough, based on the types of neurons and fiberarchitecture, "areas" can be identified within these subdivisions, including the spherical cell area(s), the globular cell area, the octopus cell area, several layers of the dorsal cochlear nucleus, the interstitial cell area, and more. The other major nuclei can, likewise, be broken down into subdivisions and areas.

Thus, the CAS is immensely complex in its anatomical organization.

It has become clear that most of the anatomical complexity has functional importance as well (see, for example, Irvine, 1986). The neurons in the AVCN, PVCN, and DCN send their axons to rather different targets. To take one of many examples, AVCN neurons project to areas of the superior olivary complex that appear to be involved in binaural spatial localization, whereas DCN neurons do not. Likewise, the different morphological types of neurons within subdivisions have different connections. For example, it is probable that only one type of AVCN cell, the bushy cell, is involved in certain aspects of binaural localization at the lower brainstem level.

It is reasonable to conclude that the subdivisions and areas of the CAS play different functional roles in auditory perception; they differ greatly with regard to the destination of their axons, the morphological types of neurons they possess, the spatial organization of cell bodies and fibers, and other properties (e.g., the neurotransmitters and types of inputs they receive). It follows that impairment of certain CAS regions by age and/or peripheral pathology may have unique effects on perceptual capacities (e.g., temporal resolution, frequency resolution, loudness, spatial localization, speech, etc.). Likewise, age-related dysfunction of specific neuron types would be expected to have specific functional correlates. Evidence will be provided later in this chapter to show that, indeed, subdivisions and neuronal types may differ in their vulnerability to age-related variables.

NEURONAL CIRCUITRY AND THE PROCESSING OF AUDITORY INFORMATION

The pulse-coded information carried by the auditory nerve fibers is distributed in a complex yet precise manner to a variety of targets in the cochlear nucleus, the first CAS station. Figure 6-2A shows a region of the mouse cochlear nucleus, cut in the sagittal plane, in which bundles of axons (most coming from the cochlea) are distributed in an organized spatial array. Figure 6-2B, taken from another part of the cochlear nucleus at a higher magnification, demonstrates how the axons weave their way through neurons, some perhaps supplying synaptic input, others traveling on to their ultimate destinations. Because of axonal branching the destinations can be multiple. Importantly, the position of axons in the array (Fig. 6-2A) is related to their origin in the cochlea: fibers arising in the cochlear base travel and synapse dorsally within subdivisions of the cochlear nucleus, carrying high-frequency information; those traveling ventrally arise from more apical regions of the cochlea and provide lower frequency input. This organization is maintained at higher levels of the CAS as shown by Figure 6-2D. In this histological section of the inferior colliculus, parallel sheets of neuronal processes can be seen. These sheets are tonotopically organized, with each being most sensitive to a certain frequency range, by virtue of the tonotopically organized input it receives from the lower brainstem.

Individual auditory neurons are typically designed in a manner that permits many synaptic inputs to be received, often in an elaborate (and functionally significant) spatial scheme. Figure 6-2C shows a mouse cochlear nucleus neuron at several microscopic planes of focus, revealing its three-dimensionality. The elaborate dendritic tree provides numerous sites for the reception of input. If the dendritic tree intersected different bundles of cochlear axons, it could act as an integrator of a broad spectrum of frequencies; if the tree were oriented so as to receive input from one cochlear region, it could deal with specific frequencies.

It is immediately obvious that cochlear pathology or dysfunction has the potential to disrupt this tonotopic scheme, since a significant number of nerve fibers is removed either physically by degeneration or functionally by loss of cochlear sensitivity. This is especially true for those fibers arising in the cochlear base and projecting to the dorsal regions of the CN subdivisions. The alteration of CAS circuits relying on tonotopic organization would be an example of CEPP. However, disruption of the system can also be accomplished by damaging the dendritic trees of CAS neurons, removing the cochlear fibers' target (as demonstrated later in this chapter, dendrites often do degenerate or change with aging). This could result from biological aging (CEBA) or as a secondary response to denervation (CEPP). Whether axons and/or dendrites are lost, the neural circuitry is degraded. The "integrating neuron" can no longer integrate properly; the "frequency specific" neuron may be totally relieved of its input. The responses of these neurons are, in turn, transmitted to neurons in other parts of the CAS. Those target neurons will also be deprived of their normal input, as will the neurons to which they, in turn, project. Since most CAS subdivisions send information to many other subdivisions (directly or indirectly), virtually the entire neural circuitry may be disrupted.

SYNAPSES AND NEUROTRANSMITTERS

Another level of neural circuit complexity is provided by the synapses, which may vary in form, function, and chemistry. Two types of synapses are shown in Figure 6-3A,B (there are many other types, as well), with obvious differences in the size and density of the vesicles that contain neurotransmitters. Different types of synapses arise from different sources (e.g., the primary cochlear fibers, other central neurons) and may have different effects on their target neuron (e.g., inhibition, excitation). They may also use different chemical neurotransmitters. For instance, the tissue shown in Figure 6-3C, from the inferior colliculus of a mouse, was treated with immunocytochemical techniques to reveal the presence of GAD (glutamic acid decarboxylase), a marker for the inhibitory neurotransmitter, GABA (gamma aminobutyric acid). Synaptic terminals can be seen contacting the neuronal cell bodies, indicating the presence of these inhibitory synapses; other (unstained) non-GAD staining terminals are undoubtedly present as well. Two of the three neurons shown have accepted the stain, but a third, faintly visible (arrow), did not. This example

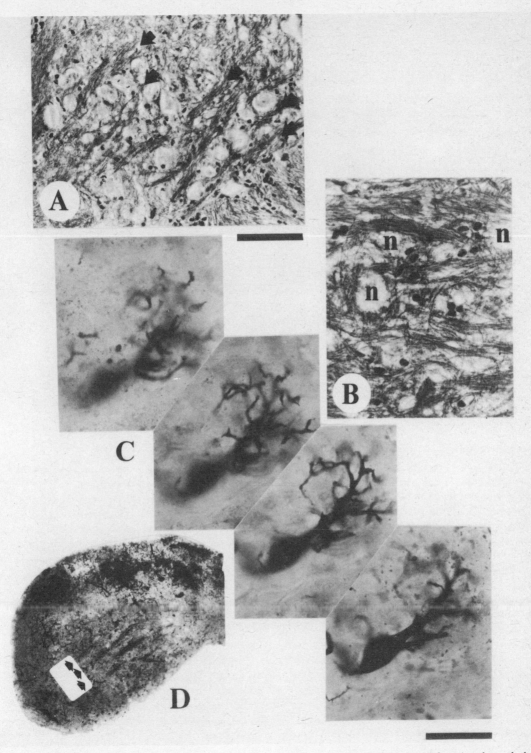

Figure 6-2. Some features of the central auditory system (Golgi and fiber stains, mouse). A. Sagittal section through the ventral cochlear nucleus showing bundles of axons (arrows), primarily of cochlear origin; dorsal is to the upper left corner (fiber stains scale bar =100 um). B. Higher power view of cochlear nucleus showing numerous axons weaving around neurons (n) (scale bar =50 um). C. A cochlear nucleus neuron at several planes of focus showing the dendritic tree (Golgi stain, scale bar = 40 um). D. Frontal section of inferior colliculus showing tonotopic laminae (arrows) (scale bar = 200 um).

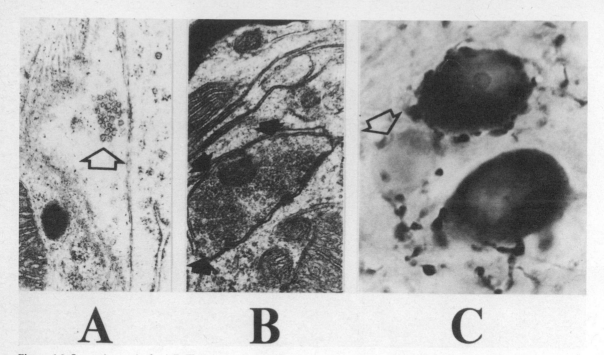

Figure 6-3. Synaptic terminals. A,B. Electron micrographs showing two types of terminals in the mouse AVCN. Note differences in the size and density of the synaptic vesicles and different appearance of the interface between pre- and post-synaptic elements (courtesy of Dr. Wayne Briner). C. Neurons in the mouse inferior colliculus immunostained for GAD. Two cell bodies are darkly stained, but a third (arrow) is not. Numerous darkly stained terminals are seen contacting the neurons (obtained in collaboration with Dr. Shao-Ming Lu).

shows how neurons differ in both the types of biochemicals they produce and the types of synaptic terminals they receive.

Because both excitatory and inhibitory neurotransmitters exist, it is impossible to predict the effects of neuronal loss or dysfunction in the CAS. For instance, if neurons using an inhibitory transmitter, such as GABA, were lost to aging, the result would be an increase in the excitability of their targeted, post-synaptic neurons. However, those target neurons could either excite or inhibit their respective target neurons, and so on throughout complex circuits.

It is clear that the fate of neurotransmitter systems must be elucidated before central presbycusis can be fully understood. This will not be easy. A review of the literature by Rogers and Bloom (1985) underscored the difficulties in attempting to understand how the brain's neurotransmitter systems change with aging. Research has often been inconsistent and contradictory. Furthermore, it is feasible that a number of facets of any neurotransmitter system may be affected, including synthesis (precursors, enzymes, cellular machinery), release, deactivation, and post-synaptic receptors. Nevertheless, there are many reports in the literature of changes in acetylcholine, norepineph-

rine, GABA, glutamate, or other transmitter systems with age. Because there is growing evidence that these neurotransmitters, among others, play roles in the auditory system (Drescher, 1985), it is possible that their decline during aging may affect the ability of the CAS to code auditory information. Changes in transmitter systems associated with biological aging would be an example of CEBA; changes in response to peripheral denervation would be CEPP.

RESEARCH CONSIDERATIONS

Three factors have conspired to hamper progress in understanding the neurobiological aspects of central presbycusis in humans. (a) It is impossible to obtain rapid and thorough fixation of post-mortem brain tissue, increasing the likelihood of autolytic artifacts. More importantly, most modern in vivo methods, required to reveal the anatomical and physiological details of neurons, cannot be used with human subjects. (b) It is possible that sensorineural pathology causes secondary morphological and physiological changes in the CAS. This would result in a confounding of the influences of peripheral impairment and biological aging, if they occur together (as is typically the case in humans). In other words, it may be impossible in practice to distinguish between CEBA and CEPP. (c) Environmental and genetic influences may interact with age-related biological events to affect the CAS in older individuals in unknown ways, making it difficult to determine the role of each.

These problems limit the usefulness of much data obtained from human subjects, and it is prudent to qualify conclusions derived from such data. The use of animal models can mitigate at least some of the problems, particularly those of a technical nature. In the author's laboratory, inbred mouse models (described in Chapter 4) are used to study aging and the CAS. The mouse models demonstrate how the problems outlined above can be addressed. (a) Sophisticated in vivo biological techniques can be humanely and ethically applied to the study of the aging CAS. (b) The central correlates of aging *with or without* significant peripheral presbycusis can be evaluated by comparing inbred strains or mutants that differ in this regard. Recall, for instance, that the CBA/J shows no peripheral impairment until late in life (Henry, 1983b; Wenngren and Anniko, 1988a; Willott, 1986), while the C57BL/6J undergoes progressive sensorineural loss with onset during young adulthood to middle age. Changes in the CAS of middle aged C57 mice would be correlated with sensorineural hearing loss (CEPP), whereas changes in the CAS of old CBA mice would occur irrespective of peripheral hearing loss (CEBA). (c) Biological variables that might affect the ear or CAS can often be predicted and accounted for on the basis of other work on inbred mice. Mice have been used in numerous experiments involving auditory physiology biochemistry, behavior, and anatomy (Willott, 1983) and are widely used in gerontological research in general. (d) The animals can be easily reared in a controlled moderate acoustic environment so that confounding by noise exposure or unknown environmental factors can be minimized. Genetic influences on aging, brain morphology, and numerous other variables can be controlled for by using inbred strains.

Most of the *physiological* findings to be dealt with in this chapter are based on research using mice; there are virtually no data from other animals. This situation should be rectified because, despite the advantages outlined, mice also have limitations as models. For instance, their range of most sensitive hearing is from about 2000 Hz to 50,000 Hz, compared to about 20 Hz to 20,000 Hz in young humans. Therefore, for some issues, such as coding of low-frequency sounds, the mouse may not be an appropriate model. In addition, when inbred mice are used , it is necessary to determine that observations on age-related changes can be generalized to other genotypes and species.

HISTOPATHOLOGY

AGING AND HISTOPATHOLOGY OF THE CENTRAL NERVOUS SYSTEM IN GENERAL

The aging brain is subject to a variety of histopathological changes that have been reviewed elsewhere (e.g., Duara et al., 1985; Willott, 1990). These include a loss of neurons, changes in neuron size (usually, but not necessarily, shrinkage), alterations of the neuronal cytoskeleton, changes in neuronal nuclei, diminution or disappearance of dendrites, alterations in myelin, proliferation of microglial cells, loss of other types of glial cells (e.g., astrocytes), gross changes of the brain and loss of weight, accumulation of lipofuscin and other intracellular inclusions, and more. In short, numerous histopathological changes can occur in the aging brain, any of which has the potential to disrupt central processing of information. Fortunately, however, pathological changes are not inevitable. Indeed, *variability* is a hallmark of neurogerontology, and it is difficult to make any generalizations about age-related histopathology of the aging brain. The effects of aging, just listed, differ as a function of species, individuals, and parts of the brain. Because of this variability, it is important to study empirically the histopathology of the CAS.

AGING AND HISTOPATHOLOGY OF THE HUMAN CENTRAL AUDITORY SYSTEM

Several studies have dealt specifically with histopathology of the human CAS. Kirikae, Sato, and Shitara (1964) and Hansen and Reske-Nielsen (1965) were among the first researchers to realize that the CAS of older individuals should be examined histologically in order to understand presbycusis fully. Dublin (1976) also stressed the importance of defining CAS pathology in presbycusis.

Kirikae et al. (1964) examined the brains of 11 older Japanese adults (68 to 87) and compared them with

20- to 30-year-olds. The brains were apparently obtained from routine autopsies, and no information was provided about post-mortem conditions. Only qualitative impressions were reported, including the following: a decrease in the number and size of neurons in auditory brainstem regions; an increase in pigmentation; "ghost-like indistinctness" and pyknotic nuclei in some cells; an increase in the ratio of nucleus to cell body size in small cells of the inferior colliculus.

Qualitative histopathological descriptions were provided by Hansen and Reske-Nielsen (1965) for a group of patients, most of whom were over 80 at the time of death. Because hearing loss appeared rather late in life in these patients, pathological changes in their CAS were presumably due primarily to aging, rather than to chronic loss of peripheral input. Hansen and Reske-Nielsen felt that the density of neurons was less than what is typically observed in the cochlear nucleus and inferior colliculus of young brains. Neurons appeared shrunken in many cases, but it is unclear whether this represents post-mortem change or a true aging effect. Since the brains were not placed in formalin until 12 to 24 hours after death, it is possible that the apparent reduction of neuron density could have resulted from cell shrinkage due to inadequate fixation of tissue.

Hansen and Reske-Nielsen (1965) reported a number of other observations. In the cochlear nuclei, "swollen" neurons were observed along with fine vacuolization and accumulation of granules. Nissl substance was displaced to the cells' periphery and was often coarsely granulated. The nuclear membrane was often folded, irregular, or displaced. Microglial cells appeared to be increased in number and elongated in shape. No consistent differences in the degree of pathology in different brainstem regions were found; however, degenerative changes in the medial geniculate nucleus appeared to be, in general, somewhat less pronounced than those in the lower auditory brainstem. Pathology was bilaterally similar in all cases.

Several examples of CAS histopathology in elderly patients were provided by Dublin (1976). He found, in one case, evidence for degeneration and loss of spherical cells and gliosis in the dorsal region of the VCN in a patient with ganglion cell pathology in the basal portion of the cochlea, which provides input to the dorsal VCN. Reduced cell density was also observed in the superior olivary complex, inferior colliculus, and auditory cortex of old patients.

Makishima (1978) described qualitative age-related changes in the central auditory system of patients over 50 years of age. Unfortunately, the observations were not compared to young patients, and it was only reported that "atrophy, degeneration of the nerve cells, spongy change, and softening were frequently noted."

These histopathologic descriptions are indicative of a number of age-related changes in the CAS. Interpretation of the observations is somewhat diminished, however, by the absence of quantitative methods. Without rigorous comparisons to material from young patients, it is difficult to assess impressions of "cell loss," changes in cell size, or other indications of pathology. Fortunately, several quantitative studies have also been performed on the aging human CAS.

THE COCHLEAR NUCLEUS

Konigsmark and Murphy (1970; 1972) evaluated the volume and number of neurons in the VCN of post-mortem patients in an age range from infancy through 90 years. They found no evidence of age-related change in the *number* of VCN neurons. Audiometric data were available for 10 of the 23 cases in Konigsmark and Murphy's (1970) study. There was no correlation between cell counts and the degree of hearing loss, suggesting that neither aging nor peripheral pathology caused a loss of VCN neurons. Despite the constancy of neural numbers, however, Konigsmark and Murphy (1972) did find a loss of CN *volume* with aging. VCN volume showed a 32 percent decrease (12.1 to 8.2 mm³) between age 50 and 90 years, which they attributed to diminution of the neuropil. Prior to the age-related decrease, volume increased from infancy through middle age. Konigsmark and Murphy's data are summarized in Figure 6-4. Several other qualitative observations of interest were reported on a subset of the cases. The average size of neurons "enlarged with increasing age;" it is not clear if any evidence of cell shrinkage was found in the oldest patients. The packing density of glial cells decreased from infancy through middle age, then "increased slightly" in the old age cases. Lipofuscin became more evident with aging. The number of small vessels and capillaries per unit area decreased with age. Finally, there appeared to be a decrease in the number of well-myelinated fibers in the VCN of old patients.

A doctoral dissertation by Crace (1970) described age-related changes in the human CN in detail. Post-mortem tissue was obtained from 18 subjects, aged 24 to 81 years, with a mean time of about 12 hours from death to immersion of the brain in formalin fixative. Crace found a statistically significant age-related decrease in the size of neurons (area) and the percentage of tissue occupied by neurons (density) (Fig. 6-5). There was not a significant change in the number of neurons with aging; however, many cells appeared degenerated in older individuals. Little evidence for an age-related change in glial cells was found, al-

Figure 6-4. The volume and number of neurons of the ventral cochlear nucleus of humans (adapted from Konigsmark and Murphy, 1970; 1972).

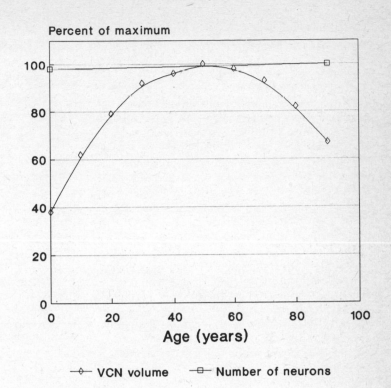

100% volume = 12 cm3
100% number = 49,000

Figure 6-5. Various morphometric measurements from the cochlear nucleus of humans (adapted from Crace, 1970).

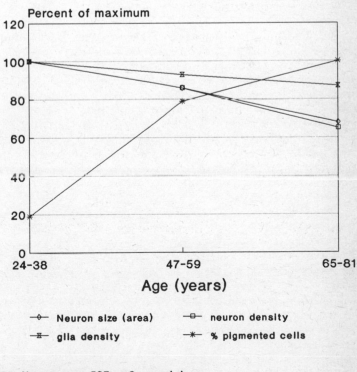

100%: Neuron area=587 um2; neural dens.=
1.7/100um2; % glia = 8.2/100 um2;
% pigmented cells=70

though a decrease in the density of glial cells occurred in parts of the CN. The most striking age-related change was an increase in the percentage of neurons containing pigment (Fig. 6-5).

Arnesen (1982) counted neurons in the cochlear nucleus in 6 brains from patients who had been diagnosed as having presbycusis. This study found a mean of 37,600 VCN neurons, somewhat fewer than in Konigsmark and Murphy's (1970) study (about 49,000 neurons) and considerably fewer than Arnesen's reference value from another study based on material from children. Arnesen concluded that a loss of cochlear nucleus neurons of nearly 50 percent (compared to the reference population) had occurred in the presbycusis patients. Clearly, Arnesen's conclusions differed from those of Konigsmark and Murphy and Crace, who found little loss of CN neurons with age. Technical difficulties may be responsible for the discrepancies. For instance, in Arnesen's study, autopsies were performed more than 24 hours after death, and young patients were not evaluated. Thus, the findings must be viewed with caution. On the other hand, it is possible that the subject populations of the different studies did in fact differ with regard to cell numbers. It is important to note that Arnesen's subjects were rather old (mean of more than 84 years) and had documented presbycusis. Only one of Crace's patients was over 80. However, Konigsmark and Murphy had 3 patients over eighty, and none showed a loss of neurons.

The "jury is still out" on the relationship between aging and the number of surviving cochlear nucleus neurons. It appears from the work of Crace and Konigsmark and Murphy that the number of neurons in the human cochlear nucleus typically does not change very much with age. However, more severe losses are indicated by Arnesen's neuron counts and by qualitative descriptions by Dublin and others. It seems safe to conclude at this time that some degenerative changes occur in cochlear nucleus neurons (with modest gliosis), particularly at advanced ages. However, a loss of neurons is not inevitable, and the degree of histopathology may vary considerably across individuals.

There is good agreement that the amount of lipofuscin increases with aging. However, the relationship between age and the size of cochlear nucleus neurons is not yet clear. Crace (1970) measured an average decrease of more than 30 percent in the cross-sectional area of neurons of elderly patients, and Kirikae and colleagues (1964) observed shrunken neurons. Hansen and Reske-Nielsen (1965) saw both shrunken and swollen cells, while Konigsmark and Murphy saw an increase in cell size, at least for part of the age range they examined. Of course, all neurons

in the cochlear nucleus may not change in size to the same extent or direction. As discussed later, differences in age-related changes in size among neuron types occur in mice.

THE LATERAL LEMNISCUS AND ITS NUCLEI

Ferraro and Minckler performed a quantitative analysis of the lateral lemniscus (LL; a major CAS brainstem fiber tract) and its nuclei (NLL) in 15 human brains, aged from newborn to 97 years. As shown in Figure 6-6, the density of LL fibers decreased a bit with aging; however, because the size (cross-sectional area) of the LL decreased, there was a correspondingly larger decline in the total number of LL fibers. The number of neurons in the nuclei of the LL, volume of the NLL, and ratio of glia to neurons showed a great deal of measured variance, with only a tendency to decrease (not shown in Fig. 6-6). The size of NLL neurons did not appear to decrease with aging ("neuron area," Fig. 6-6). With the exception of a significant loss in lemniscal fibers, age-related changes were not striking.

BRACHIUM OF THE INFERIOR COLLICULUS

Ferraro and Minckler (1977a) computed the fiber density and cross-sectional area of the brachium of the IC (the major fiber tract connecting the IC and medial geniculate body) in patients up to 97 years of age. No age-related differences were found among the 23 subjects aged 10 to 89 years, with typical fiber densities in the range of about 165,000 to 170,000 fibers per mm^2. In the two patients over 90, a decrease in fiber density of about 6 percent was found; this was accompanied by a 10 to 14 percent reduction in cross-sectional area.

AUDITORY CORTEX

Brody (1955) evaluated brains of patients ranging in age from newborn to 95 years. The brains were removed one to four hours after death. One of the areas evaluated by Brody was the superior temporal (auditory) cortex. Compared to the other cortical areas evaluated (inferior temporal, striate, precentral, and postcentral) the superior temporal cortex had the greatest loss of cells and the strongest correlation coefficient (-0.99) with age. Figure 6-7 shows the number of neurons in the superior temporal cortex as a function of age, compared to the number of cells in the striate (visual) cortex; the greater magnitude of cell loss in auditory cortex is evident.

Figure 6-6. Various morphometric measurements from the lateral lemniscus of humans (adapted from Ferraro and Minckler, 1977).

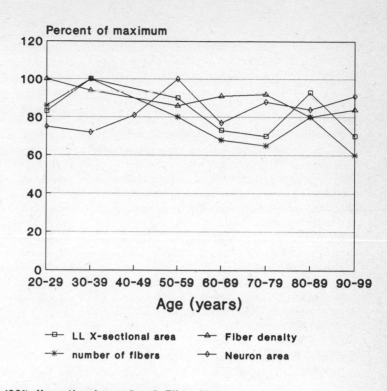

100%: X-sectional area=3mm2; Fiber dens. =87,000/mm2; # fibers=249,000; Neuron area=310um2 (length X width)

Figure 6-7. The number of neurons in the superior temporal and striate regions of the human cortex (adapted from Brody, 1955).

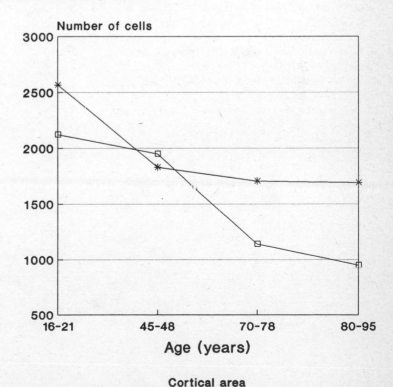

Brody's material also indicated that the thickness of the superior temporal gyrus decreased with age (3075 um in the 45- to 48-year-olds to 2592 um in the 75- to 95-year-olds). In contrast, the thickness of inferior temporal and striate cortex increased across these age groups. Cell size was not significantly affected by aging.

In the material of Hansen and Reske-Nielsen (1965), discussed previously, the temporal lobes appeared to have normal stratification, but gliosis and the accumulation of granules and amyloid (a glycoprotein that can proliferate with aging) were observed. Both "focal and diffuse" loss and degeneration of neurons were described. In the white matter, thinning and degeneration of fibers were found, and many axons were swollen and fragmented. The diameters of fibers had become abnormally heterogeneous.

Scheibel, Lindsay, Tomiyasu, and Scheibel (1975) used Golgi stains to evaluate the cerebral cortex of older patients with and without evidence of senility. The superior temporal cortex was included in their analysis. A sequence of pathological changes was observed in the pyramidal cells of the third cortical layer: swelling and "lumpiness" of the cell body and proximal dendrites, loss of dendritic spines (extensions of dendrites, believed to be sites of synaptic contacts), progressive loss of horizontally oriented dendrites, and eventual loss of apical shafts and cell death. There was some indication that the degenerative changes were more pronounced in senile patients. Scheibel and colleagues felt that the loss of dendrites was particularly important because of the loss of synaptic interactions and subtle aspects of cortical function.

CONCLUSIONS FROM HUMAN HISTOPATHOLOGY

The limited evidence available shows age-related histopathological changes in the CAS, most clearly documented in the auditory cortex and cochlear nucleus. There is an indication that the changes are not uniform across CAS nuclei and vary a great deal among individuals. In the auditory cortex, a dramatic decrease was observed in the number of neurons; in the cochlear nucleus, little or no loss was found; brainstem fiber tracts (lateral lemniscus and brachium of the IC) evidenced some loss of fibers but otherwise had minimal age-related changes. Whether these differences represent anything other than the use of different patients or fixation techniques by different researchers is unclear. It would be valuable to perform observations throughout the CAS on the same brains.

Even though some histopathological changes appear to occur in the CAS, their functional significance is yet to be determined. Because none of the studies reviewed had detailed test results of central auditory function, it is unknown if central presbycusis occurred. It would be a formidable task to obtain and evaluate thoroughly the brains of patients for whom detailed central audiometric tests have been performed. However, such endeavors will be required in order to interpret the significance of lost, shrunken, or lipofuscin-laden neurons. It may be the case that the CAS can withstand the loss of a significant percentage of its neurons without detrimental effects; it may be the case that shrunken neurons continue to function or that lipofuscin does not interfere with function. Given the variance among studies, the potential technical pitfalls, the interpretive difficulties, and the sometimes minimal magnitude of age-related changes, the evidence for functionally significant central presbycusis in humans, as indicated by histopathology, is not yet compelling.

AGING AND CAS HISTOPATHOLOGY IN ANIMAL MODELS

There has been disappointingly little work done on the histopathology of the aging CAS in animal models, despite the technical advantages outlined previously. One advantage that has been taken is the ability to induce hearing loss experimentally in young adults to elucidate the histopathological consequences. Because such experiments can help to reveal the vulnerability of the CAS to the loss of peripheral input per se (irrespective of aging), we shall briefly review them prior to addressing the literature on aging and CAS histopathology.

CAS HISTOPATHOLOGY WITH INDUCED COCHLEAR DAMAGE

The experimentally induced removal or attenuation of cochlear input in non-aged adult animals has been found to cause some histological changes in the CAS. Table 6-1 summarizes studies on this topic. Researchers have reported changes indicative of degeneration in the cochlear nucleus and in higher order CAS nuclei (transneuronal degeneration). The changes were typically undramatic, and there was no evidence of neuron loss. Since aging is typically associated with the loss of spiral ganglion cells (albeit not nearly as severe as with complete transection of the eighth nerve or destruction of the cochlea),

TABLE 6-1. STUDIES OF THE EFFECTS OF PERIPHERAL HEARING LOSS INDUCED DURING ADULTHOOD ON THE CAS OF ANIMALS: ANATOMICAL STUDIES.

Powell and Erulkar (1962). Cat, unilateral surgical cochlear ablation. Pronounced atrophy of ipsilateral VCN (smaller, paler-staining neurons, less prominent dendritic processes, gliosis, loss of VCN volume), with transneuronal degeneration of pre-olivary nuclei, contralateral MNTB and NLL; no change in the fusiform cell layer of the DCN. Most changes occur after 60 days. No evidence of cell loss, even after a year.

Gentschev and Sotelo (1973). Rat, surgical destruction of cochlea. After degeneration of large cochlear terminals (end bulbs, boutons), some AVCN neurons were reoccupied by terminals; more often, post-synaptic specializations are lost, preventing reinnervation. This may be beneficial because it prevents reinnervation by inappropriate presynaptic terminals.

Liden et al. (1973). Cat, noise-induced cochlear degeneration or labyrinthectomy. Shrinkage of perikaryon and pyknosis or chromatolysis of cochlear nucleus neurons, but no loss of neurons (the mean number of VCN cells after noise exposure was 7 percent lower than controls but was identical in the DCN for the two conditions).

Morest and Jean-Baptiste (1975). Cat, surgical deafferentation. Calycine terminals in the MNTB showed changes (filamentous hyperplasia, decreased mitochondria and synaptic vesicles). After 30 days, the post-synaptic principle neurons showed increased condensation of nuclear chromatin and 30 percent cell shrinkage, suggesting interference with a trophic effect of the calycine terminals.

Theopold (1975). Guinea pig, noise-induced cochlear degeneration. Formation of huge mitochondria in neurons of the ventral cochlear nucleus; apparently degenerating dendrites with glial reaction.

Hall (1976). Monkey, streptomycin ototoxicity or noise exposure. Degeneration (pyknosis and chromatolysis) of cochlear nucleus neurons, loss of neurons, and reduction of CN volume. Degenerated cells were intermingled with normal appearing cells. VCN multipolar and octopus cells showed vacuolizing, chromatolytic degeneration; spherical cells showed pyknotic degeneration. Loss of neurons was similar for DCN and VCN.

Morest and Bohne (1983). Chinchilla, noise-induced cochlear degeneration. IHC loss was associated with degeneration of coarse fibers in the VCN; OHC loss was associated with degeneration of fine fibers in the DCN. Some transneuronal degeneration in the SOC and IC.

Koitchev et al. (1986). Guinea pig, gentamycin ototoxic destruction. No sign of changes in AVCN neurons up to 30 days of cochlear pathology.

---

the possibility exists that similar changes may be secondary to sensorineural presbycusis (CEPP). It is also possible that age-related changes might be more severe because the period of chronicity is generally much longer (years) than that used in these experimental studies (weeks or months).

HISTOPATHOLOGY OF THE CAS DURING AGING IN ANIMAL MODELS

THE COCHLEAR NUCLEUS

This brainstem region has been examined in some detail in aging rats and mice.

Feldman and Vaughan (1979) performed histopathological evaluation of albino Sprague-Dawley rats aged up to 36 months. In this age range, no evidence of cell loss was found. Electron microscopy showed some neurons with "watery-appearing" cytoplasm and a reduction of organelles. Volume of the VCN in the oldest animals was about 25 percent less than that in young animals. An increase in lipofuscin in VCN neurons with age was significant.

The electron microscope revealed two patterns of dendritic degeneration: a "focal accumulation of mitochondria within an enlarged dendritic profile," and a loss of microtubules with prominent vacuolization. Feldman and Vaughan (1979) observed channels connecting the interior of these dendrites with extracellular environs. Another feature of aging dendrites was enlargement of mitochondria accompanied by proliferation of the intramitochondrial membranes of the cristae.

Within the nuclei of VCN neurons, Feldman and Peters (1972) observed unusual filamentous rod-like structures (intranuclear rods) that became more prominent in older animals. Through 2 years of age the widest intranuclear rod observed measured 0.96 um. In 36-month-old rats (Feldman and Vaughan, 1979) rod diameters up to 1.3 um were measured. The significance of the rods is not clear, but they appear to be positively correlated with neural activity. This seems paradoxical since afferent input from the cochlea to VCN neurons would presumably be diminished in older animals. Perhaps the aging VCN neurons increase their "nonauditory activity" as inferior colliculus neurons appear to do (see below).

The rostral pole of the AVCN was evaluated with EM in young and old Sprague-Dawley rats by Feldman (1982). In old rats (27 to 36 months), the extent of AVCN neuronal somata contacted by synaptic terminals, particularly the end bulbs of Held originating from the axons of spiral ganglion cells, was decreased. No evidence was seen for reinnervation of sites vacated by degenerated end bulbs of Held. Keithley (1989) also found fewer synapses on spherical cells in the AVCN of old Fisher 344 rats. However, the area of complex endings and the degree of complexity of the endings were greater in the old Fisher 344 rats (Keithley and Croskrey, 1990). This finding differed from Feldman's (1982) observation on Sprague-Dawley rats in suggesting that, following the degeneration of some ganglion cells in the older rats, the surviving terminals may have expanded to contact vacated post-synaptic sites.

In the AVCN of aging CBA mice, there is a small but steady decline in the size of both bushy cells (Lambert and Schwartz, 1982; Willott, Jackson, and Hunter, 1987) and multipolar cells, the major neuron types in the AVCN. A net loss of AVCN neurons is observed only in rather old mice (Willott et al., 1987). The volume of the AVCN, and of the whole cochlear nucleus (Lambert and Schwartz, 1982), decreases during the second half of the life span. In C57 mice, bushy cells increase in size (particularly in the high-frequency region of the AVCN) but multipolar cells remain unchanged or decrease slightly. A small but significant loss of neurons is seen in young adulthood, but the number of neurons remains fairly constant during aging/chronic peripheral pathology.

A recent electron microscopic analysis of the C57 AVCN (Briner and Willott, 1989) found several age-related changes in 2-year-old mice. There was an increase in the number of lipofuscin particles in neurons throughout the AVCN. However, the build up of lipofuscin was most pronounced in the high frequency region of the AVCN, which is most severely denervated in old C57 mice. The appearance of nucleoplasm changed in many neurons (a less homogeneous appearance), and nuclear invaginations developed with age. The invaginations were more pronounced in multipolar cells than in bushy cells of old mice. Overall, however, the combined effects of aging and chronic sensorineural impairment were not striking in the 2-year-old C57 mice.

Willott and Bross (1990) examined the octopus cell area (OCA) of the posteroventral cochlear nucleus in C57 and CBA mice and extended the analysis to very old mice (30 months and older). OCA neurons receive most of their synaptic input from cochlear nerve fibers, so, like AVCN bushy cells, they should reveal the effects of peripheral sensorineural pathology in C57 mice, as well as the effects of aging. In both CBA and C57 mice, the volume of the octopus cell area declines substantially (e.g., by almost 50 percent) during the second half of life. The packing density of octopus cells changes little during this time, so a loss of octopus cells is associated with the reduction in OCA volume late in life. The packing density of glial cells increases as octopus cells are lost. The size of octopus cell bodies decreases in both strains, but only as the end of the life span is approached. As seen with the Golgi stain, the condition of dendrites of octopus cells in old animals (2 years or more in age) varies from normal, to minor losses of branches, to complete loss of dendrites. Octopus cells with either normal or abnormal dendritic trees can be seen in the same animal.

The changes that occur in the OCA with aging appear to be primarily manifested near the end of the life span and are generally similar in both strains during this period. OCA histopathological changes do not appear to be exacerbated by severe, chronic sensorineural pathology. If such were the case the magnitude of aging effects should have been more pronounced in C57 mice, but this did not occur. Thus, the late changes are likely associated with CEBA, rather than CEPP.

Whereas subtle differences in age effects were observed in bushy cells of the AVCN as a function of the neurons' dorsoventral location, location-dependent differences were not detected in the OCA. It is important to note that the bushy cells receive massive synapses (end bulbs of Held) from the spiral ganglion cells whose origin is restricted to a particular part of the cochlea (re: base-apex). Octopus cells receive at least half of their synaptic input from the cochlea, but it tends to come from ganglion cells spread more widely along the cochlear turns. Octopus cells probably receive relatively more non-cochlear input than bushy cells, as well. These findings are consistent with the notion that the loss of ganglion cells in the basal cochlea, which typically occurs with sensorineural presbycusis, may affect the histopathology of bushy cells of the AVCN more than it affects some other CAS neurons.

The morphology of the dorsal cochlear nucleus of 3- and 26-month-old C57BL/6J mice was described by Browner and Baruch (1982) in what was the first thorough morphological study of the C57 central auditory system. There did not appear to be a significant loss of DCN neurons, but Golgi-stained tissue revealed age-related differences in several cell types. (a) Fusiform cells of young mice had one or two primary dendrites covered with spines; old fusiform cells had dendritic varicosities and few spines, which were short and stubby. (b) Young cartwheel neurons had elaborate dendritic trees covered with spines; old cartwheel neurons had varicosities and blunted spines (Fig. 6-8). (c) Large multipolar cells of old mice had

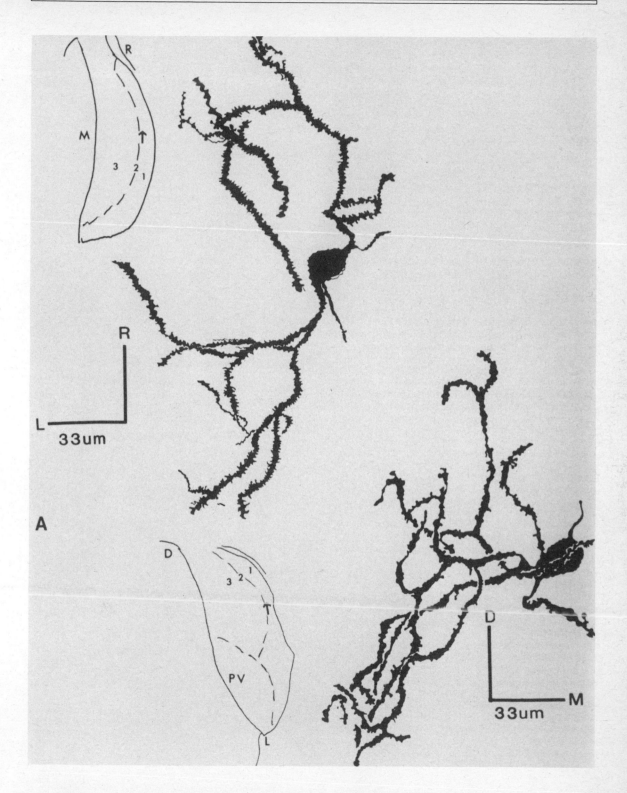

Figure 6-8. Camera lucida drawings of Golgi-stained "cartwheel neurons" from the dorsal cochlear nucleus of a 3-month-old (A) and 26-month-old C57 mouse (B). Note that the dendrites of the older neuron do not have as many spines as the dendrites of the young neuron. From Browner, R.H. and Baruch, A. (1982) The cytoarchitecture of the dorsal nucleus in 3-month and 26-month-old C57BL/6 mouse: A Golgi impregnation study. *Journal of Comp. Neurology, 211,* with permission.

thinner dendrites and more varicosities than those of young mice. Thus, Browner and Baruch found evidence of degeneration in the dendritic trees of DCN neurons, particularly fusiform and cartwheel cells. While the degree of degeneration was not dramatic, the change from many spines to fewer spines and increased varicosities indicate a loss of synaptic contacts that would be expected to have functional implications in a hearing animal.

Recent work by Willott, Bross, and McFadden (unpublished) has provided a quantitative analysis of DCN structure in aging C57 mice. There was little loss of neurons through 1 year of age (after an initial loss between 1 and 7 months, also seen in other cochlear nucleus subdivisions). However, mice aged 24 months or older exhibited a significant loss of neurons. The loss of neurons was restricted to the third DCN layer, with layers 1 and 2 showing no loss of cells. The third layer is the DCN region most heavily innervated by auditory nerve fibers (Moore, 1986), suggesting that the attrition of ganglion cells contributes to the loss of cells. The other major change in the very old mice was a significant reduction in the volume of the neuropil. In aging CBA mice, there was no significant loss of neurons through old age, supporting the notion that the loss of ganglion cells influenced the loss of DCN neurons in the C57 mice.

While many cochlear nucleus neurons survive to an old age, their usefulness depends on the integrity of axonal projections from one part of the CAS to another. In other words, the neural circuits must remain intact. The horseradish peroxidase tract tracing technique, a powerful method for tracing CAS pathways, was used to determine if pathways change in response to aging and peripheral presbycusis in C57 mice (Willott, Pankow, Hunter, and Kordyban, 1985). When horseradish peroxidase conjugated with wheat germ agglutinin (HRP/WGA) is injected into the brain, it is transported by axons back to the neuron cell bodies from which they originate. Cell bodies are thereby "labeled" with a dark reaction product that can be seen clearly in microscopic analysis. The number of labeled neurons and topography of AVCN projections was found not to differ between young and old mice. In general, pathways from the CN to IC central nucleus (ICCN) remain largely intact, even in very old, chronically deaf C57 mice. These findings suggest that CAS projections can be robust in the face of aging and chronic peripheral impairment. An example is provided in Figure 6-9 from a 26-month-old mouse, showing ample neurons projecting from each division of the cochlear nucleus to the IC.

SUPERIOR OLIVARY COMPLEX

A series of papers by Casey and Feldman (Casey and Feldman, 1982; 1985 a,b; 1988) described the me-

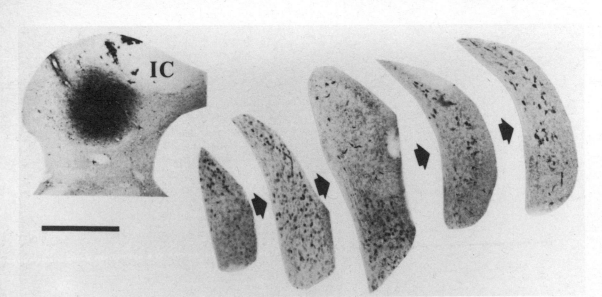

Figure 6-9. Light microscopic sections showing retrograde transport of horseradish peroxidase/wheat germ agglutinin from the inferior colliculus to the cochlear nucleus of a 26-month-old C57 mouse. The injection site is shown in the IC (upper left, scale bar = 1000 um). Frontal sections of the cochlear nucleus from anterior (left) to posterior are shown (scale bar = 400 um). Neurons that transported HRP/WGA from their axon terminals in the IC injection site are "labeled" with the black reaction product that accumulates within the cell body. Even in this old, chronically impaired animal, the circuitry between the CN and IC is intact.

dial nucleus of the trapezoid body (MNTB), one of several nuclei in the superior olivary complex. Neurons of the MNTB are innervated by huge calyce of Held terminals of axons originating in the cochlear nucleus. Casey and Feldman examined the MNTB in Sprague-Dawley rats aged 2 to 3, 6, 18, 24, and 33 months. By 24 months of age, the number of MNTB neurons was reduced by 34 percent, but some loss of neurons was already evident by 6 months of age. The loss of neurons appeared to be similar for the major types of neurons found in the MNTB, and the proportion of neurons (23 to 26 percent) receiving the calycine synapses did not change with aging. Pigment granules became larger and more numerous as the rats aged, but pigmentation was not as pronounced as that found elsewhere in the aging rat brain. Estimates of the volume of the MNTB showed a decrease from 0.176 mm^3 at 3 months to 0.124 mm^3 at 27 months (Fig. 6-10).

At the electron microscopic (EM) level, evidence of degenerating axons, dendrites, and synaptic terminals was seen in the neuropil of 24- to 33-month-olds (Fig. 6-11). Quantitative findings on terminals are shown in Figure 6-10 (percent calycine and non-calycine terminals). Casey and Feldman (1985a) suggested that the age-related loss of calycine terminals that results in a partial deafferentation of the MNTB would likely alter the processing of auditory stimuli. Apparently,

the number of non-calycine terminals remained stable with aging.

Casey and Feldman (1985b) also found a loss of vascularity in the MNTB of 24- to 33-month-old rats, as revealed by a decline in the volume density ratio of capillaries (Fig. 6-10, VDR). Two other observations were made: (a) large "cavitations," or spaces, appeared within the capillary basal lamina (Fig. 6-12); and (b) membranous debris, probably from pericyte degeneration, was seen in leaflets of the basal lamina (Fig. 6-12). The reduction in vascularity could affect the metabolic activity of aging MNTB neurons and might alter their functional properties in a significant way.

Recently, Casey (1990) counted neurons in the SOC of Fischer 344 rats and included the lateral and medial superior olivary nuclei (LSO and MSO) in his analysis, as well as the MNTB. Between the ages of 3 months and 30 months, there was no change in the number of LSO or MSO neurons, while the number of MNTB neurons decreased at 2 years of age. However, the decrease in MNTB neurons was only 8 percent, compared to the 34 percent loss measured in Sprague-Dawley rats. These findings indicate that strain differences in CAS histopathology exist and that SOC subdivisions are differentially vulnerable to aging.

The papers by Casey and Feldman did not present data on the size of MNTB neurons in rats. However, data are available from mice. Browner and Riedel

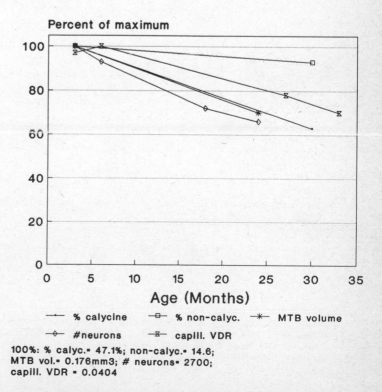

Figure 6-10. Various morphometric measurements from the nucleus of the trapezoid body of rats (after Casey and Feldman, 1982; 1985). % calycine = relative number of calycine terminals; % non-calyc. = relative number of non-calycine terminals; MTB volume = volume of the medial nucleus of the trapezoid body; capill. VDR = volume-density ratio of capillaries.

Percent of maximum

Age (Months)

— % calycine   —□— % non-calyc.   —*— MTB volume
—◇— #neurons   —x— capill. VDR

100%: % calyc.= 47.1%; non-calyc.= 14.6;
MTB vol.= 0.176mm3; # neurons= 2700;
capill. VDR = 0.0404

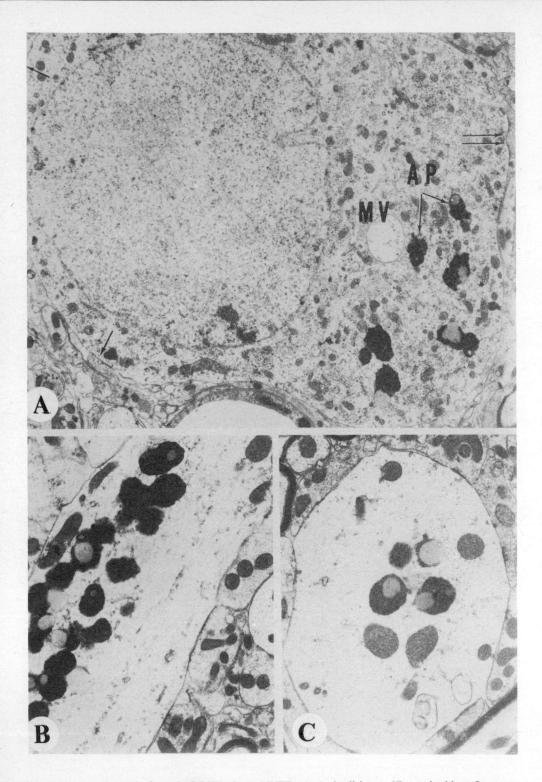

Figure 6-11. Electron micrographs from the MNTB of rats. MNTB principal cell from a 27-month-old rat. Some age pigment (AP) has accumulated; multivesicular bodies (MV) are more abundant and larger in old animals; axosomatic terminal (arrows) are reduced in number compared to young animals (not shown); the increased electron density and vesicle packing density of one terminal (double arrow) suggests an early stage of terminal degeneration. B, C. Pigment deposits in dendrites of MNTB cells of rats aged 27 months. From Casey, M.A. and Feldman, M.L. (1985a) Aging in the rat medial nucleus of the trapezoid body. II. Electron microscopy. *Journal of Comp. Neurology, 232,* with permission.

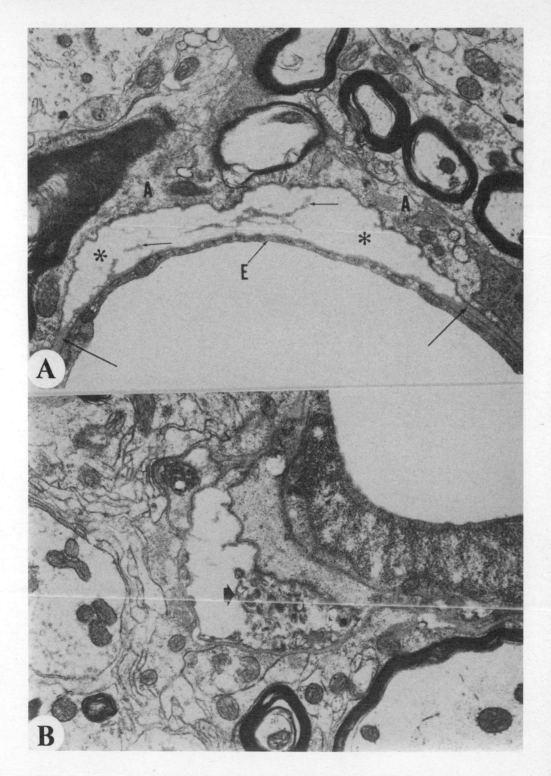

Figure 6-12. Electron micrographs showing age-related abnormalities associated with capillaries. A. Basal laminar cavitation in MNTB capillary of a 24-month-old rat. Intact portions of the basal laminae are marked by the larger arrows; the cavitations contain a floccular material similar in structure to basal lamina (small arrows); in some areas, the material has a "honeycombed" appearance (*). B. Membranous debris within capillary basal lamina (arrows). From Casey, M.A. and Feldman, M.L. (1985b) Aging in the rat medial nucleus of the trapezoid body. III. Alterations in capillaries. *Neurobiology of Aging, 6,* Pergamon Press, Inc., with permission.

(1988) measured the cross-sectional area of neurons in the MNTB of Young (30 days) and old (2 years) C57 mice. Mean cell area declined from 167.9 um² to 142.6 um² across this age range (a statistically significant difference).

INFERIOR COLLICULUS

Hoeffding and Feldman (1989) described the morphology of the IC of macaques aged 5 to 34 years. Although the general appearance of the neurons and neuropil was similar in young and old monkeys, neurons of old monkeys contained more lipofuscin, and vacuoles were seen in the cytoplasm. The size of the IC did not change with age, but the density of neurons decreased, suggesting a loss of neurons. Increased thickness of myelin sheaths and a decrease in the mean axoplasmic diameter of some axons were also observed in old animals.

The morphological properties of the CBA and C57 mouse inferior colliculus have not yet been quantified. However, it is apparent from inspection of histological sections that a loss of neurons occurs in very old (more than 29 months) mice of both strains. As seen in Figure 6-13, there is little obvious difference between colliculi of 2- and 24-month-olds, but a loss of neurons occurs in the very old animals. Another histopathological change, particularly evident in CBA mice, is the development of cyst-like holes in the neuropil of the oldest animals.

AUDITORY CORTEX

Peters, Feldman, and Vaughan (Feldman and Vaughan, 1979; Peters and Vaughan, 1981; Vaughan, 1977) found a number of age-related changes in the

C57   CBA

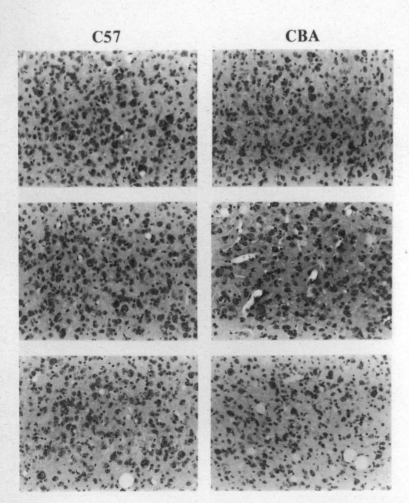

Figure 6-13. Light microscopic sections from the ventral inferior colliculus in C57 (left column) and CBA mice (right column) stained with cresyl violet. First row is from 2-month-olds; second row from 2-year-olds; third row from 30-month-olds. There is little apparent loss of neurons through 2 years in either strain. By 30 months (beyond the median life span and nearing the end of life) the density of neurons is noticeably reduced, particularly in the CBA strain.

auditory cortex of Sprague-Dawley rats. The auditory cortex of 3-year-olds was 10 percent thinner than that of young animals, although no changes in the vertical organization or horizontal lamination accompanied the thinning. The distribution of neuron sizes shifted toward smaller sizes, and lipofuscin content of older neurons increased to about 8 percent of perykaryal volume.

Within the neuropil, the morphology of most elements appeared normal in the cortex of old rats, but abnormal axon terminals (enlarged and filled with membranous material or dense and degenerated) were sometimes seen. Pathological dendrites were seen, with swollen regions filled with membranous whorls, but they were not common.

Age-related changes were also found in Golgi-stained cortical pyramidal cells. The density of the neurons' basal dendrites decreased (Fig. 6-14), with reductions of about one half the number of dendritic branches 40 um from the soma (Vaughan, 1977). The

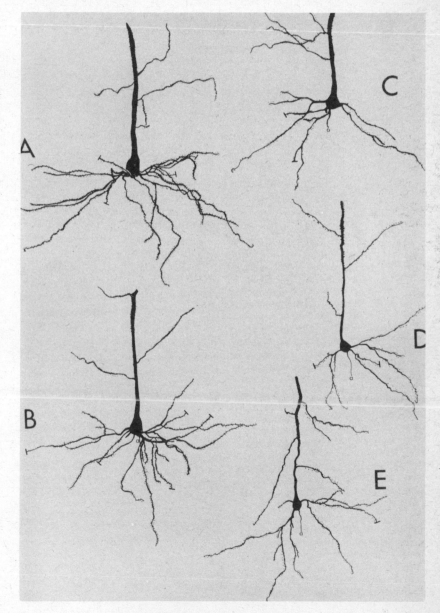

Figure 6-14. Camera lucida drawings of layer V pyramidal cells from the rat auditory cortex. A,B. from 3-month-olds; C. from a 34-month-old; D,E. from 36-month-olds. "a" = axon. From Vaughan, D.W. (1977) Age-related deterioration of pyramidal cell basal dendrites in rat auditory cortex. *Journal of Comp. Neurology, 171,* with permission.

loss of branches was associated with elimination of the parent primary or secondary dendritic trunks, not with dying back of peripheral branches. Vaughan suggested that the loss of primary dendrites was not a typical neuropathological manifestation. Rather, it may be characteristic of age-related pathology.

The number of dendritic spines on auditory cortical pyramidal cells of rats is reduced during aging (Feldman and Dowd, 1975), and appears to be a rather consistent correlate of aging (Peters and Vaughan, 1981). Age-related spine loss was also observed in the apical dendrites of layer V pyramidal cells in the CBA mouse auditory cortex by McGinn, Henry, and Coss

(1984). By obtaining thresholds electrophysiologically, they were able to divide old (460 days) mice into a group with normal hearing and a group with substantial threshold elevations. Some neurons in both groups of older mice showed dendritic varicosities, loss of dendrites, and swollen and distorted somata. The density of dendritic spines on small diameter dendritic shafts was reduced in the animals with good hearing; however, spine density was reduced on both large and small diameter shafts in the animals with diminished hearing. These findings suggest that the loss of hearing exacerbated the age-related loss of spines.

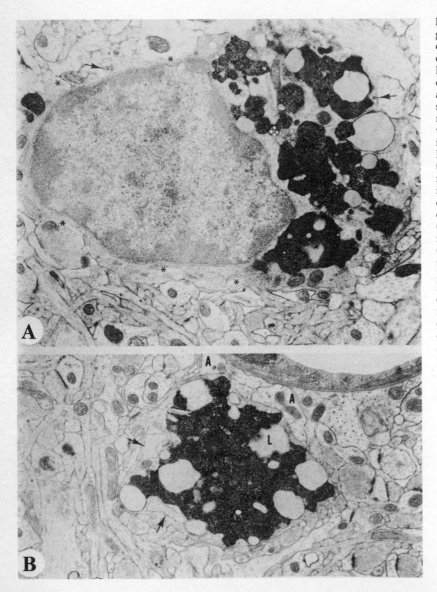

Figure 6-15. Electron micrographs showing microglial cells. A. Rounded microglial cell in a 27-month-old rat. Heterogeneous dense material dominates the cytoplasm around the nucleus; irregular spaces (*) are characteristic of many microglia; two coated vesicles at the cell surface are indicated with arrows. B. Isolated microglial process in the cortex of a 24-month-old rat containing both dense material and lipid (L); expanded cisternae of the endoplasmic reticulum (arrows) appear in some microglia; astrocytic processes (A) separate this process from the basal lamina of a capillary. From Vaughan, D.W. and Peters, A. (1974) Neuroglial cells in the cerebral cortex of rats from young adulthood to old age: An electron microscopy study. *Journal of Neurocytology, 3,* with permission.

Vaughan and Peters (1974) evaluated the glial cells of the aging rat cortex. The population of astrocytes and oligodendrocytes remained stable, but microglia, which play a macrophagic role in the aging brain, increased in density by 65 percent. The microglia also changed in shape from simple multipolar forms to elongated or spherical forms containing cellular debris (Fig. 6-15).

CONCLUSIONS FROM ANIMAL HISTOPATHOLOGY

The work on animal models demonstrates the complexity of age-related histopathological change in the CAS. First, age-related changes differ among neuron types. This was seen in the cochlear nucleus of C57 mice with regard to bushy, multipolar, and octopus cells. Second, tonotopic location can be a factor if peripheral pathology has occurred, but this depends on cell type. In aging C57 mice, bushy cells in the dorsal AVCN show slightly more pronounced changes than those in the ventral AVCN, presumably because the dorsally located bushy cells are deprived of their normal input from the (now degenerated) basal cochlea (a similar observation in human material was noted by Dublin, 1976). In contrast, histological changes in multipolar and octopus cells do not depend on dorsoventral location. Third, there are significant genetic influences on age-related histopathology. For instance, a loss of AVCN neurons was observed during the second year of life in CBA mice, but not in C57 mice, and the degree of cell loss in the MNTB differed for Sprague-Dawley and Fischer 344 rats. Fourth, within an individual, considerable variance in age-related histopathology occurs among neurons. The condition of octopus cells in aging mice ranged from normal to severely degenerated. Feldman and Vaughan (1979) noted that, intermingled with neurons exhibiting signs of pathology or degeneration, were many auditory cortical neurons of old rats, which appeared to be free of pathology. Fifth, connections between CAS subdivisions can persist despite the combined insults of aging plus chronic peripheral sensorineural impairment, as demonstrated by the projections from the cochlear nucleus to the inferior colliculus in old C57 mice.

As was the case with histopathological observations on humans, the functional significance of age-related change in animals is difficult to assess. While we can describe the histopathological changes in animals in great detail, it is more difficult to relate them to complex perceptual capacities. Behavioral studies are sorely needed to determine how far the histological changes can advance before perceptual abilities are affected.

CONCLUSIONS FROM HUMAN AND ANIMAL MATERIAL

Certain similarities emerge in comparing the histopathological material obtained from humans and other species. Thus, several conclusions can be made about age-related changes that are probably common to mammals in general. (a) Very old individuals are likely to have a reduced number of CAS neurons. However, the losses are typically modest, at least in the subcortical CAS. (b) The volume of CAS structures tends to be smaller in old individuals, with loss of neuropil contributing significantly to the reduced volume. Evidence for loss of dendrites and/or dendritic spines has been found for several species, including humans. (c) Aging CAS neurons accumulate lipofuscin in moderate amounts. (d) There is considerable variability among individuals in the number of neurons surviving to old age. Material from mice suggests that genetics plays a strong role in this regard.

These findings imply a histological basis for central presbycusis. As noted earlier, however, whether or not they cause hearing disorders is yet to be demonstrated.

The question of whether peripheral sensorineural pathology may exacerbate some age-related histopathological changes is yet to be completely resolved. While peripheral sensorineural pathology can have some central effects in young, deafferented animals, these are typically not pronounced. Likewise, peripheral pathology does not appear to greatly exacerbate age-related histopathological changes in mice, with the possible exception of dendritic spine loss (which could have very important effects on the ability of neurons to communicate with one another). Other than spine loss, the most pronounced effects of cochlear pathology probably occur in cells of the cochlear nucleus which receive substantial synaptic input from the cochlea. In C57 mice, these cells show an age-related change in size and/or number.

Taken together, the histopathological evidence for CEPP is not dramatic. However, it will become clear in the following sections that the physiological effects of peripheral impairment are considerably more cogent.

NEUROPHYSIOLOGY

The manner in which individual neurons and populations of neurons respond to sound provides a key to understanding how the CAS processes auditory information. Age-related changes in neuronal responses are, presumably, the basis of central presbycusis. Unfortunately, the techniques currently available to monitor the action potentials of individual neurons in the brain cannot be used with humans, so we must rely on animal experiments to determine how those responses are affected by aging and/or peripheral pathology. As was the case in the discussion of age-related CAS histopathology, it is necessary to consider the effects of biological aging on central neuronal physiology, as well as the effects of peripheral hearing loss. Therefore, these topics will be briefly reviewed before moving on to a discussion of aging and CAS physiology.

AGING AND THE RESPONSES OF NEURONS IN THE BRAIN

Electrophysiological recordings from neurons in the nonauditory central nervous system have indicated that neuronal response properties may change with aging. Some of the observations that have been made include: a reduction in the synaptic excitation of neurons in the caudate nucleus and an increase in the time interval required between responses in aged cats (Levine et al., 1987); reduced spontaneous activity in neurons of the locus coeruleus of old rats (Olpe and Steinmann, 1982); increased thresholds for excitation

of cerebellar neurons (Rogers et al., 1980); reduced excitability to afferent input in hippocampal neurons of old rats (Barnes, 1979); a decrease in the conduction velocity of spinal cord motoneurons and changes in several neuronal membrane properties in aged cats (Chase et al., 1985). On the other hand, little age-related change was found in the passive electrical properties of hippocampal granule cells in rats (Barnes and McNaughton, 1979). These kinds of studies indicate that the way central neurons respond can be altered by aging. However, age-related declines may not be inevitable. Consequently, the possibility must be entertained that age-related physiological changes (CEBA) may or may not occur in CAS neurons as a result of biological aging.

CAS PHYSIOLOGY WITH EXPERIMENTALLY INDUCED PERIPHERAL HEARING LOSS IN YOUNG ADULTS

Several studies, summarized in Table 6-2, have obtained physiological recordings from CAS neurons of young adults after damaging the cochlea with noise, ototoxic drugs, or surgery. Because these ototraumatic procedures result in damage that is in some ways similar to that associated with aging (Chapters 3 and 4), this research may provide insight into the effects of peripheral presbycusis on CAS responses. In these

TABLE 6-2. STUDIES OF THE EFFECTS OF PERIPHERAL HEARING LOSS INDUCED DURING ADULTHOOD ON THE CAS OF ANIMALS: PHYSIOLOGICAL STUDIES.

Koerber et al. (1966). Cat, surgical destruction of cochlea. Deafferentation resulted in a loss of spontaneous activity in the VCN but not in the DCN.

Salvi et al. (1978). Chinchilla, acute noise exposure. Tuning curve thresholds were elevated and tuning was less sharp. Some decreases in spontaneous activity were found.

Gerken (1979). Cat, surgical destruction of the cochlea. Thresholds for electrical stimulation of the CAS decreased; deafferentation resulted in an increased sensitivity to electrical stimulation.

Willott and Lu (1982). Mice, acute noise exposure. In addition to elevation of tuning curve thresholds of IC neurons, temporal discharge patterns of some neurons changed. In some cases, neurons became more excitable (lower thresholds, higher levels of evoked discharge, change from inhibition to excitation) after noise exposure.

Popelar and Syka (1982). Guinea pig, acute noise exposure. Tips of IC tuning curves were elevated, tuning became less sharp. No changes in the temporal discharge patterns or intensity functions were observed. Total number of evoked action potentials decreased and response latencies increased.

Van Heusden and Smoorenburg (1983). Cat, acute noise trauma. Frequency selectivity (sharpness of tuning curves) in AVCN neurons was decreased. Some tuning curves shifted their peak frequencies. Most sensitive tips of tuning curves were elevated, while less sensitive tail regions were not.

Woolf and Ryan (1985). Chinchilla, kanamycin to produce selective OHC loss. Some changes similar to those seen in eighth nerve fibers, but 22 percent of neurons had normal tuning curve tips despite OHC loss; first spike latency was increased; features arising in VCN (e.g., non-primary-like responses) were not affected.

Boettcher and Salvi (1991). Chinchilla, acute tone exposure. Increased maximal firing rate in AVCN at and above CF when exposure tone was above CF.

studies, damage to the inner ear affected neural responses in various ways, including a reduction in non-evoked action potentials (spontaneous activity) in the ventral cochlear nucleus (but not in the DCN), an *increase* in responsiveness to acoustical or electrical stimulation, and decreased frequency selectivity (decreased sharpness of tuning curves). Although these changes were demonstrated acutely, it is reasonable that related effects (CEPP) may be associated with the chronic loss of peripheral input that often accompanies aging.

RESPONSES OF CAS NEURONS IN AGING ANIMALS

An indication that age-related changes may occur in the responses of neurons of the inferior colliculus (IC) was provided by Malmo and Malmo (1982). In the course of obtaining multiple-unit responses from electrodes implanted chronically in rats, they obtained longitudinal records for over two years in some animals. Since their study was not specifically designed to measure auditory responses, only limited information was obtained. However, the recordings indicated a decline in the magnitude of sound-evoked activity in the IC. Age-related declines in response to nonauditory stimuli were not seen in forebrain recording sites, suggesting that nonspecific factors were not involved.

Other than the acoustically crude study of Malmo and Malmo, most of the available information on response properties of CAS neurons in aging animals has been obtained from C57 and CBA mice by the author and his colleagues. What follows is a summary of this work (Willott, 1991; Willott et al., 1988 a,b,c; Willott, Parham, and Hunter, 1991). Changes in neuronal response properties of middle-aged C57 mice should largely reflect the effects of sensorineural hearing loss (CEPP), whereas changes in responses of old CBA mice should be related to aging of the CAS (CEBA). Comparison of data from the two strains allows the effects of hearing loss and aging to be "teased apart." In all cases, the animals were anesthetized, and recordings of neuronal action potentials were obtained with extracellular microelectrodes. Brief sounds (200 msec.) were delivered to one ear while action potentials were recorded from CAS neurons.

ROLE OF ANATOMICAL LOCATION WITHIN THE IC

Measurements of thresholds of neuronal responses to tones indicate that anatomical location within the IC is a cogent variable in determining the effects of peripheral impairment on frequency coding of C57 mice. Neurons in the dorsolateral IC (normally an area responding best to low frequencies) are much less dramatically affected than neurons in the ventromedial IC (normally a high-frequency area). The severe high-frequency hearing loss in aging C57 mice is accompanied by drastic elevations of neuronal response thresholds in the ventromedial half of the IC central nucleus, but minimal threshold elevations in the dorsolateral IC, which includes part of the central nucleus and the IC dorsal cortex (a subdivision of the IC). In IC neurons of CBA mice, the magnitude of age effects is not greatly influenced by their location within the IC.

REPRESENTATION OF FREQUENCY IN THE IC

The representation of frequency within the IC (tonotopic organization) is greatly disrupted in middle aged C57 mice (Fig. 6-16). The neurons' "best frequencies" (BF, that frequency in the response area for which threshold is lowest) change; BFs of neurons in the ventromedial IC (the right portion of the abscissa of Figure 6-16), which are normally high, shift to lower frequencies. In addition, the low-frequency "tails" of tuning curves in the ventromedial IC become more responsive to low-frequency sounds. Responses of IC neurons to suprathreshold stimuli support the tuning curve data; low-frequency stimuli evoke a higher than normal rate of responses in ventral IC neurons in middle-aged C57 mice. This is shown by the response areas (number of action potentials evoked as a function of stimulus frequency and intensity) of neurons in Figure 6-17. In young mice, neurons in the ventral region of the IC typically respond in a manner exemplified by panel F: robust responses and low thresholds at high frequencies, but no response to low-frequency tones. The remaining panels (A-E) depict the response areas of middle-aged C57 neurons from the same region of the IC. The neurons respond poorly or not at all to high frequencies (due to peripheral pathology; see Chapter 4). More importantly, they now respond rather well to low-frequency sounds. In contrast, the representation of frequency in the IC of CBA mice (not shown in the figure) is not greatly affected by aging. Apparently, peripheral pathology (C57 mice) causes significant alterations in the way frequency is represented in the CAS, but aging of CAS neurons (CBA mice) does not.

The enhanced responsiveness to low frequencies in ventral IC neurons of middle-aged C57 mice could result from several possible mechanisms. First, it could reflect a change in the frequency response of the

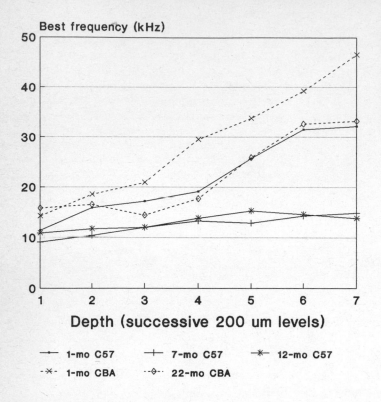

Best frequency (kHz)

Depth (successive 200 um levels)

— 1-mo C57   + 7-mo C57   * 12-mo C57
-*- 1-mo CBA   --◇-- 22-mo CBA

Figure 6-16. The mean best frequency of inferior colliculus neurons in C57 and CBA mice as a function of the dorsoventral depth within the IC. BFs are normally relatively low in dorsal regions (low depths), becoming progressively higher at more ventral depths. This tonotopic organization is lost in middle-aged C57 mice but not in old CBA mice (after Willott, 1986).

cochlea, whereby basal regions become more responsive to low-frequency sounds. This seems unlikely because the basal cochlea is severely impaired and largely nonfunctional in middle-aged C57 mice; furthermore, a similar enhancement is not seen in the AVCN (which should more closely reflect the responses of cochlear neurons). Second, the change could reflect an alteration in the anatomical projections to the ventral IC. If low-frequency regions sprouted axonal branches to innervate the region, it would become responsive to low frequencies. This is feasible, although the HRP/WGA experiments, described above, provide no evidence of altered axonal projections in aging C57 mice. Third, low-frequency input might be available to this region in young mice, but be normally suppressed or inhibited. If peripheral impairment reduced this suppressive process (or caused enhancement of the low-frequency source), the low-frequency input could emerge. One variation on this theme is that low-frequency and high-frequency inputs to some IC neurons are provided by different CAS nuclei (e.g., the DCN and AVCN, respectively), and that the low frequency source becomes relatively more "potent" as high-frequency sensitivity is diminished by cochlear

pathology. As shown below, there is evidence that the AVCN of aging C57 mice is more severely affected than the DCN.

Whatever the mechanism of altered frequency representation in C57 mice proves to be, the implications for frequency coding may be significant. The "rules" have changed in that high-frequency neurons now respond to low frequencies. This could be a source of confusion for the CAS, causing sounds to be coded inaccurately. Central alterations of coding such as this (even though caused by peripheral pathology) might account for some of the perceptual problems faced by elderly listeners (Chapters 8 and 9).

INTENSITY RESPONSES OF IC NEURONS

The percentage of neurons with "nonmonotonic" rate-level functions decreases with age in C57 mice, especially in the IC dorsal cortex. Nonmonotonic rate-level functions are characterized by an increase in evoked discharges as stimulus level is increased from threshold, but after reaching some maximal level, the rate decreases with further stimulus level increases.

The decrease in discharge rate is likely caused by neural inhibitory processes recruited at high stimulus levels. Thus, it would appear that the ability of neurons in the IC dorsal cortex of aging C57 mice to manifest such inhibitory processes is impaired. Aging CBA mice show little change in nonmonotonic intensity functions.

SPONTANEOUS ACTIVITY IN THE IC

In both C57 and CBA strains there is an age-related increase in the proportion of neurons that are spontaneously active (i.e., they produce impulses in the absence of intentional acoustic stimulation). The increase occurs in the ventral IC, suggesting that loss of peripheral input at high frequencies may be responsible. An increase in spontaneously active neurons would alter the "signal to noise" ratio in the CAS and might interfere with neural coding of sounds.

SLUGGISH AND NORMAL RESPONSES IN THE IC

In CBA mice there is an age-related increase in "sluggish" neurons (auditory, but poorly driven by sound) from 3 percent in young mice to 22 percent in old mice. In C57 middle-aged mice, the increase in "sluggish" neurons is less pronounced (from 2 percent in young mice to 11 percent by middle age). Despite the increase in sluggish neurons, most neurons in aging animals of both strains respond robustly to suprathreshold stimuli. In most respects, the non-sluggish neurons appear to have normal responses to suprathreshold stimuli. They exhibit temporal discharge patterns similar to those of young neurons in response to 200 msec tones (e.g., a sustained excitatory response, inhibition by sound, various other patterns).

COCHLEAR NUCLEUS

Response changes also occur in the cochlear nucleus. The age-related changes in response properties in C57 mice are, in general, more severe in the AVCN and PVCN than in the DCN. Compared to the DCN, VCN neurons of middle-aged mice have more severe threshold elevations in response to noise and tone stimuli, more severely reduced response area widths

(i.e., frequency ranges), and steeper increases in the slope of rate-level functions. Responses of cochlear nucleus neurons in old CBA mice are similar to those of young mice[2].

The classic cochlear nucleus response patterns originally described by Pfieffer (1966) are affected differently in middle-aged C57 mice. Many neurons in the ventral cochlear nucleus (probably multipolar cells) of young mice exhibit "chopper" responses: for short duration sounds (e.g. about 30 msec.) the time interval between action potentials is fairly constant, so that post-interval time histograms are multipeaked with the peaks separated by a consistent interval. The incidence of chopper responses decreases dramatically in the VCN of middle-aged C57 mice. In contrast, the incidence of "primary-like" responses remains high in aging C57 mice. These responses, which resemble those of cochlear nerve fibers (with varying intervals between action potentials) probably arise from bushy cells. Finally, neurons demonstrating inhibition decrease in both VCN and DCN, but the change is more pronounced in the DCN (which has much more inhibition in young animals).

SUMMARY: C57 AND CBA MICE

Because peripheral sensorineural hearing loss is severe by middle age in C57 mice, changes in the CAS of this strain should be associated with central disorders of peripheral origin. In contrast, responses of CAS neurons of old CBA mice should reflect alterations in the CAS that would produce central disorders due to biological aging.

In either strain, neural coding activities that rely on populations of neurons must do so with diminished numbers due to threshold elevations and an increase in sluggish neurons. However, important differences exist between the strains. Biological aging in CBA mice apparently levies a greater toll with respect to the emergence of sluggish neurons (22 percent incidence in aged CBAs versus 11 percent in 12- to 15-month-old C57s). By comparison, high-frequency threshold elevations in middle-aged C57 mice are much more severe. The consequence should be that functions involving populations of C57 neurons responding to high frequencies would be more deleteriously affected than those involving low-frequency

[2] Keithley (1990) obtained single-unit records from the VCN of young and old (24 to 26 months) Sprague-Dawley rats. All of the classic response types were observed in the old animals, and most units did not have greatly elongated latencies in the old rats. There was a reduction in the range of characteristic frequencies from 0.4 to 55 kHz in young rats 0.9 to 30 kHz in the old rats.

population responses; in old CBA mice the frequency-related effect should be less pronounced. This notion is supported by data on the acoustic startle response (Parham and Willott, 1988; Chapter 8). In middle-aged C57 mice responses to low-frequency tone pips persist, while responses to higher frequencies are drastically reduced in amplitude. In aging CBA mice, reductions in startle amplitude are similar for all frequencies tested.

The responses of most ("non-sluggish") *individual neurons* of CBA mice reveal a remarkable degree of "normalcy." The majority of neurons in the IC of old CBAs appear to maintain response properties typical of young animals, with regard to the repertoire of response types available and properties of rate-level functions. Thus, neural coding processes that might depend on reliable relationships among stimulus parameters and neuronal response properties (e.g., as in the notion of acoustic "feature detectors") seem to be rather resilient. Middle-aged C57 also maintain a degree of "normalcy" in temporal response patterns of individual IC neurons. However, changes in some response properties (tuning curves, intensity functions) of peripherally impaired, middle-aged C57 mice tend to be much more substantial than those occurring in very old CBA mice. In other words, even though more neurons remain "non-sluggish" in C57 mice, some of the physiological effects of peripheral pathology are more pronounced than those associated with biological aging alone.

Experiments on neurons in the cochlear nucleus of C57 mice provide some insights into the complexity of the mechanisms underlying CEPP. The finding that some response types (e.g., choppers) are more severely affected by peripheral pathology than others (e.g., primary-like) suggests a greater *physiological* vulnerability of multipolar cells compared to bushy cells. However, bushy cells are probably more severely denervated by the loss of basal cochlear neurons because of their innervation by end bulbs of Held (see earlier discussion). It may be that the chopper response pattern is more sensitive to changes in the cell's membrane properties or to the weakening of synaptic "driving" by cochlear neurons that results from damage to the inner ear. In any event, the differential vulnerability of CAS neurons to aging and/or peripheral pathology does not appear to be a simple phenomenon.

AGING AND THE METABOLISM OF GLUCOSE

Under normal conditions the brain metabolizes glucose for energy. One method of evaluating the

brain's ability to metabolize glucose is by measuring the incorporation of systemically injected, radioactive 2-deoxy-D-glucose (2DG) by brain tissue. Because 2DG is a glucose analogue, its uptake should reflect the relative degrees of glucose utilization by different regions of the brain. The relative degrees of 2DG uptake in quiet was evaluated with optical densitometry in young and old C57 and CBA mice (Willott, Hunter, and Coleman, 1988). Neither aging per se nor chronic severe peripheral impairment causes declines in the relative degree of incorporation of 2DG by the CN or IC as measured by this method.

Clerici and Coleman (1987) measured 2DG uptake in the IC of Sprague-Dawley rats under conditions of quiet and sound stimulation. Overall, age had little effect on 2DG incorporation. They found no change in 2DG uptake in quiet as a function of age. With high frequency (50 kHz) monaural stimuli at a relatively high intensity (about 70 dB SPL), stimulus-evoked levels of 2DG were slightly less than normal, while 8 kHz stimuli resulted in a slight relative *increase* in old rats. There was an indication that the bands of 2DG incorporation were less well defined in the older rats, however, and there appeared to be a greater relative representation of the 8 kHz stimulus, with a diminution of banding in response to the high frequency stimulus. This suggests a change in the loci that are responsive to specific stimulus frequencies similar to that found in the C57 mouse IC, noted above (Willott, 1986; Fig. 6-17).

The findings of Clerici and Coleman (1987) and Willott, Hunter, and Coleman (1988) are consistent with a number of studies showing stability of glucose metabolism during aging in the rodent brainstem (Duara, London, and Rapoport, 1985). The resting metabolism in the IC and cochlear nucleus suggests continued viability of the CAS during aging, with or without severe peripheral hearing loss. However, the relationship between aging and energy metabolism in humans is still not clear, and some animals (e.g., Fischer 344 rats, dogs) may show age-related declines (Duara et al., 1985). Thus, caution should be exercised in generalizing the findings from rodents.

AGING AND CAS NEUROTRANSMITTERS

It was mentioned earlier that the relationship between aging and neurotransmitter systems is confusing at present. While very little is known about the CAS in this regard, some findings have recently been reported.

Caspary, Raza, Armour, Pippen, and Arneric (1990) evaluated GABA neurotransmission in the central

Figure 6-17. Response areas in the ventral inferior colliculus of C57 mice. A-E are from 12- to 15-month-olds; F is from a 2-month-old. Many neurons in the older animals respond to low-frequency tones in this IC region, whereas neurons in the young animals rarely do. From Willott, J.F., Pathum, K. & Hunter, K.P. (1988b) Response properties of inferior colliculus neurons in middle-aged C57BL/6J mice with presbycusis. *Hearing Research, 37,* with permission.

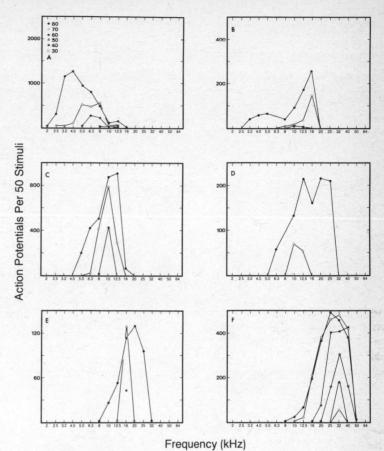

nucleus of the inferior colliculus of young and old Fischer 344 rats. The number of neurons labeled by an antibody against GABA was decreased by 36 percent in the ventrolateral portion of the central nucleus of the old rats. They also measured the release of GABA and other amino acids evoked by potassium ions. Both the basal and evoked release of GABA (but not other amino acids) were reduced in the old rats.

Willott, Lu, and Bross (unpublished observations) used an antibody for GAD (an enzyme involved in the synthesis of GABA) in an immunocytochemical study of C57BL/6J and CBA/J mice. The impression from viewing Figures 6-18 and 6-19 is that no loss of GAD-positive neurons occurred in two-year-old mice of either strain. This impression was confirmed by counting GAD-positive neurons and finding no significant age differences. It is unlikely that pockets of lost GAD-positive cells failed to be observed, since the IC was thoroughly examined. Thus, the data from mice indicate that GABAergic neurons persist during aging

whether chronic peripheral presbycusis is present (C57 mice) or not (CBA mice).

The data from Fischer 344 rats (Caspary et al.,1990) and those obtained from mice seem to be at variance. One possible explanation for the discrepancy is a basic species difference in the effects of aging on GABAergic neurons. For instance, Fischer 344 rats show an age-related decline in glucose metabolism in the IC (Duara, London, and Rapoport, 1985), but CBA and C57 mice probably do not (see above). The formation of certain neurotransmitters, including GABA, is related to glucose metabolism (Hoyer, 1988). Thus, differences in age-related declines in glucose metabolism may be involved (although other transmitters were not affected by age in the study of Caspary et al.). It is also possible that the aging curves for the loss of GABAergic neurons differ between species. Had older mice been examined, a loss may have been revealed. Finally, it is possible that the enzyme GAD is present in normal amounts, but the product, GABA, is not. In any event,

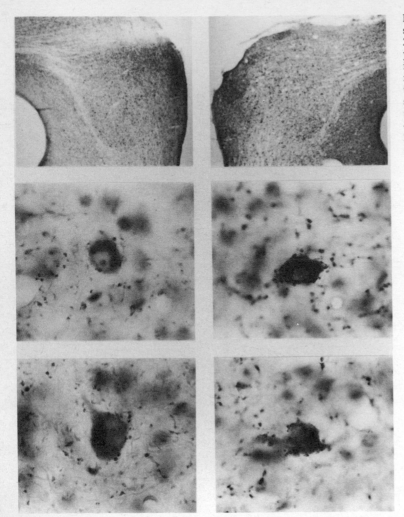

Figure 6-18. Light microscopic sections of the inferior colliculus of a 2-month-old (left column) and 2-year-old (right column) CBA mouse immunostained for GAD. The old mouse has no noticeable decline in the number of neuronal cell bodies or small forms (e.g., presumably axons/terminals). Scale bar for first row = 400 um; scale bar for rows 2 and 3 = 20 um (obtained in collaboration with Dr. Shao Ming Lu).

the GABA system does appear to be diminished in aging rats, suggesting weakened inhibitory processes in the inferior colliculus. The negative findings in mice suggest that this effect may be influenced by unknown variables.

CONCLUSIONS FROM ANIMAL CAS PHYSIOLOGY

While there is little evidence that histopathological correlates of aging are greatly exacerbated by peripheral pathology, this is not the case with regard to the physiological responses of neurons. The presence of high-frequency hearing loss in C57 mice causes marked disruption of the normal responses as a function of frequency or intensity. In contrast, aging per se (CBA mice) has less pronounced effects on neuronal re-

sponses. A good deal of variability in the degree of age-related changes is observed among neurons. "Sluggish" neurons become more common with aging, but relatively normal response properties are the rule among surviving, physiologically responsive neurons, at least in the inferior colliculus. The persistence of certain classes of neurons may depend upon factors such as the neurotransmitter system they employ (e.g., GABA versus other amino acids); however, such relationships may vary across species. Energy metabolism does not appear to be greatly affected by aging irrespective of peripheral presbycusis.

Once again, the functional significance of the age-related changes needs to be clarified. For instance, the incidence of spontaneous neural activity, decline of the inhibitory GABA system (rats), and maintenance of energy metabolism levels in quiet conditions all

Figure 6-19. Light microscopic sections of the inferior colliculus of a 2-month-old (left column) and 2-year-old (right column) C57 mouse immunostained for GAD. The old mouse has no noticeable decline in the number of neuronal cell bodies or small forms (e.g., presumably axons/terminals). Scale bar for first row = 400 um; scale bar for rows 2 and 3 = 20 um (obtained in collaboration with Dr. Shao Ming Lu).

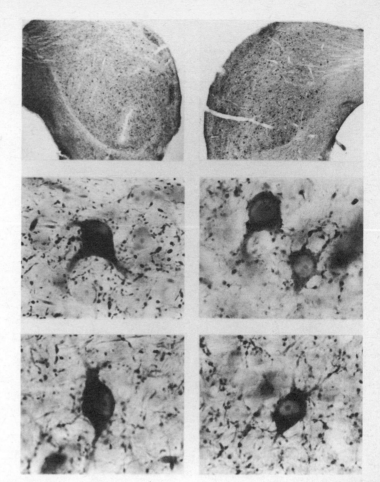

suggest that "neural noise" may be augmented in the aging CAS. It would be valuable to have behavioral/perceptual data to determine what, if any, auditory functions are affected.

Because no data are available from humans, it is unknown if similar physiological changes take place in our own species. It is intuitively reasonable that "sluggish" responses may arise from pathological neurons. Since there is ample evidence that some neurons exhibit histopathology in aging humans, it may be the case that their responses would also be "sluggish." One can speculate that such neurons would be less effective in the encoding of speech and other suprathreshold sounds, as discussed in Chapters 8–10. It is also feasible that they could be responsible for elevated thresholds for low-frequency sounds that have been attributed to central presbycusis (Hansen and Reske-Nielsen, 1965; Hayes and Jerger, 1979). The formulation of the "volley" theory of frequency coding by Wever and Bray (1930) provided a mechanism by which frequency could be represented in the firing patterns of neurons. Individual neurons respond to the phase of a low-frequency tone, firing in response to every nth cycle. Numerous neurons fire in synchrony to the stimulus phase, with the frequency of tones determining the frequency of firing. It seems reasonable that this means of coding frequency might be problematic if aging CAS neurons have become "sluggish" or completely unresponsive. Impaired ability to code low frequency sounds would be predicted, and this could result in the elevated thresholds attributed to central presbycusis.

Two changes in the physiological response properties of the C57 mouse's central auditory system have interesting implications. First, the representation of frequency (tonotopic organization) is greatly disrupted in the inferior colliculus. As discussed earlier, this reorganization would be expected to cause problems with the neural coding of frequency. It will be shown in Chapter 8 that frequency discrimination and resolution are usually diminished in older humans. The deficits are often not a simple function of the degree of hearing loss, implying central changes. Second, thresholds of neurons in the VCN of middle-aged C57 mice are more severely affected by peripheral impairment than those in the DCN. Likewise, different types of neurons (e.g., bushy and multipolar) are affected to different degrees by peripheral pathology. Since subdivisions (VCN and DCN) and neuron types appear to have different functions in hearing (see above), it follows that peripheral presbycusis may affect various auditory functions in different ways. This suggests that the impact of peripheral presbycusis and CEPP on various perceptual abilities in humans (Chapters 8–10) may be complex and multi-faceted.

COMMENTS ON HISTOPATHO-LOGICAL VERSUS PHYSIOLOGICAL CORRELATES OF AGING AND PERIPHERAL PATHOLOGY

It is apparent that the anatomical and physiological data paint rather different pictures of age-related change in the C57 and CBA mouse CAS. The histopathological changes observed in these strains are most closely correlated with old age and are not always affected by peripheral pathology. By comparison, physiological responses at the cellular level are decidedly altered by peripheral impairment (middle-aged C57 mice) but less so by biological aging (old CBA mice). If these observations can be extrapolated to humans, two cautionary notes are raised. On the one hand, some age-related central histopathology (as in old CBA mice) can occur without drastic effects on the responses of many CAS neurons; *a moderate degree of CAS histopathology may not necessarily cause perceptual difficulties.* Thus, the assumption that central presbycusis results from histopathological changes in brain cells may not always be valid. On the other hand, distortion of the incoming neural information by sensorineural impairment (as in aging C57 mice) can cause substantial problems in CAS neural coding even though the histological circuitry remains largely intact; *the central physiological ramifications of sensorineural impairment should not be underestimated.* The concept of CEPP may be extremely important in understanding central presbycusis.

THE CAS AND OTHER AGE-RELATED PATHOLOGY

Luxon (1981) reviewed the types of pathology that may affect the CAS, and often accompany aging. Chronic disorders that can affect the CAS include arteriosclerosis, anoxia, and metabolic dysfunction of kidney or liver. To the extent that chronic disorders are more likely to be manifested in older individuals, such disorders may contribute to central presbycusis.

Fisch (1970) argued that the CAS is particularly vulnerable to insults, such as anoxia or drug toxicity. Because the CAS is a relatively recent phylogenetic development and is functionally complex and active, the CAS metabolic requirements are unusually high, as indicated by its high degree of vascularity. Differences in vascularity and microcirculation among individuals, known to occur, might also lead to differences in the vulnerability of the CAS, accounting for some individual differences in hearing loss. Fisch's vulnerability hypothesis could be extended to the challenges that aging presents to the brain, implying that the CAS would be particularly vulnerable to age-related pathology.

Hansen (1968) assessed the relationship between blood pressure and audiograms in subjects over 45 years. He found no correlation between blood pressure and hearing loss, but did find that patients with hearing loss were more likely to have diffuse brain degeneration, suggesting a link between high blood pressure and central presbycusis. Uziel and colleagues (1983) observed a higher incidence of brainstem-evoked response abnormalities (e.g., prolonged interpeak latencies) in elderly patients with vascular disorders than in those without vascular disorders. It is interesting to speculate that some of the findings relating arteriosclerosis to presbycusis (Chapter 5) may have reflected a central effect on hearing.

The influences of nonauditory, age-related complications on the aging CAS are not well understood, but may be important. This is another area deserving of more research attention.

INDEPENDENT SUBSYSTEMS FOR SPEECH AND NON-SPEECH MATERIAL

Liberman (1970; 1989) has argued for many years that speech is processed in a a specialized subsystem that is partially independent from other auditory pathways. Suga (1990) has suggested that these pathways are differentiated at subcortical levels, most notably at the level of the medial geniculate body of the thalamus. He proposed that a "ventral system," involving the ventral portion of the MGB and the primary auditory cortex (AI), processes sounds that are unfamiliar or have limited biological (species specific) significance. A "dorsal system," involving the dorsal division of the MGB and non-primary auditory cortex, are specialized for species specific sounds such as speech in humans.

If Liberman's hypothesis is correct, it is feasible that age-related changes in the subsystems may differ, with important perceptual consequences. The work reviewed earlier, suggesting that CAS subdivisions are differentially vulnerable to peripheral pathology and biological aging, is of interest in this regard. The implications of the theories of Liberman might provide fresh insights into mechanisms of central presbycusis.

CONCLUDING REMARKS

When all of the human and animal data are considered, it is evident that the central auditory system undergoes some age-related changes that have the potential to deleteriously affect the perception of sound. On the other hand, some anatomical and physiological features fare rather well with age. It has been emphasized that the functional significance of these occurrences remains unclear because detailed evaluations of hearing/perception have typically not been obtained before the death of the subjects (human or otherwise). Even when data are available, only correlations—not cause and effect relationships—can be established. Nevertheless, there is a great deal of information on auditory brainstem function and auditory perception of speech and other sounds by aging humans, reviewed in the following three chapters. In addressing these issues, the reader is urged to give speculative consideration to how the findings reviewed in this chapter—and the concepts of CEBA and CEPP— might be related to the auditory performance in the elderly.

For instance, when age-related peripheral pathology has occurred in middle-aged C57 mice, neurons located in the ventral region of the inferior colliculus can no longer respond to high frequencies as they normally would. However, they now respond more robustly to middle- and low-frequency sounds (see above). In other words, the amount of central neural tissue responding to middle and low frequencies increases as the amount of tissue responding to high frequencies decreases. One would predict that this condition could result in increased behavioral responsiveness to low or middle frequencies. Thus, recent findings on humans by Hellbruck (1988) are of interest. Hellbruck used a category scale to measure the loudness of narrowband noises centered at frequencies from 125 to 8000 Hz in young and old listeners. High frequency losses were found. However, *hypersensitivity* was also observed at middle frequencies and was correlated with high-frequency loss. This outcome can be predicted by the physiological data from mice.

One final note: Research is reviewed in the remaining chapters in which tests of "central auditory function" are employed. It should be noted that these tests cannot discriminate between central disorders resulting from CEPP or CEBA. Because even those older individuals with "normal hearing" exhibit some degree of peripheral pathology (often in excess of what is revealed by the pure tone audiogram), it is virtually impossible to rule out CEPP in most cases. We shall return to this issue in Chapter 10.

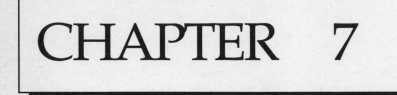

CHAPTER 7

The Acoustic Reflex, Evoked Responses, and Otoacoustic Emissions

This chapter deals with phenomena that have important research and clinical applications—the acoustic reflex and evoked electrophysiological responses including the auditory brainstem response (ABR), middle latency response (MLR), and cortical responses, and otoacoustic emissions (OAEs).

THE ACOUSTIC REFLEX

The acoustic reflex is a response of middle ear muscles (particularly the stapedius muscle) and ossicles to intense sound. It is revealed by measurements of middle ear immittance similar to those described for static middle ear properties in Chapter 2. The acoustic reflex has two modes, crossed and uncrossed, depending on whether the acoustic stimulus is presented to the contralateral or ipsilateral ear, respectively. The two modes undoubtedly involve different, albeit partially overlapping, central circuits.

The acoustic reflex can be measured routinely in the clinic and has become a powerful diagnostic and research tool. Two parameters that are readily measured are amplitude and threshold, which is typically expressed with respect to either absolute intensity levels (SPL or HL) or audiometric sensation level (SL).

RESEARCH CONSIDERATIONS

The acoustic reflex is affected by middle ear disorders (in which detection of the reflex may be squelched), and by cochlear and retrocochlear pathology (see recent review by Stach, 1987). For instance, Anderson, Barr, and Wedenberg (1969) initially showed that in patients with retrocochlear tumors the crossed reflex is elicited at elevated SLs, whereas in patients with cochlear pathology it is elicited at SLs lower than normal.

The diagnostic sensitivity of the acoustic reflex indicates that this measure may be useful in evaluating age-related changes in both the peripheral and central auditory system. However, one important caveat should be mentioned: the acoustic reflex has both sensory and motor components. The motor component (brainstem motor nuclei, neuromuscular synapses,

middle ear muscles, ossicular chain) might be affected by age-related factors altering properties of the reflex, particularly the amplitude. Therefore, caution must be exercised in concluding that the locus of age-related change lies within the auditory system.

ACOUSTIC REFLEX THRESHOLD RE: DB SPL OR HL

An early report by Jepsen (1963) measured the acoustic reflex threshold (ART) in subjects having normal hearing for their age. For tone frequencies through 4000 Hz, no age-related changes were seen relative to dB SPL. More recently, Thompson, Sills, Recke, and Bui (1980) also observed no significant age-related change in the ART (500-2000 Hz tones). Their subjects were females with air conduction thresholds of 20 dB HL or better from 250 to 4000 Hz. Osterhammel and Osterhammel (1979a) found no age difference for the ART (re: dB HL) except at 4000 Hz, where an age-related increase was seen (Fig. 7-1). In a study by Jerger, Jerger, and Mauldin (1972), thresholds at 500, 1000, and 2000 Hz decreased slightly in older, normal-hearing subjects (Fig. 7-2, continuous lines). Their finding of a precipitous decrease in thresholds in septuagenarians at 4000 Hz differed from the age-related increase observed by Osterhammel and Osterhammel (1979a).

Jerger and colleagues (1972) also tested subjects with sensorineural hearing loss [1]. ARTs for high frequencies were greater than those of normal-hearing subjects for all age groups, but there was no systematic age effect (Fig. 7-2, broken lines), and ARTs were within normal clinical limits.

The ART in response to broadband noise (BBN) shows a different age-related pattern than tone-evoked ARTs. Silman and Gelfand (1981) observed *elevation* of reflex thresholds for broadband noise but not for tones (500–2000 Hz) in normal-hearing older subjects relative to previous data on young subjects. Earlier, Silman (1979) reported ART thresholds for tones of 500, 1000, and 2000 Hz and for broadband noise in young and old (60 to 76 years) normal-hearing adults. No significant age effects were detected for tones, but noise thresholds increased by about 10 dB. Gelfand and Piper (1981) repeated this study but chose their subjects such that hearing levels were more similar across age; they

---

[1] In most of the literature to be reviewed in this chapter, "sensorineural" hearing loss or impairment is used in the general sense of cochlear and peripheral neural involvement, irrespective of age or etiology. The precise nature of the pathology underlying sensorineural hearing loss or its cause are often not known and could involve sensory and/or neural tissue. Thus, "sensorineural impairment" or "sensorineural hearing loss" in elderly listeners is not necessarily synonymous with "sensorineural presbycusis," as defined in Chapter 3, which specifically refers to hearing loss associated with age-related pathology of both the organ of Corti and spiral ganglion cells.

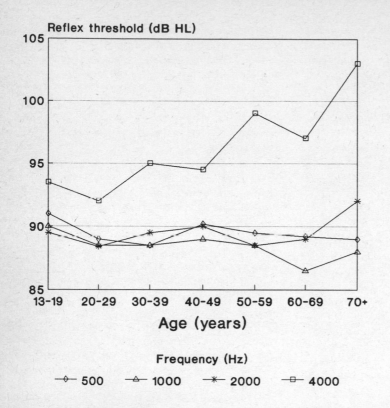

Figure 7-1. Acoustic reflex thresholds re: HL at 4 frequencies (adapted from Osterhammel and Osterhammel, 1979a). Subjects had normal hearing for their age.

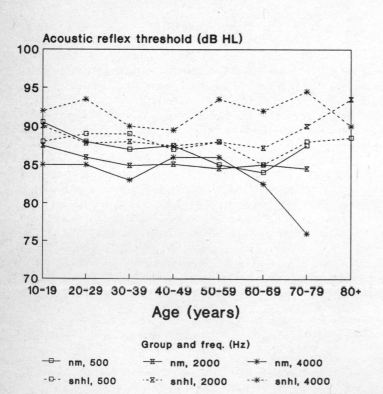

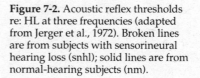

Figure 7-2. Acoustic reflex thresholds re: HL at three frequencies (adapted from Jerger et al., 1972). Broken lines are from subjects with sensorineural hearing loss (snhl); solid lines are from normal-hearing subjects (nm).

also included thresholds to 8000 Hz in meeting their criteria for normal hearing. As seen in Figure 7-3, ARTs for 500, 1000, and 2000 Hz were similar between age groups, while the ART for broad band noise (BBN) was elevated in the older group. Silverman, Silman, and Miller (1983) also found that the ART for BBN was elevated in normal-hearing older subjects, but tone-evoked ARTs (500 to 4000 Hz) were not affected. Earlier, Handler and Margolis (1977) had obtained similar results for tones. Wilson (1981) determined that ARTs of persons over 50 were elevated for high-frequency tones (4000 and 6000 Hz) and wide-band noise, but not for low-frequency tones (250-2000 Hz), compared to ARTs of subjects younger than 30. The difference between tone and noise ARTs was also reduced in the older subjects.

Somewhat different results were reported by Jerger, Hayes, Anthony, and Mauldin (1978). Their data indicated a gradual reduction in ART between 20 and 59 years with tone stimuli but no change with noise (although the normal difference between tone and noise ARTs, about 20 dB, was diminished).

Margolis et al. (1981) speculated that the reason Jerger and colleagues did not find an increase in the noise ART may have been methodological. Their findings were derived from clinical data, and ARTs for noise were unusually high in the young subjects. This may have minimized age differences. Another methodological difference may be that Jerger and colleagues used stimulus intensity steps of 5 dB, compared to 1 dB steps in other studies. The poorer resolution of the 5 dB steps may have obscured age-related changes in noise ARTs (Silverman, Silman, and Miller, 1983). In any event, the consensus favors the conclusion that noise-evoked ARTs are elevated with age, but tone-evoked ARTs are minimally affected.

A recent study by Jakimetz, Silman, Miller, and Silverman (1989) obtained ARTs for multi-component tonal complexes of varying bandwidth and spectral density in young and old (60- to 71-year-old) normal-hearing subjects. ARTs decreased as spectral density (number of tonal components) increased. However, a plateau was reached with seven components in the young listeners compared to five for older listeners

Figure 7-3. Acoustic reflex thresholds and absolute audiometric thresholds in young and old subjects (adapted from Gelfand and Piper, 1981). ARTs (in dB SPL) for young and old subjects (tones and broadband noise) are solid lines; audiometric thresholds (dB HL) for tones are broken lines.

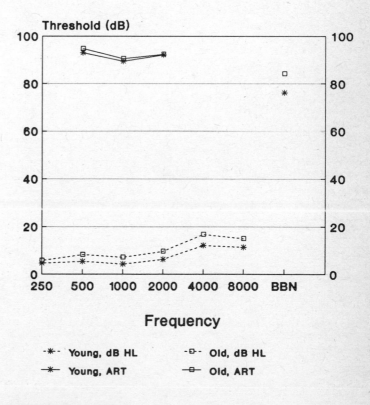

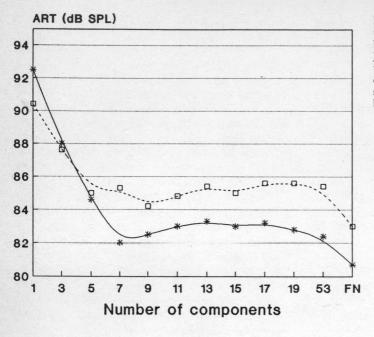

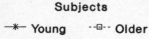

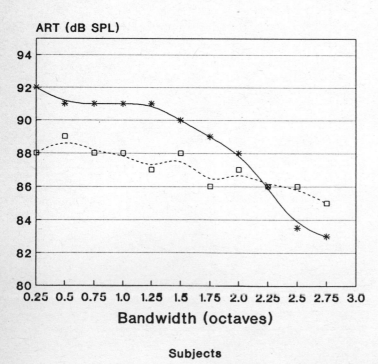

Figure 7-4. Relationship of acoustic reflex threshold (dB SPL) to spectral density and bandwidth of stimuli (adapted from Jakimetz et al., 1989). Upper panel: ART versus the number of components in multi-component stimuli in young and old subjects; lower panel: ART versus the bandwidth in octaves.

(Fig. 7-4 upper panel). Furthermore, the plateau was reached at a higher SPL in the older subjects. The "band width effect" was reduced in the older listeners, as indicated by plotting the ART as a function of band width (Fig. 7-4 lower panel). This study suggests that the elevated broadband ARTs characteristic of elderly listeners is related to this reduced band width effect.

THE ART RELATIVE TO SENSATION LEVEL

Although Jepsen (1963) found no age-related change in the ART with respect to SPL, a decrease did occur relative to SL. A number of subsequent studies have confirmed this observation.

Silman's (1979) older subject group had elevated sensory thresholds ranging from 6 dB at 500 Hz to 10 dB at 4,000 Hz. Comparing sensory thresholds and ARTs for tones, it appears that tone ARTs decreased relative to SL, but were unchanged relative to HL. The same conclusion can be made from inspection of Fig-

ure 7-3 (Gelfand and Piper, 1981) because hearing levels become elevated more than SRTs across age.

Osterhammel and Osterhammel (1979a) discerned a decrease in ART for tones with age (3.5 dB per decade) as a function of SL (Fig. 7-5), having found no age difference as a function of HL except for 4000 Hz (Fig. 7-1). Otto and McCandless (1982b) found evidence of a reduced range between absolute sensory thresholds and ARTs in 80 percent of their subjects with presbycusis. Finally, Habener and Snyder (1974) measured acoustic reflex thresholds in normal-hearing subjects and found an age-related decrease in threshold relative to sensation level in their oldest subjects (Fig. 7-6). The decreases in reflex thresholds were most pronounced for higher frequencies.

In the study of Jerger and colleagues (1972) little age-related change occurred in the ART of subjects with sensorineural hearing loss when threshold was expressed in dB with respect to audiometric zero (HL) (Fig. 7-2). However, absolute sensory thresholds of these subjects (not shown) increased with age, so that ART decreased with respect to sensation level.

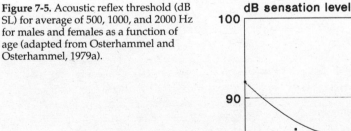

Figure 7-5. Acoustic reflex threshold (dB SL) for average of 500, 1000, and 2000 Hz for males and females as a function of age (adapted from Osterhammel and Osterhammel, 1979a).

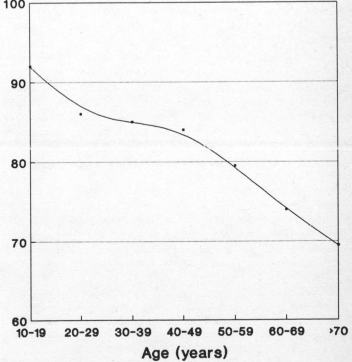

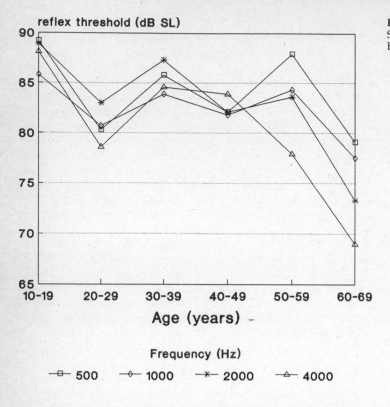

Figure 7-6. Acoustic reflex threshold (dB SL) at 4 frequencies (adapted from Habener and Snyder, 1974).

SUMMARY

For *normal-hearing subjects* there is general agreement that ARTs for frequencies of 2000 Hz and below show either no change with age or a small age-related decrease when expressed as dB SPL or HL. For 4000 Hz stimuli, the data conflict, with increases, decreases, or no change being reported (this may simply be an aspect of the general difficulty in eliciting reliable acoustic reflexes with high-frequency sounds). There is also general agreement that broadband noise requires higher SPLs with increasing age and that the normal difference in ARTs for tones versus noise is diminished. ARTs tend to remain within clinically normal limits if presbycusis is minimal.

The trends relating ART and age were exemplified by Margolis, Popelka, Handler, and Himelfarb (1981), who computed best fit functions for ARTs (dB SPL) in response to tones and noise in children and adults through the seventh decade of life. The difference between ARTs for the three lower frequencies versus the noise decreased from about 20 dB in the youngest

subjects to about 10 dB in the oldest subjects (Fig. 7-7). This was a function of a slight decrease in tone ARTs for 500, 1000, and 2000 Hz, a flat function for 4 kHz, and a slight increase for wide-band noise.

The changes in ART that do accompany aging, in particular the elevation of broadband noise ART and lowering of ART with respect to SL, imply an influence of peripheral hearing loss because similar effects occur in young listeners with sensorineural loss (see Silman, 1979 for references). Such changes may be found in "normal hearing" older listeners because they typically have some degree of hearing loss compared to young listeners, albeit not sufficient to affect tone ARTs.

A role of hearing loss in altering the ARTs of older listeners for tones versus noise is further supported by the Handler and Margolis (1977) study. They determined the ART in response to tones versus several types of noise. The ART increased with age for 4 kHz tones, but not for lower-frequency tones where threshold elevations are smaller. Furthermore, the ART for a lowpass noise did not differ between age groups but older subjects had increased ARTs for

Figure 7-7. Best fit functions for age versus acoustic reflex threshold (dB SPL) for 4 tone frequencies and wideband noise (adapted from Margolis et al., 1981).

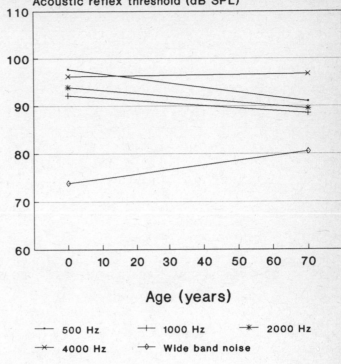

Best fit functions (y= ax+b)

broadband noise and a highpass noise. Thus, stimuli with high-frequency components (for which peripheral presbycusis is typically most severe) are associated with elevated ARTs. Indeed, when sensorineural hearing loss is clinically significant, ARTs for tones may be somewhat elevated particularly at high frequencies (Jerger et al., 1972, Fig. 7-2; Silman and Gelfand, 1981).

AMPLITUDE OF THE ACOUSTIC REFLEX

A number of studies have shown that the amplitude of the acoustic reflex and its rate of growth as a function of stimulus intensity decrease with age. Because sensorineural impairment may reduce reflex growth (Peterson and Liden, 1972; Beedle and Harford, 1973) particular care must be used in interpreting the

role of biological aging versus peripheral presbycusis in these findings.

Habener and Snyder (1974) measured acoustic reflex amplitudes in normal-hearing subjects. After reaching a developmental peak in the 20- to 29-year-old group, amplitudes evoked by stimuli with intensities 10 dB above the ART declined with age (Fig. 7-8). Wilson (1981) found smaller reflex amplitudes and a decrease in the the rate of reflex growth in older subjects. This occurred when stimulus level was expressed as SPL or relative to reflex threshold. Thompson, Sills, Recke, and Bui (1980) (Fig. 7-9) also observed an age-related reduction in the growth of the acoustic reflex despite the absence of a change in ART.

The magnitude of age-related changes in the acoustic reflex also depends upon the reflex mode, with respect to the *crossed versus uncrossed reflex*. Gersdorff (1978) reported decreased ipsilateral and contralateral tone-evoked reflex amplitudes and increased recovery

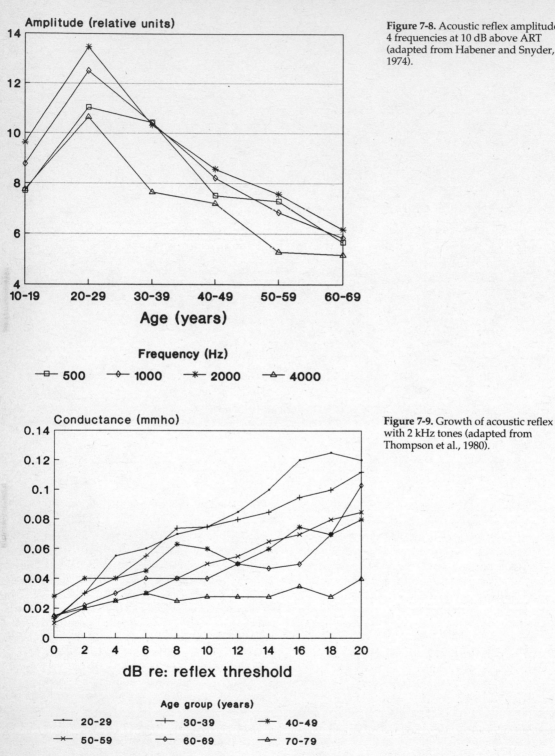

Figure 7-8. Acoustic reflex amplitude for 4 frequencies at 10 dB above ART (adapted from Habener and Snyder, 1974).

Figure 7-9. Growth of acoustic reflex with 2 kHz tones (adapted from Thompson et al., 1980).

2000 Hz (similar results were also obtained with 500 Hz, 1000 Hz, and noise)

Figure 7-10. Acoustic reflex amplitude at 1 kHz (crossed and uncrossed)(adapted from Gersdorff, 1978).

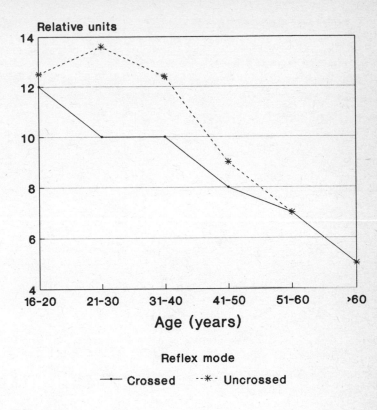

1 kHz tones

times as a function of age in normal-hearing subjects. However, the uncrossed reflex amplitudes showed a greater relative decline (Fig. 7-10). In young subjects, the uncrossed reflexes had larger amplitudes than crossed reflexes. With age, the more pronounced decline of the uncrossed amplitudes resulted in similar amplitudes for both reflex modes.

Hall (1982a) controlled for a number of possible factors that might have influenced the findings of Gersdorff (1978), including hearing sensitivity, ear canal volume, static compliance, and minor middle ear dysfunction. In three age groups matched for these variables, the uncrossed reflex amplitude decreased by 56 percent between 20 and 80 years, and amplitude growth was reduced (Fig. 7-11). The age-related decline was less pronounced for the crossed reflex. (In addition, there was a pronounced sex difference in the old group; amplitude growth was greater in females.)

Decreased acoustic reflex amplitudes for 1000 Hz tones were observed by Jerger and Oliver (1987) in older subjects. In addition, the uncrossed reflex amplitude decreased more than the crossed reflex in older

subjects. Their hypothesis to explain these findings is discussed later.

The significance of reflex mode was also implicated by Quaranta, Cassano, and Amoroso (1980). They used 1,000 and 2,000 Hz tones to measure the acoustic reflex in subjects aged 60 to 90 years and diagnosed as having presbycusis. Abnormal differences in crossed versus uncrossed reflex thresholds occurred in a number of these subjects (although the direction of those differences was not clearly stated).

THE EFFECT OF SENSORINEURAL HEARING LOSS ON REFLEX AMPLITUDE IN ELDERLY PEOPLE

Silman and Gelfand (1981) evaluated the effect of sensorineural hearing loss on the growth of crossed reflex amplitudes of 61- to 76-year-old listeners. For tone stimuli, when intensity was expressed relative to ART, growth functions for both normal-hearing and impaired older subjects were reduced compared to those of young normal-hearing subjects (Fig. 7-12,

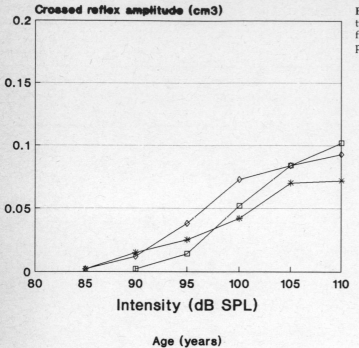

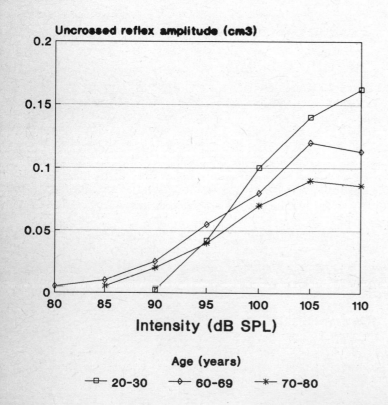

Figure 7-11. Growth of acoustic reflex amplitude at 1 kHz (crossed and uncrossed)(adapted from Hall, 1982a). Upper panel: crossed; lower panel: uncrossed.

Figure 7-12. Growth of acoustic reflex re: ART for 2 kHz tones and broadband noise (adapted from Silman and Gelfand, 1981; Silman et al., 1978).

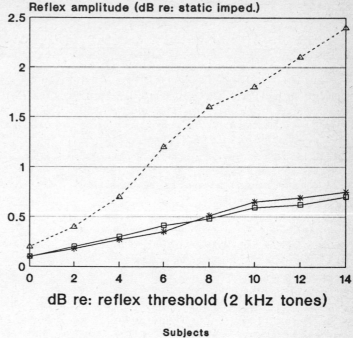

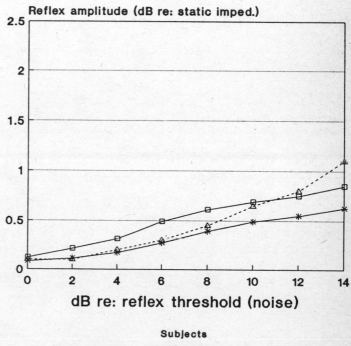

upper panel). In contrast, with noise stimuli there was little difference in growth functions as a function of age (Fig. 7-12, lower panel). Comparing the two groups of older subjects, those with sensorineural hearing loss exhibited reduced amplitudes for broadband noise and a slightly steeper growth functions that was not statistically significant. The growth functions for 500 Hz (not shown) are similar to those for noise in that amplitudes were reduced in the subjects with hearing loss, whereas for 1000 Hz tones, the relationship between amplitudes was intermediate between noise and 2000 Hz tones. Slopes of tonal growth functions did not differ between normal-hearing and hearing-impaired older subjects.

When reflex growth was expressed relative to dB SPL (Fig. 7-13), growth functions of older subjects with hearing loss (broken lines) were shifted to the right of the curves of normal-hearing elderly subjects (solid lines), reflecting an elevation of ARTs. The slopes of the growth functions of the two groups were similar for 500 Hz tones, rising monotonically with increasing SPL. However, slopes of the functions for broadband noise and 1000 and 2000 Hz tones "saturated" at high intensities in normal-hearing, old subjects, an effect that had not been seen in the earlier work on young subjects.

Hall (1982b) investigated the relationship between reflex amplitude in older subjects as a function of age-related middle ear dysfunction and sensorineural hearing loss. Minor middle ear dysfunction (as revealed by impedance abnormality) was associated with marked reduction in acoustic reflex amplitude and "flattening" of the amplitude-intensity function in older subjects, despite the fact that hearing thresholds were equivalent, no air-bone gaps were observed, and acoustic reflex thresholds differed little. Hall speculated that the differences were related to changes in the mechanical efficiency of the ossicular chain related to middle ear muscle function. He noted the clinical implications, should undetected minor middle ear dysfunctions have significant effects on the acoustic reflex. For instance, central dysfunction, which has similar effects on the acoustic reflex, might be mistakenly diagnosed.

While Hall's (1982b) study revealed that reflex amplitude for noise decreased in older subjects when sensorineural impairment was present (Fig. 7-14), this was not the case for 4kHz stimuli (not shown). A different pattern was observed with young subjects. Reflex amplitudes for noise did not differ between sensorineural and normal-hearing subjects, but the uncrossed reflex amplitude for 4 kHz was reduced in

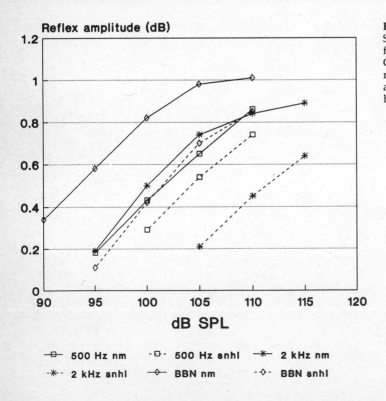

Figure 7-13. Growth of acoustic reflex re: SPL for broadband noise and 2-tone frequencies (adapted from Silman and Gelfand, 1981). Solid lines are from normal-hearing subjects (nm); dotted lines are from subjects with sensorineural hearing loss (snhl).

Figure 7-14. Growth of acoustic reflex amplitude (crossed and uncrossed) in older subjects re: hearing impairment (adapted from Hall, 1982b). Solid lines are uncrossed reflex; dotted lines are crossed reflex.

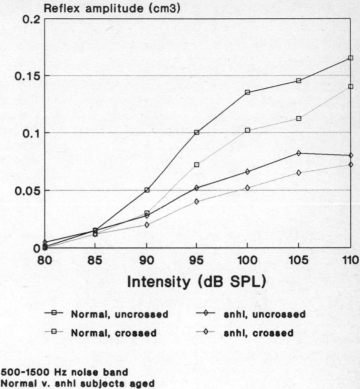

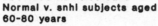

500-1500 Hz noise band
Normal v. snhl subjects aged
60-80 years

young, sensorineural patients. One possible explanation for this finding, suggested by Hall, is that older subjects have greater neural loss in the auditory system, and that noise band stimuli tax this impaired system. If this view were correct, comparison of the acoustic reflex amplitude in response to higher-frequency tones versus noise may have value in assessing neural presbycusis.

AGING AND OTHER REFLEX PARAMETERS

Jerger and Oliver (1987) measured the *offset latency* of the crossed and uncrossed acoustic reflex in young and old subjects. In old subjects, the offset latencies were prolonged relative to those of young subjects. This effect was more pronounced for the crossed reflex, especially at shorter ISIs. As seen in Figure 7-15, the crossed reflex offset latencies for young and old subjects (dot symbols) diverged at smaller ISIs, but the offset latencies for the uncrossed reflex (asterisks) did so to a much lesser degree.

Reflex decay in response to sustained, lower-frequency stimuli is exaggerated in non-elderly listeners if auditory nerve or lower brainstem neural pathology is present (Jerger, 1980). Thus, tests of reflex decay could provide an indication of age-related auditory nerve or central dysfunction. Despite this potential, little work appears to have been done on reflex decay in elderly listeners. Habener and Snyder (1974) found no evidence for age-related change in reflex decay as indicated by the "half-life time" and slope (rate of decay) through the seventh decade in normal hearing subjects (thresholds from 250–8000 Hz $\leq$ 25 dB HL). In this one study, then, reflex decay provided no evidence for lower auditory brainstem disorders.

SUMMARY

Ample evidence has been cited to show that acoustic reflex amplitude and its growth are diminished with aging and that the diminution is more pronounced for the uncrossed reflex. Possible causes of reduced amplitudes are impairment of the motor side of the

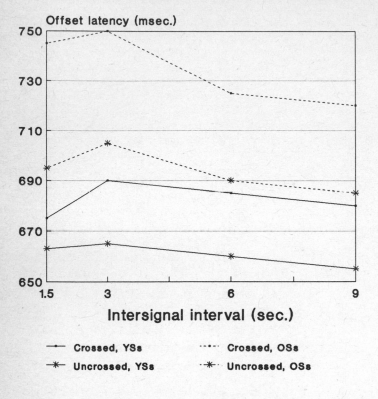

Figure 7-15. Acoustic reflex offset latency (crossed and uncrossed) re: intersignal interval (adapted from Jerger and Oliver, 1987).

reflex due to weakening of the stapedius muscle response (Hall, 1982b; Quaranta et al., 1980; Thompson et al., 1980; Wilson, 1981) and/or dysfunction of the neural circuitry that mediates the reflex (Hall, 1980b; Wilson, 1981). Alternately, retrocochlear pathology, which is known to diminish reflex amplitudes, could explain the findings. The explanations, of course are not mutually exclusive.

Jerger and Oliver (1987) provided an interesting possibility to explain the differences between crossed and uncrossed reflexes. They suggested that the smaller amplitudes in crossed reflexes are due to central inhibitory processes that are more potent than in the shorter, uncrossed neural circuit. They further suggested that aging may be associated with a weakening of central inhibitory mechanisms (a suggestion that has empirical support in the animal literature, discussed in Chapter 6). If this were the case, two opposing influences on reflex amplitude could accompany aging: a decrease in amplitude of both crossed and uncrossed reflexes (perhaps acting at or near the auditory periphery) and an enhancement of the crossed reflex due to reduced central inhibition. This would account for the relatively greater age-related reduction in the amplitude of the uncrossed reflex.

Jerger and Oliver (1987) also addressed the possibility that hearing loss, rather than aging, caused the reduction in reflex amplitudes in the elderly subjects. They rejected an important role of hearing loss on two grounds. First, the fact that crossed and uncrossed reflexes were affected differently suggests that some central factor was operating. Second, they cited other studies showing that the degree of hearing loss present in their older subjects would not be expected to affect reflex amplitude for the 1000 Hz tones they used.

These arguments may very well be valid, but it is difficult to rule out a possible role of peripheral impairment. With regard to their first point, it is possible that peripheral presbycusis would not have identical effects on crossed and uncrossed reflexes, since they involve different central pathways. Sensorineural hearing loss can affect central pathways differently (Chapter 6). With regard to their second point, the audiogram may not adequately reveal peripheral neural loss in the elderly (Chapter 3) and may underestimate peripheral neural pathology. Peripheral sensorineural pathology might result in reduced synaptic driving of the central inhibitory system suggested by Jerger and Oliver, having the same result as a loss neurons in the central circuit. Alternatively, the crossed reflex pathway may be more convergent or redundant than the uncrossed pathway (i.e., central neurons receive converging input from pathways involving a number of spiral ganglion cells). If this were the case, a degree of ganglion cell loss could be better tolerated by the crossed reflex circuitry. Surviving, redundant ganglion cells could still activate the circuit, so that age-related reflex decline would be reduced.

The difficulty in ruling out a role of peripheral neural pathology underscores the importance of considering the potential of central effects of peripheral presbycusis (CEPP), discussed in Chapter 6. Even though the differences between crossed and uncrossed reflexes are mediated centrally, the ultimate cause of the central dysfunction might be peripheral.

THE AUDITORY BRAINSTEM RESPONSE

The auditory brainstem response (ABR) reflects short latency (<10 msec.) synchronous neural activity evoked by brief, rapidly presented acoustic stimuli. Four or five major waves can typically be identified in the ABR, with wave I arising from the eighth nerve and wave V from the midbrain. As a noninvasive, commonly used clinical tool, the ABR provides our richest source of electrophysiological data on the human auditory brainstem, with the potential to gain insights into CEPP and CEBA, the central effects of peripheral presbycusis and biological aging (Chapter 6).

RESEARCH CONSIDERATIONS

Published work on the ABR in older human subjects is summarized in Table 7-1. There are several aspects of this body of literature that tend to limit interpretation of findings.

Data are often limited to the latency or amplitude of wave V. Without the benefit of data on earlier waves, it is impossible to determine if age-related changes in wave V are associated with other central changes (in which case waveform anomalies or differences in interpeak latencies may result) or peripheral changes (in which case latencies of all waves may be altered).

Other interpretive difficulties arise due to the potential effects of auditory system pathology (irrespective of age) and inconsistencies in these effects. For instance, cochlear pathology (irrespective of age) can cause changes in the ABR, such as increased latencies

(Attias and Pratt, 1984; Fialkowska et al., 1983; Jerger and Johnson, 1988; Mitchell, Phillips, and Trune, 1989); however, normal latencies have been found in patients with permanent noise-induced hearing loss (Almadori et al., 1988). The interpeak latency (time elapsed between waves) has been found to be *unaffected* by cochlear pathology (Attias and Pratt, 1984), *reduced* (Coats and Martin, 1977; Sturzebecher et al., 1985), or *prolonged* (Sturzebecher et al., 1985). Retrocochlear pathology is typically accompanied by large interaural wave V latency differences (prolonged on the pathological side), increased wave V latency, or absence/abnormality of waves (Clemis and McGee, 1979). However, false diagnoses of retrocochlear pathology can be made on these bases, as well (Bauch, Rose, and Harner, 1982).

It is also the case that systemic problems, such as reduced cerebrovascular circulation, may result in prolonged latencies of wave V (Mills and Ryals, 1985).

Difficulties also arise in interpreting the *underlying cause* of latency and amplitude changes. (a) The absolute latency may increase in subjects with high-frequency impairment because the basal cochlea normally responds with the shortest latencies, and sensorineural damage would remove this short-latency response. Alternatively, undetected changes in the difference between the intensity used to evoke an ABR versus absolute sensory threshold might affect latency. It is also conceivable that age-related deficiencies in peripheral transductive or synaptic processes could affect the latency of auditory nerve responses. (b) The interpeak latency is generally taken as a sign of central conduction speed (e.g., the speed of synaptic transmission and axonal action potentials). However, changes in neural recovery processes and/or synchrony of neural responses might alter the shape of waves, including the wave peak used to identify latency. Another possibility is that changes in central circuitry (e.g. selective attenuation of faster circuit components with fewer synapses) might contribute as well. (c) Amplitude is potentially a function of the number of neural units activated, the synchrony of their activation by brief sounds, and the magnitude of the individual bioelectrical events that are summed to produce the ABR wave. Changes in any or all of these factors might affect ABR amplitudes.

It is probably impossible to determine the underlying causes of age-related changes in ABR latencies and amplitudes, and caution is advised in doing so. Perhaps the best we can do is to conclude that "something has changed" in the auditory brainstem and generate reasonable hypotheses about the meaning of the changes.

EFFECTS OF AGING ON ABR LATENCY

Most studies obtaining ABR latency measures have concluded that *absolute latencies*—at least for wave V—increase with aging (Table 7-1). A study by Chu (1985), summarized in Figure 7-16, is typical. Modest trends toward increased latencies of waves I,III, and V are seen, with the increase in wave V being most strongly correlated with age. However, in some studies showing increased latencies (Table 7-1), the increases were only "trends" and not always statistically significant, and data were not always obtained from older subjects whose hearing was shown to be normal. Thus, it is important to note that some studies have found no evidence for increased latencies in older subjects with good hearing (Table 7-1). For instance, as shown in Figure 7-17, Beagley and Sheldrake (1978) observed no

TABLE 7-1. STUDIES OF AGING AND THE AUDITORY BRAINSTEM RESPONSE IN HUMANS

Findings from older subjects

Reference	Latency	Interpeak latency	Amplitude	Hearing loss
Fujikawa & Weber '77	V:+			normal for age (Fig. 7-25)
Beagley & Sheldrake '78 *	all:n	n	V:-	normal (Figs. 7-17)
Thomsen et al. '78 *	V:n (+ trend)			normal ear of neuroma patients
Rowe '78	all:+	I-III:+ III-V:n		click thresholds elevated by 8 dB (Figs. 7-18,27)
von Wedel '79	IV:+		IV:-	normal for age
Jerger & Hall '80 *	V:+		V:-	normal & impaired (Fig. 7-20,26)
Kjaer '80*	I:-	I-III,IV, V:+ (men)	all:-	some hearing loss
Rosenhammer et al. '80 *	I,III,V:+ (females)	some:+		hearing loss
Shanon et al. '81		I-IV:+		unspecified (Fig. 7-25)
Harkins '81	all:+	n	all:-	normal range
Patterson et al. '81 *	some:+	I-III:+		normal at 2kHz and below
Maurizi et al. '82	V:+	I-IV:+		range of hearing loss (Figs. 7-21)
Otto & McCandless '82b	all:+	n		normal & impaired (Figs. 7-19,29)
Allison et al. '83 *	all:+	some:+		normal for age
Uziel et al. '83		I-V:+ trend		

significant age effects on latency of any waves with subjects as old as 70 to 80 years.

An age-related increase in *interpeak latencies* has been found by some researchers using subjects screened for normal hearing. In the study of Chu (1985), for example, wave I-V interpeak latency increased progressively with age (Fig. 7-16). Rowe (1978) obtained ABRs from young and old subjects. The upper range of click stimulus thresholds was 8 dB higher in the old sub-jects, and stimulus intensity was referenced to the average click threshold of some *young* subjects. Thus, ABRs were obtained at lower SLs for Rowe's older subjects. With this qualification, interpeak latencies increased at several combinations of click rate and intensity (Fig. 7-18). Increased interpeak latencies in normal-hearing subjects were also reported by Allison and colleagues (1983; 1984) and Sturzebecher and Werbs (1987).

TABLE 7-1. (CONTINUED)

Findings from older subjects

Reference	Latency	Interpeak latency	Amplitude	Hearing loss
Allison et al. '84 *	all:+	some:+		normal for age
Johannsen & Lehn '84	III,IV,V:+	+ & -	n	normal range
Kelly-Ballweber & Dobie '84	V:+			young and old had hearing loss
Chu '85 *	V:+	I-III:n I-V:+		normal range (Fig. 7-16)
Rosenhall et al. '85 *	I,III,V:+	I-V:n		normal range
Rosenhall et al. '86 *	I,III, IV,V:+	some:+		hearing loss
Sturzebecher & Werbs '87 *	I,III:n; V:+ (females) III,V:+ (males)	I-V,III-V:+ (males)		normal range (Fig. 7-22)
Jerger & Johnson '88*	V:+			range of hearing loss
Psatta & Matei '88*			I-V:-	10 dB HL for clicks
Lenzi et al. '89 *	V:+;			normal range
Mitchell et al. '89*	I,III,V:+		I,III,V:-	range of hearing loss
Soucek & Mason '90	I,III,V:+		I,III,V:-	some hearing loss
Wharton & Church '90*	I,III,V:+	I-V,III-V: + trend, (females)	I:- III,V:- (females)	normal range

*Gender differences found
Note: I,II,III,IV,V, "some, or "all" indicate ABR waves;
"+" = increase in older subjects; "-" = decrease in older subjects;
"n" = no age effect.

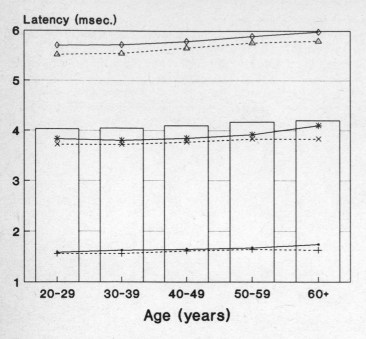

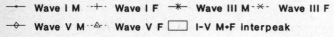

Figure 7-16. ABR latency in men and women (adapted from Chu, 1985). Solid lines are men; broken lines are women.

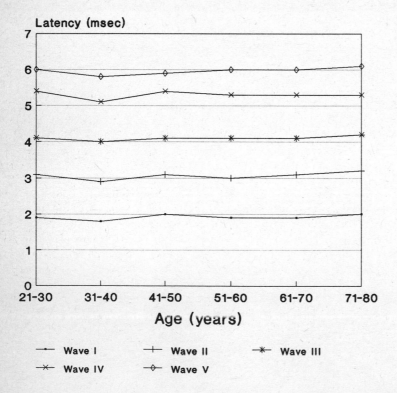

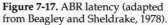

Figure 7-17. ABR latency (adapted from Beagley and Sheldrake, 1978).

80 dB clicks, 20/sec, males + females

Figure 7-18. ABR interpeak latency in young and old subjects at two click rates and SPLs (adapted from Rowe, 1978).

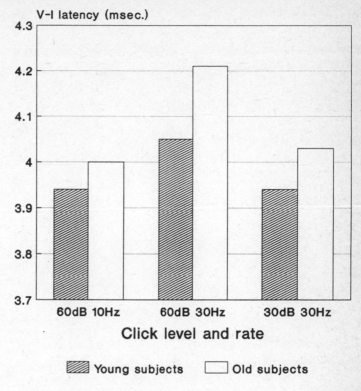

However, the relationship between age and interpeak latency is not a simple one. Patterson et al. (1981) observed increased interpeak latencies in older subjects for waves I-III at 70 and 80 dB SL, but not at 60 dB SL. The older group had significant high-frequency hearing loss (>2 kHz) compared to the younger subjects, suggesting that hearing loss and stimulus intensity may interact to determine interpeak latency.

Indeed, some researchers have found no evidence for age-related changes in interpeak latency (Table 7-1). For example, despite longer latencies for waves III and V in normal-hearing older listeners (some of whom had some high-frequency loss), there was no change in the wave I-V interval in the study by Rosenhall, Bjorkman, Pedersen, and Kall (1985). Similarly, latencies of waves I, III, and V were longer in the older men and women studied by Wharton and Church (1990), but interpeak intervals did not differ significantly.

THE INFLUENCE OF SENSORINEURAL HEARING LOSS ON ABR LATENCY IN ELDERLY PEOPLE

Otto and McCandless (1982b) matched young and old subjects for hearing loss (Fig. 7-19) and found that latency increased as a function of both age and hearing

loss. Latency of wave V increased as hearing loss became more severe but was always longer in the older subjects. The age difference decreased when hearing loss was severe, perhaps representing a ceiling effect for prolongation of latency. Rosenhall, Pedersen, and Dotevall (1986) measured ABR latencies in young and older people with sensorineural hearing loss. Older subjects tended to have longer latencies, and, except for individuals with severe loss, the I-V interpeak latency was prolonged in comparison to young subjects.

Kelly-Ballweber and Dobie (1984) compared latencies in young and old subjects whose high-frequency (4, 8 kHz) thresholds were greater than 40 dB HL. Older subjects had longer wave V latencies. Because young and old subjects were matched for hearing loss, they concluded that this variable was not responsible for the age effect. The latencies they obtained were 6.40 in older subjects and 6.01 in younger subjects. Thus, young and old subjects had longer latencies than some other studies have obtained (e.g. Fig. 7-16), presumably related to their sensorineural hearing loss. This suggests a combination of the effects of age and sensorineural hearing loss.

Male subjects aged 40 to 59 with sensorineural loss, tested by Jerger and Hall (1980), had longer wave V latencies than their normal-hearing counterparts (Fig. 7-20), although such was not the case for women. At

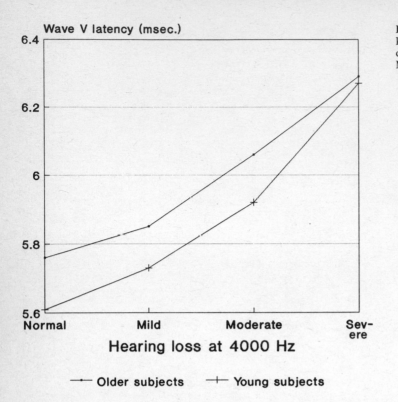

Figure 7-19. ABR wave V latency at 4 kHz in young and old subjects re: degree of hearing loss (adapted from Otto and McCandless, 1982b).

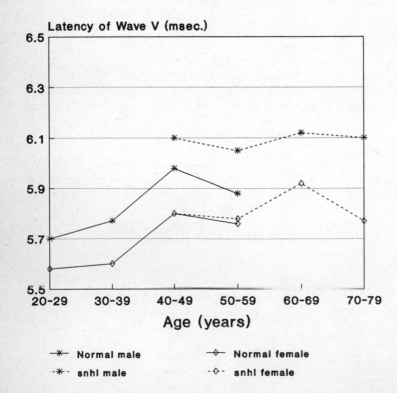

Figure 7-20. ABR wave V latency in normal-hearing and hearing-impaired men and women (adapted from Jerger and Hall, 1980). Solid lines are normal-hearing; broken lines have sensorineural hearing loss (snhl).

older ages, further increases in latency were not observed in hearing-impaired subjects of either sex, again suggesting a ceiling effect.

Maurizi and colleagues (1982) recorded ABRs from male subjects aged 60 to 86 with different degrees of hearing loss. They analyzed the data according to age or hearing loss, but not their interaction. In either case, absolute latencies (at least for later waves) and the I-V interpeak latencies were prolonged (Fig. 7-21).

In summary, sensorineural hearing loss—and by implication, peripheral presbycusis—is a potent factor in prolonging the latency of wave V in elderly

Figure 7-21. Upper panel: ABR latency as a function of age, irrespective of hearing level. Lower panel: ABR latency as a function of hearing level, irrespective of age (adapted from Maurizi et al., 1982).

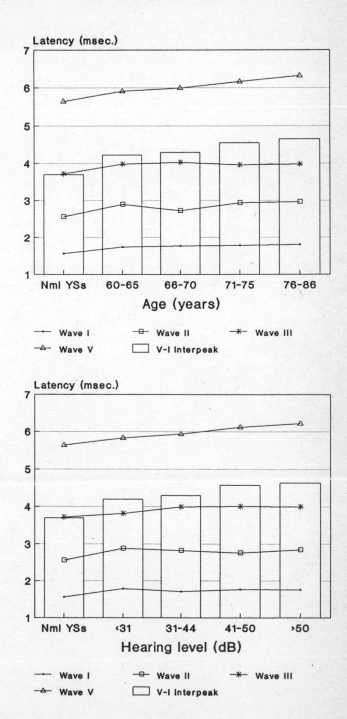

persons (especially males). However, other age-related factors may also contribute to increased latencies, since older people with sensorineural hearing loss tend to have longer latencies than like-hearing young subjects.

THE GENDER EFFECT AND ABR LATENCY

Many of the studies summarized in Table 7-1 (asterisks) have found latencies of ABR waves to be shorter in women, irrespective of age. Examples were presented earlier in Figures 7-16 (Chu, 1985) and 7-20 (Jerger and Hall, 1980), and below in Figure 7-23 (Jerger and Johnson, 1988).

Sturzebecher and Werbs (1987) computed regression lines for latency of waves I, III, and V as a function of age in men and women. As shown in Figure 7-22, slopes were steeper for males. A significant correlation with age was obtained for all three waves in males but only for wave V in females. The fact that the regression lines intersect the latency axis at similar values at age 0 led Sturzebecher and Werbs to hypothesize that the gender differences were determined postnatally as a function of greater age-related changes in males (be-

ginning at the youngest of ages). A later report with additional data (Sturzebecher and Werbs, 1988) supported their hypothesis to a degree but also concluded that age-related divergence of latency was not sufficient to account for the gender differences.

Support for an age-by-gender interaction is provided by some investigations of the ABR. The data of Rosenhall et al. (1985) indicate a greater age-related increase in males than in females for waves III and V, but not for wave I. Allison et al. (1984) computed the slopes for latency change as a function of age. Slopes were steeper for males for waves II through V. Kjaer (1980) found greater age-related increases in interpeak latencies for males. For instance, the I-V latency increased from 4.10 to 4.51 msec. in males, compared to 4.02 to 4.12 in females (20 to 29 years versus 50 to 69 years). Chu's (1985) age-latency curves for men and women diverge for waves I and III, but appear to run parallel for wave V (Fig. 7-16).

Other work provides partial support for an age-by-gender interaction, but indicates that the relationship is not simple and interacts with stimulus intensity. In the Beagley and Sheldrake (1978) study, at 60 dB SL, latencies for the genders diverged with age through the seventh decade, but by the eighth decade they merged; at 80 dB SL the curves ran parallel across age.

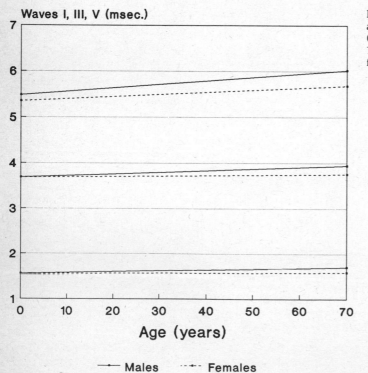

Waves I, III, V (msec.)

Age (years)

——— Males   ····· Females

Figure 7-22. Regression lines for ABR latency as a function of age in men and women (adapted from Sturzebecher and Werbs, 1987). Solid lines are males; broken lines are females.

Figure 7-23. ABR wave V latency in young and old men and women as a function of "effective click level" (adapted from Jerger and Johnson, 1988). Solid lines are males; broken lines are females.

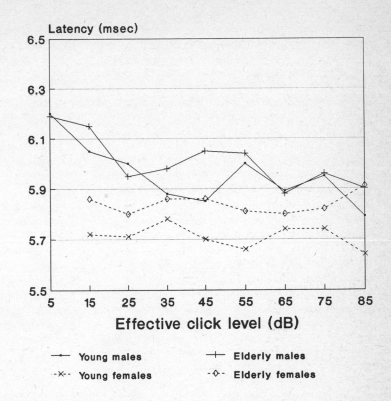

In contrast, Patterson et al. (1981) found a larger gender difference with 80 dB SL clicks in 60- to 79-year-old subjects than in young subjects (0.12 msec. in young versus 0.17 msec. in old) and a decrease in the gender difference between young and old subjects with 60 dB SL clicks (0.10 msec. in young versus 0.5 msec. in old).

Still other research findings provide no support for, or contradict, the notion of an age-by-gender interaction. Jerger and Hall's (1980) wave V curves run parallel for normal hearing males and females (Fig. 7-20), while the gender difference decreased slightly with age in the work of Lenzi and colleagues (1989). Rosenhamer and colleagues (1980) found significant gender differences in young, but not in old, subjects, suggesting a diminution of the gender effect with age. In a study by Wharton and Church (1990), the age difference in latency of wave V was *greater* in females than males.

In summary, there is little doubt that females tend to have shorter latency ABR waves than males, and that gender is an important variable with regard to ABR latency. It is also clear that the interaction of age and gender is not a simple one.

Jerger and Johnson (1988) noted three factors that have been suggested to explain the gender effect: a difference in head/brain size, whole body temperature, or hormonal milieu. The latter variables might interact with age (although the linear trends in the aging curves do not suggest a correlation with menopause). The gender effect may also be confounded by unspecified variables such as hearing loss and gender-related noise exposure. These various factors may account for the lack of a clear-cut consensus on the age-gender interaction.

AGE, GENDER, AND HEARING LOSS INFLUENCE ABR LATENCY

Two recent studies have used regression analysis to evaluate the roles of age, gender, and hearing loss on the ABR. Mitchell, Phillips, and Trune (1989) found that wave I latency was best predicted (in order of relative importance) by hearing threshold at 8000 Hz, gender, and age; wave III latency was best predicted by hearing threshold at 4000 Hz, age, and gender; and wave V latency was best predicted by gender, age, and head diameter, with a minor influence of threshold at 4000 Hz. The interval between waves I-V depended on head diameter and threshold at 8 and 4 kHz, with age being of minor importance. Latencies and amplitudes of different waves were affected by hearing loss at different frequencies, making the overall relationship between hearing loss and the ABR complex.

Jerger and Johnson (1988) found that age, gender, and the degree of sensorineural hearing loss interacted to determine the latency of wave V. This is shown in Figure 7-23 in which the wave V latencies of young and old males and females are plotted as a function of the "effective click level" (ECL; the difference between the click level used to elicit the response and subject's hearing threshold at 4 kHz). High ECLs are associated with normal high-frequency sensitivity. Females showed shorter latencies than males, but their wave V latencies were less affected by hearing loss (low versus high ECLs). In males, hearing loss was associated with increased latency. It is also evident that the curves for young and old females differ more consistently than those of young and old males (this was supported by a significant gender effect).

Jerger and Johnson (1988) were somewhat puzzled by their findings, since hormonal milieu or other variables seemed unable to account for the interaction between gender and hearing loss in their study. They speculated that differences may have occurred in the nature of sensorineural hearing loss between the males and females of their study, perhaps related to noise-induced cochlear damage.

ANIMAL RESEARCH ON ABR LATENCY

ABRs can also be obtained from animal models, with the advantage of being able to control for noise exposure and other variables that might confound age effects.

Several studies have found no effect of age or moderate hearing loss on absolute or interpeak latencies. Dum and von Wedel (1983) performed longitudinal ABR measurements on guinea pigs between the age of 6 months and 3 years (not very old). Threshold elevations of about 20 dB, across a broad range of frequencies, were observed by two years. These were not accompanied by changes in latencies. Harrison and Buchwald (1982) measured the ABR in young and old cats. Despite elevations of threshold, latencies and interpeak latencies did not differ as a function of age. Hunter and Willott (1987) observed no significant age effect on latencies of CBA mice through 18 months of age (when a small degree of hearing loss is exhibited).

Other researchers have obtained mixed results. Simpson and colleagues (1985) measured ABRs in unanesthetized Fischer 344 rats in two groups: young (mean 8.5 months) and aged (mean 25 months). The older animals had click thresholds about 20 dB higher than the young animals. For 80 dB SPL clicks, older animals had longer latencies for waves I and IV, but no difference in the I-IV interpeak latency. For clicks presented at 35 dB above threshold, there were no differences in absolute or interpeak latencies. They did find prolongation of the negative wave that followed ABR wave IV for both 80 dB SPL and 35 dB SL clicks. Click-evoked ABRs were obtained by Feldman and Burkard (1991) from young and old (26 months) Sprague-Dawley rats, either fed ad-lib or on a restricted diet. ABR thresholds were about 10 dB higher in the old rats. Mean latencies increased in the older rats and variability was greater, as well. The I-IV interpeak latency showed no consistent age effect. Cooper, Coleman, and Newton (1990) obtained ABRs from young and old (24 to 29 months) Sprague-Dawley rats using tone pips of 3, 8, and 40 kHz. Latencies of waves I through V increased significantly with age at 3 and 40 kHz but not at 8 kHz. Age effects on interpeak latencies depended in part on frequency. The wave III-V latency increased by 0.41 msec. at 3 kHz, 0.17 msec at 8 kHz, and *decreased* by 0.05 msec. at 40 kHz. The wave I-III latency increased at all three frequencies.

A decrease in interpeak latencies was also reported by Church and Shucard (1986). This was found to accompany the progressive elevation of thresholds in aging BDF1 mice. Latency-intensity functions also became increasingly steep, suggesting recruitment, characteristic of hair cell damage. In C57 mice (Hunter and Willott, 1987; see Fig. 7-24) I-V interpeak latencies likewise tended to decrease, but only during the first five months of life when hearing impairment was not severe. However, as hearing loss became more severe in older mice, the I-V interval increased.

The data from C57 mice suggest a relationship between peripheral presbycusis and longer latencies. The trend toward prolonged latencies in aging C57 mice observed by Hunter and Willott (1987) paralleled the progressively elevated thresholds characteristic of this strain (Fig. 7-24). Both ABR latencies and sensory thresholds begin to rise by 6 to 7 months in C57 mice and continue to do so until severe threshold elevations preclude further ABR testing after 16 months of age.

EFFECT OF STIMULUS RATE ON ABR LATENCY

Another variable that might interact with age to affect ABR latency is the rate of stimulation, since it is conceivable that an aged auditory system might not be capable of responding as rapidly as a young one. Fujikawa and Weber (1977) and Shanon, Gold, and Himelfarb (1981) varied the click rate in young and old subjects. As seen in Fig. 7-25, the latency increased more in older subjects as click rate increased.

Figure 7-24. ABR latency in the C57 mouse (adapted from Hunter and Willott, 1987).

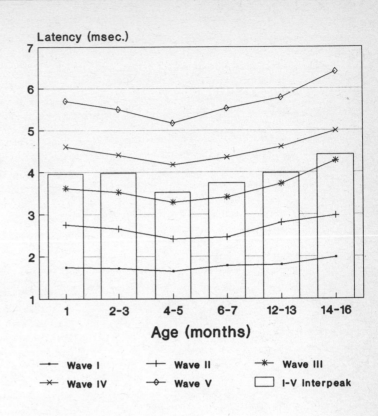

80 dB SPL noise pips

Figure 7-25. ABR latency in young and old subjects re: click rate (adapted from Fujikawa and Weber, 1977 and Shanon et al., 1981). Solid lines are from the Fujikawa and Weber study; broken lines are from the Shanon et al. study.

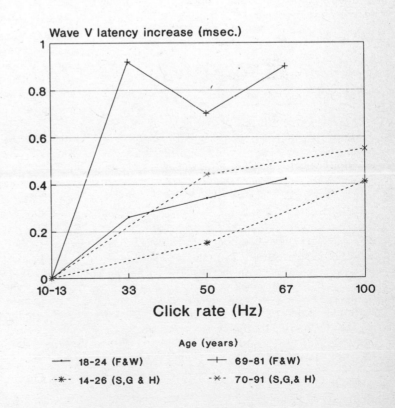

Other studies have not replicated this type of finding. The latency data of Harkins (1981) suggested a mild interaction between rate and age for waves I and III, but this was not strongly supported by the statistical analysis. Soucek and Mason (1990) obtained ABRs, as well as electrocochleographic (ECochG) measures (including the compound AP), from normal-hearing young subjects and from older subjects (mean age of 75 years) with some hearing loss. Latencies of the AP and ABR were prolonged in the older group, but the shift in latency as stimulus rate was increased (5 to 200 per second) was similar for both age groups.

The interaction of click rate and age has also been evaluated in cats. In the study by Harrison and Buchwald (1982), which included rather old cats, varying the rate of presentation (10-100 Hz) affected the ABRs of young and old animals similarly.

The latter studies indicate that the effects of rate on ABR latencies are not necessarily altered in older people or cats. Perhaps peripheral hearing loss played a role in the findings shown in Figure 7-25. Fujikawa and Weber (1977) used young and old subjects whose hearing was normal for their age (i.e., older subjects had some hearing loss), whereas the Shanon et al. (1981) used a group of unscreened older subjects which, presumably, contained individuals with significant hearing loss. Thus, the exaggeration of the relationship between stimulus rate and ABR amplitude in the elderly may be a function of peripheral presbycusis, and an example of CEPP.

SUMMARY: AGING AND ABR LATENCY

Absolute latencies of ABR waves typically increase slightly with age in humans. Both peripheral presbycusis and other age-related variables appear to contribute, and it may be futile to attempt to discern the relative contributions of these factors since they co-vary so strongly.

Some studies have found little or no age effect on absolute or interpeak latencies in humans and animals that retain relatively good hearing. Similarly, ABR latencies of older subjects are not necessarily more susceptible to prolongation by rapid rates of stimulation. Thus, it appears that aging need not result in significantly prolonged ABR latencies.

On the other hand, some findings have indicated latency changes in old subjects when hearing loss is accounted for. This suggests the presence of CEPP and/or CEBA.

EFFECTS OF AGING AND HEARING LOSS ON ABR AMPLITUDE

There is a general consensus in the literature that amplitudes of ABR waves decrease with age (Table 7-1). Several research groups have reported data on ABR amplitudes in aging humans with near-normal audiograms, but the decreases were minimal. For example, Beagley and Sheldrake (1978) found small decreases in wave V amplitude of normal-hearing older subjects. The age effect was characterized by an increase in the prevalence of small waves with a concomitant decrease in prevalence of larger waves. Wave V amplitudes measured by Jerger and Hall (1980) tended to be smaller in subjects over 30, but no consistent age-related trends were evident in normal-hearing people through the sixth decade (Fig. 7-26, solid lines).

Other studies have found more convincing age-related declines in ABR amplitude. However, as was the case with ABR latency, it is difficult to determine the effects of peripheral presbycusis on ABR amplitude, since many elderly subjects have some degree of hearing loss. Harkins (1981) reported that amplitudes of waves I, II, III, and V decreased in older subjects who had a 17 dB mean hearing loss at 4 kHz compared to the young subjects. Kjaer (1980) observed decreased amplitudes of all waves of 50- to 69-year-olds compared to 20- to 29-year-olds, but some of the older "normal-hearing" subjects had audiometric thresholds 20 to 30 dB higher than the young subjects. Recently, Psatta and Matei (1988) and Wharton and Church (1990) observed smaller amplitudes across waves in older men and women with a small amount of hearing loss.

Jerger and Hall (1980) examined ABR amplitudes in aging people with documented significant sensorineural hearing loss (Fig. 7-26, broken lines). In both men and women aged 40 to 59, sensorineural loss did not appear to affect the amplitude of wave V significantly, as judged by the means (and SEMs of their original figure). There was some additional decrease in amplitude at older ages (especially in women), but the contributions of age versus hearing loss cannot be determined.

Taken together, the evidence indicates that older individuals with presbycusis have lower ABR amplitudes. Hearing loss probably contributes to this, but ABR amplitudes decline with age even when hearing loss is minimal. Indeed, the regression analysis of Mitchell and colleagues (1989) indicated that both hearing loss and age are negatively correlated with amplitudes of ABR waves.

Figure 7-26. ABR wave V amplitude in normal-hearing and hearing-impaired men and women (adapted from Jerger and Hall, 1980). Solid lines are normal-hearing; broken lines have sensorineural hearing loss (snhl).

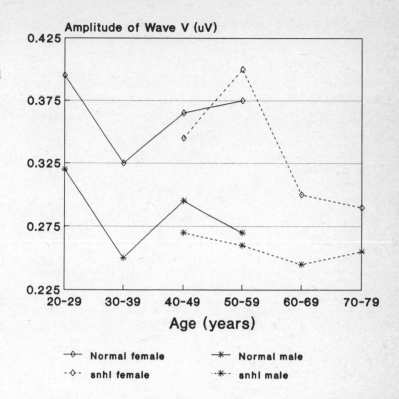

ANIMAL RESEARCH ON ABR AMPLITUDE

ABR amplitudes of aging CBA mice (in the presence of only minimal age-related hearing loss) decrease (Fig. 7-27, broken lines), with little change in amplitude ratios among different waves. The amplitude of wave IV in aging C57 mice (Fig. 7-27, solid lines), likewise, shows a decrease accompanying sensorineural impairment. The obvious difference in age-related changes between the strains is the marked reduction in wave I in C57 mice compared to CBAs. These observation are consistent with earlier work by Henry and Lepkowski (1978).

Henry and Lepkowski (1978) were the first researchers to obtain ABR data from an animal model of presbycusis, employing C57 mice 200 days old. Like-aged CBA mice were also used. Amplitudes of all waves declined in the middle-aged C57 mice, but the decline was greatest in the earlier waves. Amplitude changes in CBA mice were less pronounced. Later

ABR waves in middle-aged C57 mice exhibited a "recruitment profile," in that increased click stimulus intensity was associated with exaggerated decreases in wave latencies and increases in wave amplitudes. CBA mice did not demonstrate the recruitment profile.

Dum and von Wedel (1983) observed a decrease in amplitude of all waves in aging guinea pigs, and Harrison and Buchwald (1982) noted that amplitudes were generally smaller in old cats. However, the variability was considerable and statistically significant differences were not obtained. In old Sprague-Dawley rats studied by Feldman and Burkard (1991), absolute amplitude of wave II and the negative leg of wave III were smaller than those of young rats when clicks were 60 dB SPL. However, the age effect was not present for wave II at 90 dB SPL.

While the evidence indicates that ABR amplitudes decrease with age in animals, at least one study found no effect. Simpson and colleagues (1985) saw no age differences in wave IV amplitudes of rats.

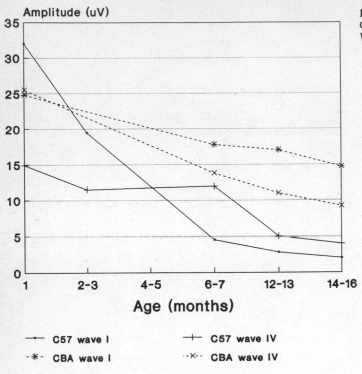

Figure 7-27. ABR amplitude in C56 and CBA mice (adapted from Hunter and Willott, 1987).

80 dB SPL noise pips

AMPLITUDE OF EARLY VERSUS LATE ABR WAVES

The amplitude data for C57 and CBA mice (Fig. 7-27) suggest that early and late waves may be differently affected by cochlear pathology. Specifically, amplitudes of early waves decline more than later waves in C57 mice as sensorineural pathology progresses. Examination of the ABR literature indicates that the same differential relationship for early and late waves may hold for humans. This relationship is reflected by the recognizability of waves and the relative amplitudes.

Otto and McCandless (1982b) were able to recognize wave V in all of their normal-hearing, young sensorineural, and elderly subjects. In contrast, earlier waves were less often detected in the latter two groups, particularly the old subjects (Fig. 7-28). Similarly, Rosenhall et al. (1986) were able to recognize wave V in almost all young and old hearing-impaired subjects irrespective of the degree of high-frequency hearing loss (45–85+ dB at 4–8 kHz). Recognizability of earlier waves declined as a function of hearing loss (but not as a function of age in subjects matched for hearing loss).

For instance, the recognizability of wave I in men with 85 dB or greater high frequency loss was only about 60 percent. In normal-hearing subjects, the same researchers (Rosenhall et al., 1985) were able to identify wave I in almost 90 percent of their cases through age 75. Rowe (1981), reviewing clinical data, pointed out that wave I is often low in amplitude or absent in patients with high-frequency hearing loss, particularly the elderly. Similar findings were recently reported for subjects in the 60- to 80-year range (Ottaviani et al., 1991).

Harkins (1981) computed the ratio of amplitudes for wave V to wave I. At each of the stimulus rates used, the ratio was higher in the older subjects (e.g., for stimuli presented at a rate of 10 per second, the ratio for young subjects was 3.05 compared to 3.23 in the old, who had a 17 dB loss at 4 kHz compared to the young subjects). The ratio of mean amplitudes for wave IV-V versus wave I computed from the paper by Kjaer (1980) was 1.52 in young men and 1.64 in older men. A more impressive difference was found in women with a ratio of 1.13 in young subjects and 1.92 in older subjects. Psatta and Matei (1988) determined wave V/I ratios and found an increase from 1.9 in 30-year-olds

Figure 7-28. Recognizability of ABR waves (adapted from Otto and McCandless, 1982b).

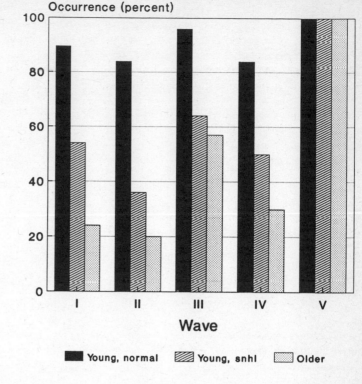

Occurrence (percent)

Wave

■ Young, normal   ▨ Young, snhl   ▢ Older

to 2.6 in 70-year-olds with 80 dB HL clicks but an increase of only 0.5 with 60 dB HL clicks. Ratios of waves V to I can also be computed from the data of Wharton and Church (1990). At 80 dB, the ratios in young and older women were 2.2 and 2.63, respectively, whereas those for young and older men were 1.6 and 3.67, respectively.

Wave V/I ratios of patients with retrocochlear lesions are often less than 1.00, whereas ratios associated with normal ears or ears with cochlear pathology are almost never below 1.00; the cochlear patients' ratios are typically higher than those of normals (Musiek, Kibbe, Rackliffe, and Weider, 1984). Thus, the amplitude ratio data of Harkins (1981), Kjaer (1980), Psatta and Matei (1988), and Wharton and Church (1990) are consistent with the manifestation of cochlear sensorineural hearing loss, rather than age-related retrocochlear pathology.

These observations have practical and theoretical implications. On a practical level, wave V is more reliable and generally more detectable than the other waves in the human ABR; thus, it is often the only wave evaluated. Wave V amplitude by itself would be inappropriate to discern the presence of peripheral pathology. However, the ratio of waves V and I might be of clinical interest regarding hearing and aging.

Indeed, evaluation of wave I or the compound action potential (CAP) might prove useful in evaluating the condition of the spiral ganglion, aiding in the identification of neural presbycusis. In a recent experimental study using rats, Hall (1990) determined that the number of surviving ganglion cells and the amplitude of the electrically-evoked CAP/ABR wave I were highly positively correlated (confirming the theoretical relationship between ganglion cells and the amplitude of summed measures of peripheral neural activity). Later ABR waves were less highly correlated with the number of ganglion cells. Extrapolation of these findings suggests that acoustically evoked CAP or ABR wave I amplitudes may be indicators of peripheral neural pathology in the elderly (perhaps in conjunction with otoacoustic emissions as a test of OHC condition; see below).

On a theoretical level, the data suggest that different levels of the auditory system vary with respect to the effects of peripheral presbycusis. One might speculate that relatively larger amplitudes of later waves could reflect divergence of ascending circuits. For example, peripheral sensorineural pathology would result in a reduction in the number of responding neurons at the auditory nerve or lower brainstem levels and a consequent lowering of early ABR wave amplitudes. The ascending axons of neurons that remain capable of producing output may branch sufficiently to innervate a relatively large pool of post-synaptic neurons at higher brainstem levels, resulting in a lesser diminution of the ABR amplitude in the upper brainstem. The effects of aging on the CAS in the absence of pronounced sensorineural pathology would presumably have a similar effect on all brainstem levels and the ABR waves they generate (see Chapter 6). Other hypotheses can also be entertained, such as impairment of central inhibitory circuits (see Chapter 6) that would enhance later ABR amplitudes. However, this would imply that the relative enhancement of later waves would be more closely associated with aging than with sensorineural hearing loss, which is not supported by the data from C57 mice.

EFFECTS OF AGING AND PERIPHERAL IMPAIRMENT ON ABR AMPLITUDE-INTENSITY FUNCTIONS

It appears that no published work has specifically investigated amplitude intensity functions in ABRs of elderly individuals. However, Rowe (1978) provided data on wave V amplitude of older persons at 30 and 60 dB above the mean threshold for clicks of young subjects (Fig. 7-29). Comparing amplitudes for 30 Hz click rates, it appears that the slope (30 to 60 dB) of the mean intensity function for older subjects is steeper than for younger subjects. However, in subjects with good hearing (20 dB HL or better) in the study of Wharton and Church (1990) no consistent age effects were evident in comparing amplitudes of waves I, III, and V at 40, 60, and 80 dB HL.

Hunter and Willott (1987) found increased slopes of amplitude-intensity functions in late waves (relative to wave I) of aging C57 mice but not in CBA mice (Figs. 7-30, 7-31). These data along with the findings of Rowe (1978) versus Wharton and Church (1990) suggest that peripheral presbycusis, but not aging per se, is associated with steepening of the intensity functions of later waves.

Conclusions about the relationship between peripheral presbycusis and the steepness of early versus late ABR waves await further corroboration, but have interesting implications. An increase in slopes of waves IV and V in aging C57 mice, but not in earlier waves, suggests that the effects of peripheral dysfunction on intensity coding vary depending on the brainstem level. For a given increment in intensity, the amplitude of later waves grows much more than that of earlier

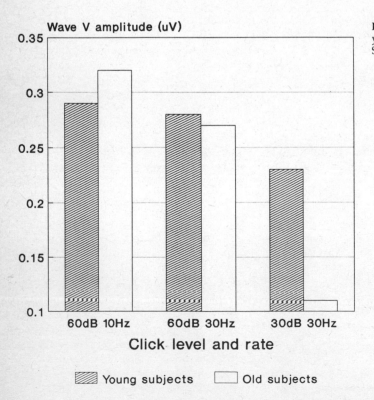

Figure 7-29. ABR wave V amplitude in young and old subjects at two click rates and SPLs (adapted from Rowe, 1978).

Figure 7-30. ABR amplitude-intensity functions in C57 mice (adapted from Hunter and Willott, 1987). Amplitudes are expressed relative to the amplitude of wave I of 1-month-olds at 80 dB SPL. Solid lines are 6- to 7-month-olds; broken lines are 1-month-olds.

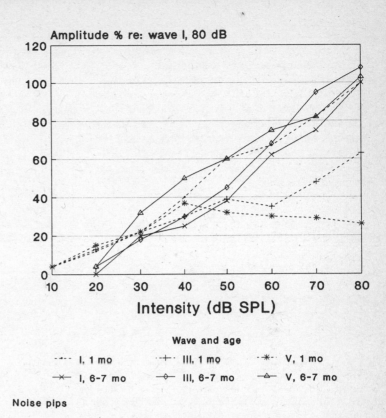

Figure 7-31. ABR amplitude-intensity functions in CBA mice (adapted from Hunter and Willott, 1987). Amplitudes are expressed relative to the amplitude of wave I of 1-month-olds at 80 dB SPL. Solid lines are 6- to 7-month-olds; broken lines are 1-month-olds.

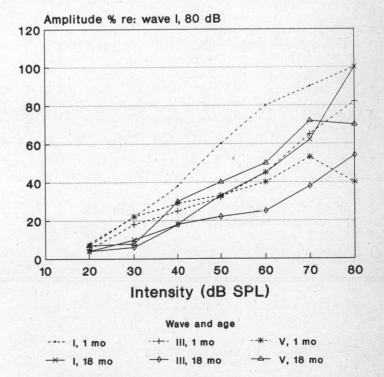

waves. On the basis of these data, it might be predicted that "loudness" of sounds grows more rapidly in older C57 mice and that this is primarily a function of central processes. It is tempting to speculate that the present findings are related to loudness recruitment, which is sometimes found in humans with sensorineural hearing loss (Hallpike, 1976; see also Chapter 8). This would suggest that loudness recruitment has a central component, a conclusion consistent with that of Henry and Lepkowski (1978), based on ABR data obtained from aging C57 mice.

EFFECTS OF STIMULUS RATE ON ABR AMPLITUDE

At present, no clear picture emerges regarding the effect of stimulus rate on ABR amplitude. Several variables appear to be significant, including the specific rates used, stimulus intensity, and the ABR wave examined.

Harkins (1981) varied click rate and observed that clicks presented at ten per second resulted in lower amplitudes in older subjects. However, compared to young subjects, their amplitudes did not decrease as much with faster click rates. Therefore, at a rate of 100 Hz, amplitudes differences were diminished.

The study by Rowe (1978) suggests that the effect of stimulus rate on ABR amplitude is dependent upon stimulus intensity. As seen in Figure 7-29, clicks presented at 60 dB resulted in minimal age differences for stimuli presented at 10Hz or 30 Hz, whereas older subjects' amplitudes were substantially reduced with 30 dB clicks at a rate of 30 Hz. Since levels were referenced to click threshold for young subjects (who had better thresholds than old subjects on the order of 10 dB), the stimuli were presented at lower SLs for the older subjects, confounding the observations.

In the study by Soucek and Mason (1990), referred to earlier, the amplitude of ABR wave III and the AP decreased more with increased stimulus rates in old, impaired subjects than in young, normal-hearing subjects. The rate effect was not significant for wave V amplitude. Because the effect of rate was similar for the AP and wave III of the ABR, Soucek and Mason concluded that cochlear pathology was responsible.

SUMMARY: AGING AND ABR AMPLITUDE

The amplitude of ABR waves tends to decrease with advancing age. Specific contributions of aging and peripheral hearing loss are difficult to tease apart, but

both probably are significant (e.g., Mitchell et al., 1989). The presence of sensorineural hearing loss appears to have pronounced effects on the amplitude and recognizability of wave I, but minimal effects on wave V. Increased V/I amplitude ratios may be characteristic of peripheral presbycusis (and, perhaps CEPP), but not of aging per se (CEBA).

OTHER ELECTROPHYSIOLOGICAL RESPONSES

THE MIDDLE LATENCY RESPONSE (MLR)

The middle latency response is characterized by components in the 10-50 msec. range, indicating that they arise from thalamic and cortical regions of the brain. The components are indicated by their positive or negative polarity and temporal order (e.g., No, Po, Na, Pa, Nb).

LATENCY AND AMPLITUDE

Woods and Clayworth (1986) recorded middle latency responses in young (20- to 40-year-old) and older (60- to 80-year-old) subjects with normal hearing. They observed increased latency and *enhanced* amplitude for the Pa wave in the older group, even when young and old individuals were matched for hearing loss. They pointed out that Pfefferbaum and colleagues (1979) had also reported enhanced amplitudes in a 45 msec. positive-evoked response component of older subjects. Kelly-Ballweber and Dobie (1984) also found enhanced amplitude and increased latency of the Pa component. The young and old subjects were matched for hearing loss in this study, suggesting that the Pa enhancement is not due to peripheral differences but may be of central origin. Whether the enhancement of Pa amplitude is due to a change in some central inhibitory system such as GABA (Woods and Clayworth, 1986) or some other factor remains to be determined. Amplitudes of Pa in elderly adults tested by Jerger, Oliver, and Chmiel (1988) were nearly twice the size of those in young adults at stimulus rates of 2 to 12 per second. Chambers and Griffiths (1991) recorded MLRs from women at various ages from 22 to 68 years; pure tone thresholds were less than or equal to 25 dB HL but older women had greater mean hearing losses than young women. Pa amplitudes increased linearly with age. The increase in amplitudes were most pronounced at higher intensities, and there was a corresponding increase in the steepness of amplitude-intensity functions by a factor of two. The increase Pa amplitudes were due in part to a positive shift in the baseline voltage, but also were due to increased peak-to-peak amplitudes, irrespective of the baseline.

Lenzi, Chiarelli, and Sambataro (1989) also found increased latencies in MLRs of older subjects with normal hearing. In contrast to other studies, they reported that amplitudes of the MLR components were reduced, with morphological changes in the waves. They did report a high level of variability in their amplitudes but did not present any data, making it difficult to compare their observations with those described above.

A study by Ryan (1989) utilized tones, rather than clicks, to elicit the MLR in young and old (greater than 60 years) subjects with relatively good hearing. She observed rather smaller increases in the latency of waves but no age difference in wave amplitude. Ryan's findings, contrasted with those cited above, suggest that the stimulus used to elicit MLRs (e.g., tones versus clicks) may be a key variable in determining age effects.

OTHER OBSERVATIONS

While Woods and Clayworth (1986) did not detect differences in binaural responses as a function of age, Kelly-Ballweber and Dobie (1984) noted an age difference in binaural responses for their young and old sensorineurally impaired subjects. Young subjects showed a reduction in binaural Pa amplitude compared to the sum of monaural responses (as is normal), but many of the older subjects did not. This suggests some abnormality in binaural processing of the MLR in older individuals with cochlear pathology.

Jerger et al. (1988) observed a rate effect in Pa amplitude of older subjects, with amplitudes decreasing as rate increased. For example, at 2 per second, mean amplitude was about 1.7 uV; at 12 per second, mean amplitude was about 1.2 uV. By comparison, Pa amplitudes of young adults were about 0.75 UV at both rates. However, a great deal of individual variance in rate effects occurred in the elderly subjects, with some subjects showing marked effects (e.g., a 75 percent reduction between 2 and 12 per second).

Jerger and colleagues also presented a case study of MLRs in a 71-year-old woman with evidence of central auditory dysfunction (e.g., poor synthetic and dichotic sentence identification scores). A Pa wave was evoked by stimuli to one ear, but not the other.

SUMMARY

The MLR appears to be significantly altered in some older people. In particular, an increase in the latency and amplitude of Pa occurs rather reliably, at least when clicks are used as stimuli. The enhanced amplitudes at higher intensities has led to speculation about the possible involvement of impaired inhibitory systems that "release" the responses (e.g., Woods and Clayworth, 1986). As indicated in Chapter 6, physiological studies of neural responses in the mouse IC and the GABA system in the rat IC are consistent with this notion, which is discussed further in Chapter 10. Thus, the MLR may reflect changes in CAS processing associated with biological aging and/or peripheral presbycusis (CEBA or CEPP).

LATE AUDITORY EVOKED RESPONSES

Evoked responses with latencies of 50–250 msec. presumably arise from cortical regions. Goodin et al. (1978), Pfefferbaum et al. (1979, 1980), and Picton et al. (1984) found increased latency of the second positive peak (P2) with little or no age effect on the first positive and negative components (P1 and N1).

Papanicolau, Loring, and Eisenberg (1984) used a two-tone stimulation paradigm to evaluate age-related recovery rates of cortical auditory evoked potentials. Tone pairs separated by 350 msec. were presented with different interpair intervals (IPIs). It was reasoned that recovery from the first tone should affect the amplitude of the second tone; by the same token, recovery from the second tone of a pair should affect the amplitude of the first tone of the next pair if the IPI fell within the recovery period. As seen in Figure 7-32, at shorter IPIs (650 and 1650 msec.) no age effects were found in the N1-P2 amplitudes (nor were they found for P1-N1). At the slowest rate (4650 msec. IPIs), however, an age effect was found. The N1-P2 amplitudes for both tones of the pair were larger in the young subjects. Furthermore, in young subjects the first tone of a pair was enhanced greatly, but this was not the case in older subjects. They concluded that the recovery cycle of young subjects was shorter than that of older subjects, which accounted for the larger amplitudes.

EVENT RELATED POTENTIALS: THE P300

The P300 is a positive scalp recorded potential occurring around 300 msec. in young adults. It is an

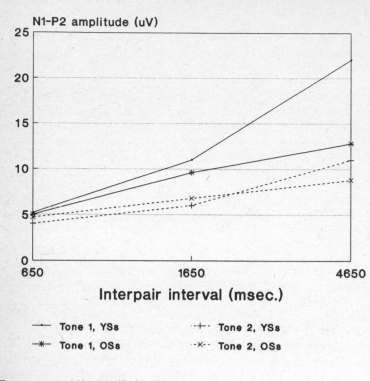

Figure 7-32. Recovery of the cortical evoked response in young and old subjects (adapted from Papanicolaou et al., 1984). Solid lines are for Tone 1; broken lines are for Tone 2. At short interpair intervals, amplitudes are small due to the inability of the responses to recover. At longer intervals, the response to tone 1 recovers fast enough in the young subjects (but not in old subjects), so that amplitudes become larger. See text for an explanation of methodology.

Tones were 1 kHz, 75 dB SL, 50 msec. duration, binaural, with fixed intertone interval of 350 msec.

"endogenous," event-related potential that occurs when information is actively processed, and it is independent of stimulus parameters and modality. Squire and Hecox (1983) suggested that the latency of the P300 may provide a means of detecting deficits in central auditory processing. Such deficits might involve evaluation time, perception of relevant acoustic features of stimuli, or processing of complex stimuli. Polich, Howard, and Starr (1985), for instance, introduced background noise with their test stimuli and observed increased P300 latencies. Squires and Hecox (1983) found the P300 to be eliminated in a young woman when background noise was introduced; yet audiometric and other electrophysiological measures were normal. The P300 in this case revealed cortical pathology that was not detected by other measures.

Aging has been shown to be associated with increased P300 latencies (Brown, Marsh, and LaRue, 1983; Ford et al., 1979a, b; Goodin et al., 1978; Pfefferbaum et al., 1980a, b; 1984; Picton et al., 1984; Syndulko et al., 1982). However, the potential of the P300 in evaluating central presbycusis has only recently been specifically addressed. Pollock and

Schneider (1989) reported that P300s of elderly subjects elicited by a 2000 Hz target tone had longer latencies and smaller amplitudes than those elicited by a 500 Hz target tone, whereas younger subjects did not show such latency differences. Sandridge (1988) measured the P300 in patients diagnosed as having central or peripheral presbycusis. While the "central" group also had high-frequency hearing loss that might have influenced their performance, the P300 of this group had a longer latency than that of the "peripheral" group. The introduction of noise also affected the two groups differently, with the "central" group performing better. Although these findings might best be considered preliminary, they suggest that the P300 may prove valuable as an adjunctive test of central auditory functioning in the elderly.

SUMMARY: IMPLICATIONS OF EVOKED RESPONSE FINDINGS

The various evoked response measures—ABRs, MLR, late responses, P300—provide indications of age-related changes in some physiological properties of the central auditory system. In many cases peripheral presbycusis may be sufficient to account for the findings. However, the presence of CEPP and/or CEBA are also suggested by some evoked response studies. Absolute latencies and amplitudes, interpeak latencies of ABRs, amplitude intensity functions, rate and recovery effects, and other measures sometimes indicate differences between young and old subjects that cannot be adequately accounted for by peripheral hearing loss alone.

Unfortunately, interpretation of the significance of these central effects with regard to *presbycusis* is impossible at this time. Just because "something is happening" to CAS responses of older listeners, it does not necessarily follow that auditory perception is significantly affected. This issue is discussed further in Chapter 10.

OTOACOUSTIC EMISSIONS (OAES)

Since they were first reported by Kemp (1978) OAEs have received a good deal of attention. Subsequent work has indicated that OAEs reflect the active mechanism involving OHC motility (see Bonfils, Bertrand, and Uziel, 1988). Bonfils and colleagues measured OAEs in subjects aged 2 to 88 years. Audiograms showed mean thresholds of 20 dB HL or better from 125–1000 Hz for all age groups, with higher frequency thresholds become progressively worse with age. Subjects older than 60 had means HLs of 30 dB at 2 kHz, 43 dB at 6 kHz, and 52 dB at 8 kHz. Emissions were present in all ears younger than 60; beyond this age, however, the incidence of measurable OAEs dropped to 35 percent. Threshold of evoked OAEs increased linearly after age 40. A plot of the mean absolute evoked OAE threshold in dB HL as a function of the mean hearing threshold for clicks showed a linear relationship between OAE threshold and click threshold, with a slope greater than 1. In other words, when HL was below 10 dB, OAE thresholds were below the hearing threshold for clicks; above 10 dB HL, OAE threshold were above click thresholds.

Bonfils (1988) also related evoked OAEs to speech audiometric data in older subjects with sensorineural impairments. OAEs were never observed when the speech reception threshold (SRT) was equal to or greater than 35 dB HL, but were always observed when SRT was 25 dB HL or less. Furthermore, the detection threshold for click-evoked OAEs was correlated with SRT. However, evoked OAE detection threshold and speech recognition (measured 35 dB above SRT) were not significantly correlated.

Cutler, Lonsbury-Martin, and Martin (1990) and Lonsbury-Martin et al. (1990) measured distortion-product OAEs at the 2f1–f2 frequency in young and old subjects with good hearing (20 dB HL or better). Reduced amplitudes and increased "thresholds" of the distortion-product OAEs revealed systematic age-related decline in cochlear function, particularly for high frequencies. Stover and Norton (1990) also reported that OAEs changed with age in "normal hearing" subjects aged 20 to 80 years. The prevalence of spontaneous and evoked OAEs decreased, magnitude of evoked OAEs was diminished, and the input-output functions were shallower.

The data from these studies indicate that OAEs and psychophysical thresholds co-vary with cochlear damage, presumably because of diminution of OHC function. They also suggest that the active OHC mechanism is impaired in many elderly listeners and may contribute to peripheral presbycusis. There is some indication (Bonfils, 1988) that OAEs (and, presumably, OHC functioning) are not good predictors of suprathreshold speech recognition performance.

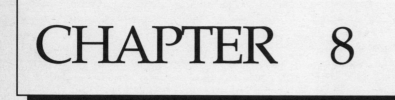

CHAPTER 8

Psychophysical Aspects of Aging and Presbycusis: Non-speech Material

It is obvious that adequate detection of sounds is a prerequisite for hearing, and that pure tone audiograms are essential indicators of hearing potential in the elderly. However, effective auditory perception also requires the listener to deal with the intensity, frequency components, temporal aspects, duration, location, and other parameters of acoustic stimuli. This chapter assesses the relationship between aging and the perception of suprathreshold, non-speech stimuli, as well as absolute tone thresholds. Chapter 9 focuses on aging and speech perception.

RESEARCH CONSIDERATIONS

Perception of suprathreshold sounds relies on both peripheral and central auditory processing. It will become evident, as the literature is reviewed, that peripheral sensorineural hearing loss—irrespective of age—disrupts performance on many psychophysical tasks[1]. Thus, peripheral presbycusis is likely to be a key factor in most psychophysical measures of suprathreshold hearing capacities. By the same token, central presbycusis also has the potential to interfere with the neural processing of various aspects of sound (Chapter 6). Psychophysical research on older listeners has emphasized the study of hearing-impaired individuals; in using older subjects, the work typically has utilized patients diagnosed as having presbycusis. Elderly subjects with "normal hearing" have been used much less often than was the case in research on the acoustic reflex or evoked responses (Chapter 7). This makes it more difficult to differentiate between the effects of peripheral dysfunction per se, the central effects of peripheral presbycusis (CEPP), or the central effects of biological aging (CEBA) on psychophysical performance.

An additional concern of psychophysical tests with elderly subjects is the potential for nonauditory variables that might influence performance. These could include age differences in practice effects (e.g. reaching optimal performance levels), motivational and attentional factors, and cognitive abilities that might impact test performance (WGSUA, 1988). The poten-

tial of variables such as these to affect experimental results are difficult to evaluate but should always be considered.

THRESHOLDS FOR PURE TONES

Numerous studies have described the relationship between pure-tone audiograms and aging, and many are cited elsewhere in this book. We have seen in Chapter 3 that peripheral pathology is associated with a variety of audiometric profiles, ranging from flat across frequencies to various degrees of high-frequency loss. Many elderly individuals, of course, do not suffer from clinically significant presbycusis or other types of hearing loss and have rather good thresholds at most frequencies. However, even these nonclinical individuals are likely to have some hearing loss, at least at high frequencies, and it is a fair generalization that some elevation of thresholds can be found in virtually all elderly listeners.

The differences in audiometric thresholds as a function of age are evident in numerous surveys that have addressed this topic. Pioneering work was published in 1929 by Bunch (Figure 8-1). In listeners screened for the absence of subjective indications of hearing loss, it was clear that thresholds for low-frequency tones changed little with age, while in sharp contrast, high-frequency sensitivity was greatly diminished. Similar findings have been obtained in a variety of subject populations over the years by numerous researchers. The results of several of these studies were compiled by Spoor (1967), as shown in Figure 8-2. A number of additional surveys are are summarized at the end of this chapter in Appendix 8-1 (Figs. 8-19 to 8-27). An important aspect of age-related hearing loss is apparent in examining the data of Spoor (Fig. 8-2) and others (Figs. 8-20, 8-23, 8-24, 8-27): men have somewhat greater age-related loss of high-frequency hearing than women. This observation is made explicitly in Figure 8-3. While aging men tend to exhibit greater losses at high frequencies, some surveys have observed a gender difference in which men have lower mean thresholds than women at low frequencies (Figs. 8-19, 8-20, 8-23, 8-24, 8-27).

---

[1] In most of the literature to be reviewed in this chapter, "sensorineural" hearing loss or impairment is used in the general sense of cochlear and peripheral neural involvement, irrespective of age or etiology. The precise nature of the pathology underlying sensorineural hearing loss or its cause are often not known in audiological and psychophysical studies and could involve sensory and/or neural tissue. Thus, "sensorineural impairment" or "sensorineural hearing loss" in elderly listeners is not necessarily synonymous with "sensorineural presbycusis," as defined in Chapter 3, which specifically refers to hearing loss associated with age-related pathology of both the organ of Corti and spiral ganglion cells.

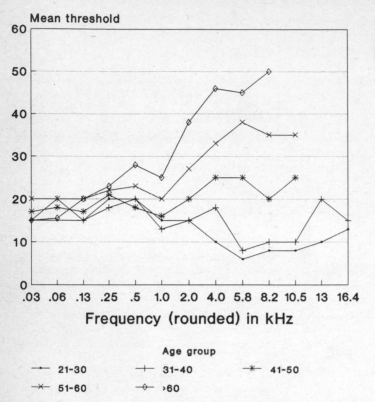

Figure 8-1. Pure tone thresholds (adapted from Bunch, 1929). Subjects were hospital patients in Baltimore, screened to eliminate those with obvious hearing problems. Thresholds in dB re: audiometer settings.

Several studies have obtained aging curves with a generally accelerating shape (Fig. 8-2, 8-21) suggesting that the loss of sensitivity increases more rapidly with advancing age. The rate of change was examined by Erlandsson et al. (1982) (Fig. 8-4), who summarized previous studies to demonstrate this aspect of presbycusis through 55 to 60 years. Indeed, the amount of hearing loss per year increases with age through 60 years.

Longitudinal studies indicate some flattening of the rate of high-frequency threshold changes beyond age 65. Milne (1977b) reported longitudinal follow-up data, summarized in Figure 8-5 for men. This study showed that hearing loss continues beyond age 65. At low frequencies (250-1000 Hz), men originally tested at 70 to 90 years of age exhibited more additional threshold change after 5 years than those originally tested at 62 to 69 years (the white bars are taller than the cross-hatched bars). In other words, the rate of hearing loss continued to increase. In contrast, the 5-year follow-up losses at 6 and 8 kHz were greater for men in the younger age group (the cross-hatched bars are taller than the white bars). This suggests that the rate of hearing loss decreased at high frequencies. An earlier longitudinal study by Eisdorfer and Wilke (1972) suggested flattening of the rate of age-related change. Over a 7-year period, subjects who advanced in age from 67 to 74 years had magnitudes of hearing decline similar to those who were tested from 75 to 82 years (about 10 dB at most frequencies).

Recent longitudinal studies have extended these findings. Pedersen, Rosenhall, and Moller (1989) reported longitudinal data on randomly selected men and women tested between the ages of 70 and 81. Figure 8-6 provides a representative example of their findings showing continued loss of sensitivity over this age range. Comparison of the successive differences in thresholds indicates that the rate of change is stable for high frequencies. For low frequency thresholds, the greatest change occurs between 79 and 81 years, suggesting continued acceleration of hearing loss. Fifteen-year longitudinal changes were reported

Figure 8-2a. Pure tone hearing level (adapted from Spoor, 1967). a. men; b. women. Compiled from eight different studies performed between 1938 and 1963, using rural, random, professional, and industrial populations. Thresholds in dB re: young subjects' mean thresholds.

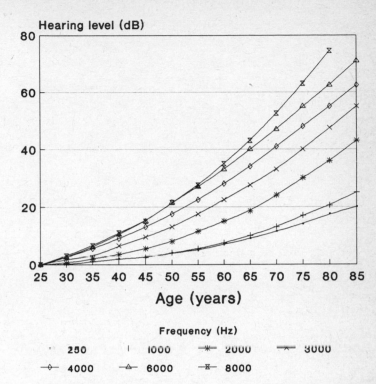

Figure 8-2b.

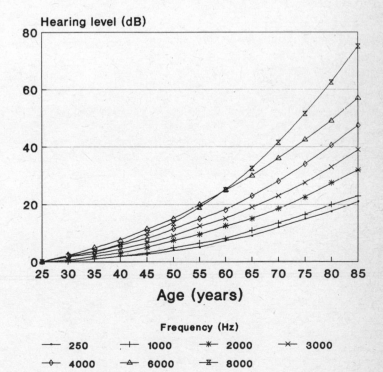

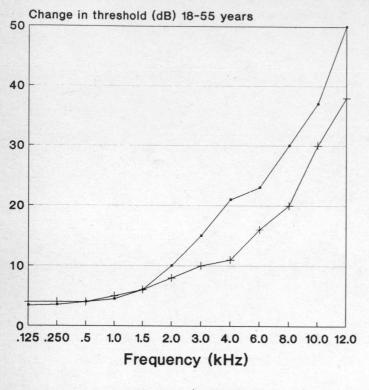

Figure 8-3. Change in pure tone threshold (adapted from Robinson and Sutton, 1979). Data were compiled from seven studies conducted between 1959 and 1970 from various types of subject populations.

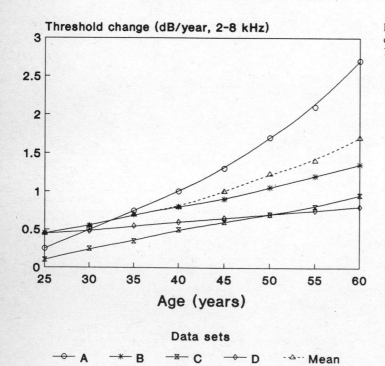

Figure 8-4. Rate of pure tone threshold change (adapted from Erlandsson et al., 1982). Data are from several studies.

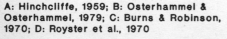

A: Hinchcliffe, 1959; B: Osterhammel & Osterhammel, 1979; C: Burns & Robinson, 1970; D: Royster et al., 1970

Figure 8-5. Longitudinal follow-up for male subjects (pure tone threshold change)(adapted from Milne, 1977).

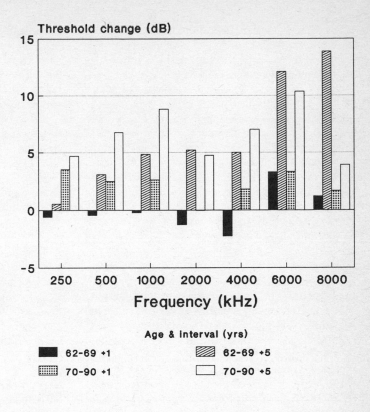

Figure 8-6. Longitudinal pure tone threshold change (adapted from Pedersen et al., 1989).

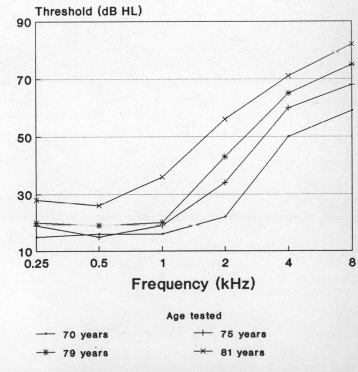

by Brant and Fozard (1990). At lower (speech) frequencies the magnitude of 15-year threshold changes increased sharply after 60, whereas the rate of change for higher frequencies decreased (see Appendix 8-1, Fig. 8-28). Keay and Murray (1988) reported the findings of a 17-year longitudinal study in which the subjects' ages extended well into the ninth decade. Hearing loss continued to progress, but the average yearly rate of change was stable at high and low frequencies in the eighth and ninth decades.

To summarize, most of the longitudinal data indicate flattening or decrease in the rate of progression of high frequency loss at advanced ages. Slowing of the rate of change is less evident at lower frequencies; in fact, hearing loss may accelerate at older ages. One explanation of these findings is that a ceiling effect may be reached at high frequencies because thresholds can only rise so much. The low-frequency thresholds have "more room" to become increasingly elevated.

High-frequency audiometry has been performed on older listeners by several investigators. Osterhammel and Osterhammel (1979b) obtained thresholds up to 20 kHz using a free field system. Age-related threshold elevations of about 10 dB were already evident for 16–20 kHz tones when comparing 20- to 29-year-olds with 10- to 19-year-olds. Substan-

tial age differences were also evident for 14 kHz tones in the 30- to 39-year decade, with successive decades showing increasing involvement of lower frequencies. Stelmachowicz and colleagues (1989) used a prototype high-frequency audiometer to obtain thresholds in subjects aged 20 to 59. The largest change in sensitivity occurred between the fifth and sixth decades of life (Fig. 8-7). Threshold shifts expressed in HL were greatest in the 13-17 kHz range and were evident even in the 20- to 29-year-old group. The region of maximum hearing loss shifted to lower frequencies with advancing age. At the lower frequencies minimal threshold elevation occurred before the 40's, and little shift occurred at the highest frequencies (a possible ceiling effect).

The data from these and other audiometric studies provide parameters for age-related hearing loss in a "typical" person. Threshold elevations are seen by the 30's, but are rather mild and restricted to high frequencies. By the 40's, thresholds for tones of 1000 Hz and below are still within 5 dB of optimal levels; however, thresholds for 3–4 kHz and 6–8 kHz may have risen by 15 dB and 20 dB, respectively. This trend progresses. By the 70's, sensitivity for tones of 1 kHz or less may be reduced by 15 dB, with concomitant losses of 30 dB at 3-4 kHz and 45 dB or more at 6–8 kHz.

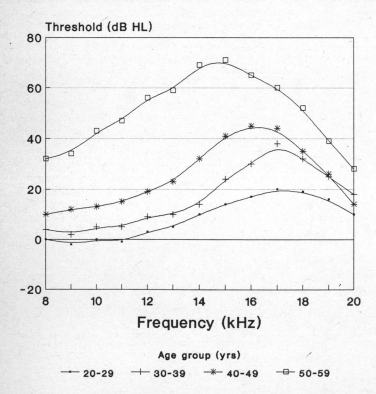

Figure 8-7. High-frequency audiometric thresholds (adapted from Stelmachowicz et al., 1989). Subjects were screened so that thresholds for 250 to 8000 Hz were normal for age and sex re: Corso (1963).

THE EAR EFFECT

Various surveys have indicated that in males (but not females) the right ear has slightly lower thresholds than the left (Chung, Mason, Gannon, and Wilson, 1983). The latter authors investigated this "ear effect" as a function of age. They found that the ear effect increased with age (into the fifties) for frequencies of 2 kHz and above, but for 500 and 1000 Hz, the ear effect tended to decrease with age. Borod, Obler, Albert, and Stiefel (1983) also evaluated pure tone thresholds as a function of age and found that the right ear advantage for pure tone average thresholds became more pronounced (by about 3 dB) in their 65- to 84-year-old males (but not females). Perhaps the most likely explanation for the ear effect is noise exposure. Automobile drivers are typically exposed to noise through the window on the left and the muzzle of rifles are toward the left side (although Chung et al., 1983 tested only non-shooters). Since men have tended to drive more and shoot more, noise-induced threshold elevations, accruing over the years, could account for the ear effect. However, Chung and colleagues noted that the ear effect is also observed in teen-agers, suggesting that some intrinsic factor may contribute to susceptibility of the left ear to hearing loss.

INTENSITY AND LOUDNESS

The key question with regard to loudness and hearing disorders is how the growth of loudness is affected. Recruitment of loudness (Fowler, 1937) refers to the abnormally steep growth of the loudness function that often accompanies cochlear impairment; relatively small increments in sound intensity are perceived as disproportionate increases in loudness. Loudness recruitment can be demonstrated by loudness balancing procedures, Bekesy audiometry, determination of intensity difference limens (DLI), magnitude estimation, the Short Increment Sensitivity Index (SISI), loudness discomfort level, temporal integration (see below) and, perhaps, electrocochleography and the middle ear reflex. There has been some disagreement in the literature regarding the prevalence of loudness recruitment in elderly listeners.

LOUDNESS BALANCING

Pestalloza and Shore (1955), using loudness balancing, concluded that 50 percent of the older subjects they tested had no recruitment, 30 percent showed partial recruitment, and 20 percent had almost complete recruitment. They interpreted the low prevalence of complete recruitment as being consistent with the prevalence of ganglion cell (as opposed to hair cell) damage.

Some information on recruitment was obtained by Goetzinger and colleagues (1961) using monaural and binaural loudness balance tests in 60- to 90-year-olds. Of 80 male ears tested, 27 showed complete recruitment, 41 showed incomplete recruitment, and 12 exhibited no recruitment. For females, of 40 ears tested, 7 had complete recruitment, 16 incomplete, and 17 no recruitment. Harbert et al. (1966) found no recruitment (monaural loudness balancing) in 70 percent of presbycusis subjects and minimal recruitment in the remaining 30 percent.

BEKESY AUDIOMETRY

Jerger (1960) obtained Bekesy audiometry tracings from a variety of subject groups, including individuals diagnosed as having presbycusis. Most presbycusis subjects demonstrated either Type I (55 percent) or Type II (34 percent) Bekesy tracings. A Type I tracing is characteristic of normal hearing listeners and is identified by interweaving of responses to continuous and interrupted tones and a tracing width of about 10 dB that is constant across frequency. In Type II tracings, the response to continuous tones drops moderately below the response to interrupted tones at high frequencies and the width of the tracings is often small (e.g., 3–5 dB) at the higher frequencies. The narrowing width of the tracing is an audiological sign of loudness recruitment. On the basis of these findings, about one-third of Jerger's cases of presbycusis were associated with recruitment of loudness. However, Jokinen (1970) found little evidence of recruitment from Bekesy tracings, with excursion amplitudes being normal and relatively constant over time in patients diagnosed as having presbycusis.

MAGNITUDE ESTIMATION

Knight and Margolis (1984) used alternate binaural loudness balancing and magnitude estimation to measure loudness in young adult listeners with normal hearing, adult listeners with asymmetrical sensorineural loss, and older listeners with bilateral, symmetrical sensorineural loss (presbycusis). In the asymmetrical group, both tests of loudness indicated recruitment and provided similar results, suggesting that the magnitude estimation technique was valid. Normal and presbycusis subjects were tested using magnitude estimation (because loudness balancing methods require either asymmetrical impairment or normal thresholds at some frequencies). There was a tendency toward steeper loudness functions in the older group, but it was significant only at 6 kHz (Fig. 8-8). Knight and Margolis pointed out that the absence of loudness recruitment, despite sensory cell damage (which accompanies presbycusis in most cases), suggests the presence of neural pathology.

INTENSITY DIFFERENCE LIMEN (DLI)

Data on intensity difference limens for listeners aged 60 to 89 years were reported by Konig (1957) for frequencies of 125–4000 Hz. Using the method of Luscher and Zwislocki (1948), complete or partial loudness recruitment was "usually present" when hearing loss exceeded 30 dB (usually the case at high frequencies). This method measures the listener's ability to detect small differences in tones that are rather abruptly modulated in amplitude.

THE SHORT INCREMENT SENSITIVITY INDEX (SISI)

The SISI involves the introduction of small increments of loudness during the testing period; listeners with sensorineural hearing loss detect more of these changes than normal hearing individuals. Jerger, Shedd, and Harford (1959) found a high degree of variance among subjects with presbycusis compared to consistently high scores typical of noise-impaired subjects. In their older subjects, scores ranged from zero (indicative of retrocochlear disorders) to 100 (indicative of cochlear disorders). Subjects with presbycusis in Otto and McCandless's (1982a) study tended to have lower SISI scores than young sensorineural subjects, particularly for 1 kHz stimuli. Young and Harbert (1967) and Konig (1969), however, found similar performance for presbycusis and other types of impaired subjects. Marshall (1981), reviewing these studies, suggested that the SISI would be affected by a

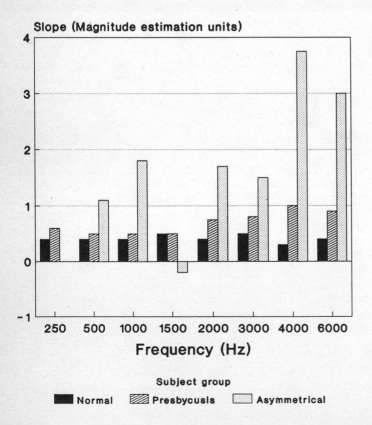

Figure 8-8. Magnitude estimation: loudness slope (adapted from Knight and Margolis, 1984).

conservative response criterion and, consequently, may be flawed as a test with elderly listeners. Nevertheless, the variance in the findings suggests a higher prevalence of neural involvement in the elderly impaired population than in the young impaired population.

ELECTROCOCHLEOGRAPHY

Bergholtz, Hooper, and Mehta (1977) used electrocochleography to measure the latency and waveform of the compound AP in patients with presbycusis. "Recruitment" of the AP (rapid rise in amplitude) was observed in 22 percent of the patients. Additional subjects with presbycusis had partial recruitment of the AP.

MIDDLE EAR REFLEX

While there is some disagreement as to the relationship of the acoustic reflex to the perception of loudness, it was shown in Chapter 7 that the acoustic reflex threshold often occurs at a lower than normal SL in older individuals, even when hearing loss is minimal. This may reflect loudness recruitment or a closely related phenomenon.

SUMMARY: LOUDNESS RECRUITMENT

Most tests of loudness recruitment in older listeners have involved subjects diagnosed as having presbycusis. In this group, some degree of loudness recruitment occurs in a sizable proportion ranging from about 20 to 50 percent of listeners. Undoubtedly, factors such as the type of cochlear disorder (e.g., sensory versus neural) and the degree of hearing loss have much to do with the occurrence of recruitment and the variance of findings across studies.

ADAPTATION

Adaptation refers to the decline in the sensation of a sustained sound. Abnormal adaptation is taken to be a sign of retrocochlear pathology, although cochlear pathology may also be a cause (Carhart, 1957). Abnormal adaptation can be demonstrated with tone decay tests or Bekesy audiometry.

TONE DECAY

Tone decay refers to a phenomenon in which listeners have difficulty in maintaining audibility for sustained tones presented at threshold, or even suprathreshold, levels.

Several groups of researchers have found little evidence of tone decay in older subjects, with or without presbycusis. In a study by Goetzinger et al. (1961) no significant age effects were obtained for tone decay. The largest range of tone decay in older subjects was at 2000 Hz, suggesting that some subjects may have exhibited decay at this frequency. Low prevalence of tone decay is also indicated by the data of Olsen and Noffsinger (1974). With several different tone decay tests, the incidence of test scores indicative of abnormal tone decay was 12 percent or less in patients diagnosed as having presbycusis (age 64 to 83). In a test battery evaluation by Otto and McCandless (1982a), 6 of 30 subjects with presbycusis had tone decay of 20 dB or more, and one showed suprathreshold adaptation. Gang (1976) and Quaranta, Salonna, and Longo, found little evidence of abnormal tone decay in older subjects with normal hearing for age. Harbert et al. (1966) concluded that tone decay in older, impaired subjects was within "clinically acceptable normal limits," but at high frequencies, decay was often near or slightly above the clinical limit.

Indeed, when high frequencies have been tested, stronger evidence of tone decay has emerged. Jerger and Jerger (1975) used a suprathreshold tone decay test on hearing-impaired patients of middle to old age. Significant tone decay occurred at 4000 Hz. Stephens and Hinchcliffe (1968) also found a high correlation between tone decay and age at 4000 and 8000 Hz (frequencies at which hearing loss is most pronounced, of course).

Tone decay was measured by Gjaevenes and Sohoel (1969) in various diagnostic groups, including patients identified as having presbycusis. In these subjects, peripheral hearing loss appeared to influence tone decay, although decay was never highly prevalent. Gjaevenes and Sohoel classified tone decay patterns. The absence of tone decay (a threshold change of 5 dB or less) was classified as Type Ia. Figure 8-9 summarizes the results of tone decay tests with 2000 Hz in subjects with normal hearing or with presbycusis, all of whom had normal tone decay performance with 500 Hz tones. Most normal hearing subjects of all ages were Type Ia (few normal hearing 80-year-olds were available). The majority of subjects with presbycusis were also classified as Type Ia. Decay of 6–10 dB was classified as Type Ib, while Types IIa, IIb, and III identified progressively more severe tone decay. These types increased in older subjects with presbycusis, although only about 25 percent of octogenarians exhibited one of the three most severe types.

BEKESY AUDIOMETRY AND ADAPTATION

Adaptation is also measured using Bekesy audiometry by examining the threshold performance over time for continuous and interrupted tones. Jerger (1960) used Bekesy audiometry to assess numerous individuals with hearing loss, including individuals with presbycusis (Fig. 8-10). Most of these individuals had Type I (normal) tracing and Type II (cochlear loss). The Type II tracings indicate moderately enhanced adaptation at high frequencies. Very few people with presbycusis demonstrated Type IV tracing (response to continuous tone drops well below the response to interrupted tones, including low-frequency tones), indicating abnormal adaptation typical of retrocochlear pathology.

Subjects diagnosed as having presbycusis were tested for adaptation by Harbert and co-workers (1966). They demonstrated only a small increase in the separation of thresholds to pulsed and continuous tones compared to normal hearing subjects, particularly for high frequencies (Fig. 8-11). This difference was similar to a Type II tracing (asterisks), indicative of cochlear pathology, but was very different from the Type III tracing (retrocochlear pathology). The authors also noted that the subjects with presbycusis performed similarly to a group of patients with Meniere's disease at frequencies above 1000 Hz when hearing levels were similar.

Jokinen performed a series of studies assessing adaptation in patients diagnosed as having presbycusis. Jokinen (1969) compared performance of older individuals on continuous and pulsed tones. As shown in

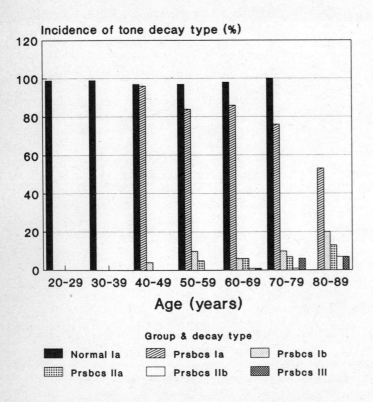

Figure 8-9. Tone decay for 2000 Hz tones (adapted from Gjaevenes and Sohoel, 1969). Tone decay type Ia is normal, Ib, IIa, IIb, and III indicate progressively more pronounced tone decay.

Figure 8-10. Types of Bekesy tracings for presbycusis and other diagnostic categories (adapted from Jerger, 1960). Type I is normal, Type II indicates cochlear impairment, Types III and IV indicate auditory nerve disorders.

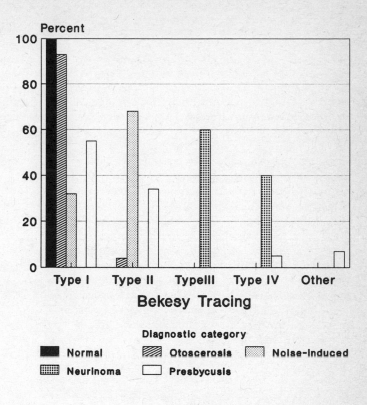

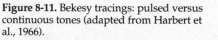

Figure 8-11. Bekesy tracings: pulsed versus continuous tones (adapted from Harbert et al., 1966).

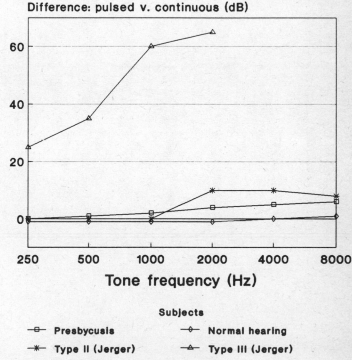

Figure 8-12, presbycusis patients with or without a 4000 Hz "dip" in the audiogram, indicative of noise-induced hearing loss (NIHL), performed more poorly on continuous tones (all differences above 3.5 were statistically significant). The presence of NIHL exacerbated abnormal adaptation at high frequencies, but not at low frequencies. Jokinen (1970) extended this study by measuring adaptation to continuous tones 3 minutes long; adaptation exceeding 30 dB was not found in any subject with presbycusis. However, the adaptation that did occur was greater at 2000 and 4000 Hz than at lower frequencies, with about 25 percent of the subjects having adaptation of 11–30 dB (compared to 8 percent with 1000 Hz tones). There was no appreciable age effect within the 59- to 86-year range of subjects' ages. Jokinen and Karja (1970) evaluated adaptation using both forward and reverse frequency sweeps. Presbycusis was not associated with abnormal adaptation with either sweep direction. Jokinen's data indicate that some listeners with presbycusis exhibit abnormal adaptation but the magnitude of abnormality tends to be small.

SUMMARY: ADAPTATION

Taking all of this together, it appears that abnormal adaptation, as revealed by tone decay or Bekesy tracings, is not a major correlate of aging. Nevertheless, moderately abnormal adaptation is observed in some subjects with presbycusis, particularly at high frequencies. Severely abnormal adaptation, as found with retrocochlear lesions, does not typically accompany aging or presbycusis.

DISTORTION OF COCHLEAR OUTPUT: AURAL OVERLOAD

Aural overload refers to the relationship between the occurrence of suprathreshold distortion (e.g., the pro-

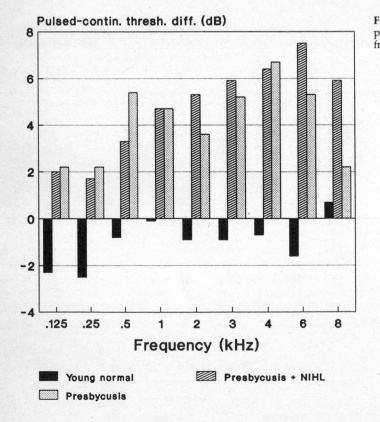

Figure 8-12. Threshold differences for pulsed versus continuous tones (adapted from Jokinen, 1969).

negative = poorer pulsed threshold

duction of harmonics by the ear) and the suprathreshold intensity (Lawrence and Yantis, 1957). If aural harmonics are present in response to a tone, a second "probe" tone of twice the frequency will result in the perception of beats. The point of distortion may be nearer to threshold in pathologic ears, reducing the undistorted dynamic range (Lawrence, 1958). For instance, Ross, Huntington, Newby, and Dixon (1965) found a decrease in the dynamic range of undistorted hearing for 500 and 2000 Hz in their hearing-impaired subjects, many of whom were older.

Bergman (1980) used the aural overload test of Humes (1978) on young (20 to 29) and middle-aged (40 to 49) subjects and found a lowered threshold for overload in the latter group, relative to sensation level. He suggested that the occurrence of abnormal overload in a normal-hearing group of middle-aged subjects might be a pre-clinical sign of presbycusis.

Harbert et al. (1966) tested for aural overload in subjects aged 60 to 85. The point of overload increased with age relative to audiometric zero. For instance, at 1000 Hz the point of overload was 65–70 dB for ages 60 to 65, while the point of overload was 90–95 dB in subjects over 75. The median point of overload for all their presbycusis subjects was 80 dB at 1000 Hz, 17 dB above the median of their normal hearing group. The median absolute threshold for this group was 35 dB (re: 1950 ASA standard). Thus, it is likely that the overload point decreased relative to sensation level in the elderly group as a whole. Their statistical analysis revealed that the change in overload point was correlated more closely with age than with absolute threshold. They suggested that an age-related increase in basilar membrane stiffness might be responsible for this.

As Bergman (1980) suggested, the measurement of aural overload may be valuable in revealing peripheral dysfunction in the elderly. However, little attention has been given to this question.

FREQUENCY DISCRIMINATION AND RESOLUTION

The ability of the auditory system to repond to the frequency components of sound impacts on several aspects of hearing. These include frequency discrimination (the ability to discern changes in frequency), and frequency resolution (the ability of the auditory system to respond selectively to the frequency components of a complex sound). Moore and Glasberg (1986)

reviewed the literature on frequency discrimination and frequency resolution and noted that the two are not always affected in the same way by cochlear impairment. For instance, poor frequency resolution is not always accompanied by poor frequency discrimination. Thus, frequency discrimination and frequency resolution appear to involve different mechanisms.

FREQUENCY DISCRIMINATION

A number of studies have shown reduced frequency discrimination (e.g., increased frequency difference limens, DLF) with cochlear hearing impairment in young listeners (Marshall, 1981; Turner and Nelson, 1982). Thus, the role of peripheral presbycusis must be considered in assessing age-related changes.

Konig (1969) noted that many years ago, Stucker (1908) recognized that older listeners had impaired frequency discrimination. Somewhat later Meurman (1954) found increased frequency difference limens in older persons. Tilling (1958; cited by Marshall, 1981) obtained increased DLFs in older listeners for frequencies of 125 to 8000 Hz. However, the older subjects also had significant hearing loss.

Konig (1957) assessed the relationship of age to difference limens across frequencies (Fig. 8-13). The method of constant stimuli was used at about 40 dB above each subject's threshold. Frequency discrimination decreased linearly between 25 and 55 years and then became markedly worse at older ages, particularly at high and low frequencies. While subjects younger than 60 had rather good hearing, the older subjects had a degree of hearing loss. For example, compared to young subjects, thresholds of the two oldest age groups for 125–500 Hz were elevated by at least 10 dB, and thresholds from 2000–4000 Hz were elevated by more than 30 dB. Thus, hearing loss might have contributed to the results in the old subjects, at least at high frequencies. Nevertheless, the fact that the greatest changes in DLFs were at low frequencies (for which threshold elevations were smallest) and the appearance of increased DLFs at all frequencies as early as 30 to 39 years (before hearing loss was significant) suggests that age-related factors other than hearing loss contributed to diminished frequency discrimination.

Two other studies indicate that both peripheral presbycusis and other age-related factors interfere with frequency discrimination. Using the method of constant stimuli, Ross and colleagues (1965) determined that the DLF was greater in their hearing-impaired group than in their normal-hearing group. Within the groups, age was positively correlated with

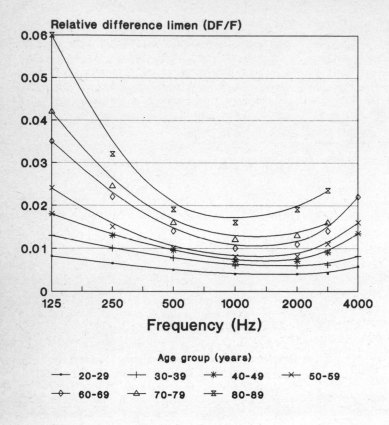

Figure 8-13. Relative difference limens for pure tones (adapted from Konig, 1957).

an increase in the DLF for their normal hearing subjects (30 to 56 years) but not for their hearing impaired group (22 to 72 years). Thus, the effects of peripheral hearing loss on DLFs may have obscured the age effect. Abel, Krever, and Alberti (1990) tested subjects who varied as a function of both hearing loss and age. Aging without concomitant hearing loss was associated with increased DLFs at both 500 Hz and 4000 Hz. Hearing loss, unconfounded by age, was associated with increased DLFs at 4000 Hz only.

In summary, frequency discrimination tends to decline in older listeners. The results of several studies converge in indicating contributions of peripheral presbycusis as well as other age-related factors, probably involving the CAS (e.g., central presbycusis).

FREQUENCY RESOLUTION AND THE MASKING OF TONES

Frequency resolution is dependent upon the frequency selectivity of the ear and involves the notion of cochlear bandpass filters, appreciated since the time of Helmholtz (1863). The filter characteristics (frequency selectivity) of the cochlea have typically been defined by masking experiments. Information about filter characteristics can be gleaned from the critical band width (the band of frequencies surrounding a pure tone; one way of defining the "filter bandwidth" of the cochlea around the center frequency), critical ratio (CR; the ratio of intensity per Hz of a noise and the intensity of a pure tone just masked by the noise), psychophysical tuning curves (see below), and other methods.

Tyler (1986) reviewed the literature on the effects of cochlear pathology (in most cases, other than age-related) on frequency selectivity. A great deal of evidence indicates that many listeners with sensorineural hearing loss have reduced frequency resolution; however, large between-subject differences are found even when audiograms are matched. Reduced frequency selectivity is manifested by various tests. Florentine, Buus, Scharf, and Zwicker (1980) measured frequency selectivity using psychophysical tuning curves, narrow-band masking, two-tone masking, and loudness summation (an increase in loudness when stimulus band width exceeds the critical band). In listeners with several types of hearing loss (none of which was presbycusis), frequency selectivity was reduced at affected frequencies, irrespective of the test levels used, and was correlated with the degree of hearing loss. The authors cited numerous other studies showing reduced loudness summation, broader psychophysical tuning curves, an increased spread of masking, and shallow two-tone masking functions in hearing-impaired listeners (pp. 662-663). Thus, it is probable that presbycusis would, likewise, result in reduced frequency resolution.

PSYCHOPHYSICAL TUNING CURVES (PTCS)

PTCs are obtained with a "probe tone" of fixed frequency and intensity that is masked by a tone whose frequency is made to vary; the result is a V-shaped threshold curve reminiscent of tuning curves obtained from auditory nerve fibers. PTCs are abnormal in hearing impaired subjects, typically being sharply tuned in regions of normal absolute thresholds and abnormally broad in regions of threshold elevations (Florentine et al., 1980; Tyler, 1986).

Zwicker and Schorn (1978) obtained psychophysical tuning curves from several diagnostic categories of hearing pathology including presbycusis. Subjects with average hearing losses of 35 and 50 dB at 500 Hz and 4000 Hz, respectively, had PTCs that had shifted upward and were very shallow at these frequencies (showing a loss of frequency selectivity). In a later, similar study (Zwicker and Schorn, 1990), frequency resolution in presbycusis subjects was further reduced by the addition of background noise at 4000 Hz (but not at 500 Hz).

Psychophysical tuning curves were obtained by Matschke (1991) in subjects aged 20 to 70 who had normal hearing for age and had medical histories that would not affect their hearing. For subjects over 60, a decline in frequency selectivity at 4 kHz was observed. Since "normal hearing" for people over 60 involves some elevation of high-frequency thresholds, a contribution of hearing loss to these findings cannot be ruled out.

CRITICAL BANDS AND CRITICAL RATIOS

These measures are not always affected greatly by cochlear pathology, although some studies have found them to increase with high-frequency loss (see Marshall, 1981 for references). Margolis and Goldberg (1980) assessed frequency selectivity using the detectability of tone signals as a function of the cutoff frequency of a low-pass, computer-generated noise masker. This method appeared to provide an estimate of the width of critical masking bands. They tested four hearing-impaired subjects aged 63 to 70 years with no history of exposure to excessive noise or ototoxic drugs. A simple relationship between hearing impairment and frequency selectivity was not found. Three of the four had elevated critical ratios; however normal frequency selectivity was observed in some despite elevated critical ratios.

Bonding (1979) used loudness summation to determine critical bands in older subjects with fairly flat hearing loss, presumed to have strial presbycusis. Most of these subjects, irrespective of the degree of hearing loss (e.g., greater or less than 50 dB HL), had normal critical bands. The same was true of young patients with sensorineural hearing loss. However, mean data obscure the fact that several elderly subjects had extremely broad critical bands.

Critical ratios of young and older (55 to 65 years) subjects were compared by Miller (1981). The subjects had normal thresholds at the frequencies employed, 483 and 2954 Hz. No significant differences in the width of critical ratios were found. However, when the older subjects were divided into two subgroups on the basis of their audiograms (better or worse than 15 dB HL) the groups did differ.

It was suggested by Jakimetz and colleagues (1989) that frequency resolution was decreased in older subjects they used in acoustic reflex experiments. This was based on their finding that the acoustic reflex threshold was less affected by increased spectral density compared to young subjects (see Chapter 7; Fig. 7-4). They felt that the number of effective frequency components was related to the number of critical bands within the multi-tonal complexes they used. Since the older subjects had a smaller number of components at which the spectral density effect reached a plateau (5 compared to 7 in young subjects), wider critical bands are implied.

Properties of *auditory filters* in older listeners have been inferred from masking experiments. Patterson, Nimmo-Smith, Weber, and Milroy (1982) measured frequency selectivity as indicated by derived auditory filters from experiments that masked speech or tones with a stopband noise centered around a center frequency (500, 2000, or 4000 Hz). As the noise stopband was widened, performance improved, but the improvement was diminished in older listeners. Patterson and colleagues derived filter shapes from their data and found that the auditory filter broadened with age (23 to 75 years) at each center frequency, with the greatest loss of selectivity occurring at 4000 Hz. The dynamic range of the filter decreased with age as well, and the critical ratio increased at all three center frequencies. Lutman et al. (1991) noted that, while the subjects in this study met criteria for normal hearing, there was a confounding correlation between age and hearing loss.

The shape and symmetry of the auditory filter at 2000 Hz was determined in subjects ranging from 22 to 74 years of age by Glasberg, Moore, Patterson, and Nimmo-Smith (1984). The filters had steeper slopes on the high-frequency side, but the degree of asymmetry varied among subjects. The bandwidth of the filter increased with age and the slope of the lower skirt decreased. The slope of the upper skirt was more highly (and negatively) correlated with threshold. The dynamic range and sharpness of the filter tended to decrease in the older listeners.

SUMMARY: FREQUENCY RESOLUTION

The research on frequency resolution in older listeners presents evidence for an age-related decline. Peripheral hearing loss is largely responsible, but other age-related factors also play a lesser role. This conclusion is supported by the results of the National Study of Hearing in Great Britain recently reported by Lutman and colleagues (Lutman, 1991; Lutman, Gatehouse, and Worthington, 1991). PTCs, obtained from more than 1100 adult subjects, revealed that frequency resolution declined as hearing loss increased. When hearing level was accounted for, there was only a minor decline in frequency resolution that depended on age. Similar results were obtained with a notch-noise method to estimate filter band width. There was no significant interaction involving age and hearing loss.

OTHER ASPECTS OF MASKING

THE EFFECTIVENESS AND SPREAD OF MASKING

Jerger, Tillman, and Peterson (1960) obtained masked thresholds at several frequencies above and below narrowband noise maskers. The maskers were present so as to produce 10 or 30 dB of masking within the band. In the latter condition, subjects with presbycusis showed an abnormally large amount of masking for frequencies above and below the masker frequencies. In other words, there was an increased spread of masking. Increased spread of masking was replicated with impaired listeners by Rittmanic (1962), Harbert and Young (1965), Martin and Pickett (1970), de Boer and Bouwmeester (1974), Leshowitz (1977), and others. In the latter study, subjects with presbycusis—but not those with noise-induced hearing loss—had in-

creased masked thresholds for frequencies below the masker frequency.

Other studies have investigated masking in cochlear-impaired subjects, albeit not necessarily elderly. Smits and Duifhis (1982) measured masking in (non-presbycusis) sensorineural listeners. Compared to normal-hearing subjects, masked thresholds of the impaired listeners were higher at frequencies for which a hearing loss occurred and at frequencies for which sensitivity was near normal. The masker did not need to be very intense. Masked thresholds for tones in the presence of different levels of broadband noise were obtained by Tyler, Fernandes, and Wood (1982) from subjects with impaired cochleas (average age 51 years). Several of the impaired listeners had higher masked thresholds than normal-hearing subjects. The growth of masking as the masker level was increased was linear for normal listeners, but was disproportionate and nonlinear for some impaired subjects. Thresholds in noise could not be predicted from thresholds in quiet (as has also been found in other studies). They concluded from their study, and from reviewing the literature, that a great deal of between-subject variance exists; some peripherally impaired listeners have increased masked thresholds, while others do not. Furthermore, some impaired listeners have enhanced growth of masking, in that increases in masking level have disproportionate masking effects.

A recent study by Klein, Mills, and Adkins (1990) determined that young and elderly listeners with normal hearing had similar upward spread of masking, as indicated by masked thresholds. Hearing loss was associated with greater upward-masked thresholds, but young and old subjects with similar audiograms performed similarly. A good deal of variability was seen in older listeners, and some had lower upward-masked thresholds than young subjects.

From these studies it would be expected that peripheral presbycusis would be associated with abnormal spread of masking. Aging per se does not appear to be an important factor. However, there is considerable variance among individual elderly listeners with regard to the occurrence, magnitude, and even direction of change in upward masking.

REMOTE MASKING

Remote masking refers to a rise in threshold for low-frequency tones when the ear is exposed to a high-intensity noise band of high frequency (Bilger and Hirsh, 1956). It has been attributed to a mechanical distortion in the cochlea, implying that mechanical changes in the cochlea (e.g., mechanical presbycusis) would reduce the remote masking. Therefore, Quaranta, Amoroso, and Cervellera (1978) evaluated remote masking in subjects with presbycusis. In older listeners with hearing loss, remote masking was reduced by more than 10 dB in 60- to 70-year-olds and by an additional 4–8 dB in subjects older than 70. More recently, Quaranta, et al. (1991) reported that remote masking was almost always abnormal in aged subjects, even though their audiograms were within normal limits for age. While these findings might be accounted for by mechanical changes in the cochlea, it is not clear whether other factors (e.g., central) could be responsible for changes in remote masking.

MASKING LEVEL DIFFERENCE (MLD)

The difference in detection level of a binaural signal presented in phase (homophasic) and detection of the signal presented out of phase (antiphasic) is the MLD (Hirsh, 1948). Although the MLD is presumably mediated by the central auditory system (CAS), a number of studies have shown that, in the presence of wideband noise, the MLD is reduced in cochlear impaired listeners (Hall and Harvey, 1985, Marshall, 1981).

An effect of peripheral presbycusis on the MLD is indicated by the work of Olsen, Noffsinger, and Carhart (1976). They measured MLDs for 500 Hz tones (and

spondee words; see Chapter 9) in a variety of patients. Those diagnosed as having presbycusis tended to have reduced MLDs for both types of stimuli. Kelly-Ballweber and Dobie (1984) found that MLDs of older subjects did not differ significantly from those of young subjects with matched audiograms, indicating that effects of age-related factors were not in evidence. These studies suggest that the presence of peripheral presbycusis is sufficient to interfere with the MLD. The topic of MLDs and aging, with respect to speech perception, is discussed further in Chapter 9.

MASKING BY "INTERNAL NOISE"

The MLD is usually measured with the addition of an external noise, but Novak and Anderson (1982) measured it with 500 Hz tones in noise and in quiet to assess the presence of "neural noise." MLDs were obtained from normal-hearing young and old subjects, subjects diagnosed as having sensory, neural, or strial presbycusis, and other groups of young or old subjects. The subjects in the three presbycusis groups had similar sensitivity (within 6 dB at all frequencies). The neural and sensory subjects were a bit older than the old normal and strial groups. Figure 8-14 summa-

Figure 8-14. Masking level difference in quiet and noise for several types of presbycusis (adapted from Novak and Anderson, 1982).

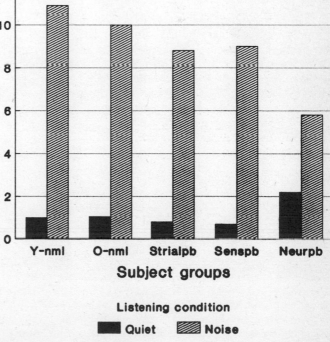

Subject groups: young normal; old normal; strial presbycusis; sensory presbycusis; neural presbycusis

rizes the findings. The neural presbycusis group performed differently from the other old subjects. Using a MLD of 7 to distinguish normal from abnormal MLDs in noise (after Olsen et al., 1976) five of six subjects in the neural group were abnormal, whereas only one of six subjects in the strial group and no subjects in the sensory group were abnormal. By contrast, in quiet, MLDs of the neural group were larger than the other groups. The findings of smaller MLDs in noise and larger MLDs in quiet in the neural group were supported statistically.

Novak and Anderson cited earlier propositions by Gregory (1974), Crossman and Szafram (1956), and Talland (1968) that aging is associated with an increase in "neural noise" (i.e., spontaneous activity). They interpreted their findings in this framework, concluding that the loss of neurons (peripheral and/or central) in neural presbycusis might enhance the neural noise. This hypothesis accounts for the increase in MLDs in quiet; they are more similar to what occurs with external noise. The reason for the decrease of MLDs in noise is less clear, but Novak and Anderson proposed an interaction between internal and external noise; the internal noise may lessen the effectiveness of the external noise. It may also be the case that the reduced number of auditory nerve fibers resulted in a lesser overall input to the CAS from the external noise, diminishing its effectiveness as a masker.

The concept of internal masking may be manifested in other ways as well. Gregory (1974) measured the differential threshold for intensity as a function of the intensity level in older listeners with and without hearing loss. The constant relationship of $\Delta I/I$ broke down at lower signal levels. With increased hearing loss the increase in $\Delta I/I$ was not proportional to the increase in ΔI. The change in older persons with hearing loss was mimicked by an externally introduced masking noise. Gregory interpreted the change in older persons to be related to internal "neural noise" that occurs in the aging brain.

TEMPORAL PARAMETERS OF SOUND AND PERCEPTION

The relationship between the temporal parameters of sound and hearing ability may be manifested in several ways, including discrimination of time intervals for brief stimuli (both monaurally and binaurally) and temporal integration (the absolute threshold as a function of the duration of a sound). Sensorineural hearing loss is typically associated with poorer temporal performance in young, hearing impaired subjects (see Marshall, 1981 for references), so once again, peripheral presbycusis in older listeners is likely to be a key element in temporal processes.

TEMPORAL DISCRIMINATION

MONAURAL TEMPORAL DISCRIMINATION

The Wichita Auditory Fusion Test was administered to elderly listeners by McCroskey and Davis (1976) and McCroskey and Kasten (1980). This test is comprised of pairs of short duration tones (250–4000 Hz), with a method of limits to determine fusion points. The tones are separated by increasing or decreasing durations and the point is determined where they no longer are perceived as continuous. The ability to detect short, silent intervals began to decline in the mid-50's and deteriorated with further aging (Fig. 8-15). The mean auditory fusion time for older subjects increased most at 250 Hz, followed by 4000 Hz, and 1000 Hz. Because the age effect was observed well above threshold (60 dB SL) and was strongest at 250 Hz, hearing loss alone cannot adequately account for these findings.

Zwicker and Schorn (1990) and Schorn and Zwicker (1990) reported that subjects diagnosed as having presbycusis showed impaired temporal resolution at 4000 Hz but not at 500 Hz (measured with a technique based on masking period patterns), with and without background noise. Similar results were obtained with other cochlear-impaired patient groups.

Ludlow, Cudahy, and Bassich (1982) tested gap detection and temporal order performance in subjects aged 18 to 70 years. The gap was embedded in broadband noise and the temporal order task involved 1000 and 2500 Hz tones, using a go-no-go vigilance paradigm. Both gap detection and temporal order thresholds became elevated with age, especially beyond 50 years. It should be noted that sensorineural hearing loss (irrespective of age) results in increased gap detection thresholds (Glasberg, Moore, and Bacon, 1987). This may account for the findings of Lutman (1991), who assessed gap-detection in subjects aged 50 to 75. Within this age range, hearing threshold level, but not age, was correlated with poorer performance.

On the other hand, age but not hearing loss was associated with increased duration DLs for some stimuli in a study by Abel et al. (1990), in which the ability of subjects to discern a difference in the duration of noise bands was assessed.

Figure 8-15. Auditory fusion point for 1000 Hz stimuli at 60 dB SL (adapted from McCroskey and Kasten, 1980).

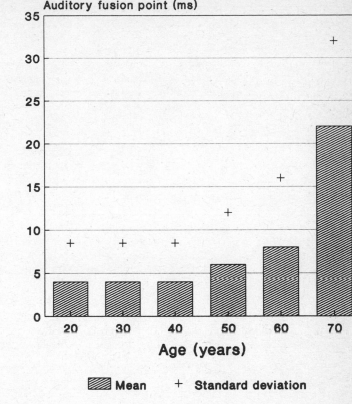

BINAURAL TEMPORAL DISCRIMINATION

Making temporal discriminations of sounds presented to two ears requires the CAS to compare binaural time cues. Thus, both peripheral and central portions of the auditory system are taxed by these tasks. Binaural time cues, of course, are important for the localization of sounds, discussed later. Herman, Warren, and Wagener (1977) tested the ability of young and old men (60 to 72 years) to identify the apparent left or right location of a train of clicks presented binaurally through headphones. The old subjects had normal hearing at 2000 Hz and below, but high-frequency sensitivity was substantially poorer than that of young subjects. Two types of cues were used: interaural click onset asynchrony and interaural differences in intensity. The older listeners required longer time delays to "lateralize" the sound; however, their performance equaled that of the younger listeners when using the interaural intensity cues. Because a forced choice technique was used, Herman and colleagues felt that possible age differences in response criteria probably did not influence the results.

These studies are consistent with an earlier study by Matzker and Springborn (1958), which determined the minimal interaural time delay required to report that the apparent source of a click train was not located in the center of the subject's head (summarized by Herman et al. 1977). Subjects in their 20's required 21.6 usec whereas subjects in their 60's required 52.2 usec (corresponding to an increase in the minimal audible angle from about 2.5 degrees to about 6.0 degrees).

TEMPORAL DISCRIMINATION: SUMMARY

On the basis of these few studies, aging appears to be correlated with reduced ability to utilize time cues, including binaural cues used in spatial localization. Peripheral presbycusis appears to contribute importantly to the deficits in temporal perception. However, other age-related changes (e.g., central) are probably relevant as well, particularly with regard to binaural discrimination of time cues.

TEMPORAL INTEGRATION

Sensorineural hearing loss, irrespective of aging, is sufficient to produce deficits in temporal integration and must be considered as a factor with older listeners (Pedersen and Elberling, 1973; Chung and Smith, 1980; Marshall, 1981).

Corso, Wright, and Valerio (1976) obtained threshold-duration functions in an older group (51 to 57 years) using brief-tone audiometry (varying the duration and intensity of sounds to obtain thresholds). Compared to a theoretic curve for young listeners (Fig. 8-16), the older subjects had depressed threshold-duration functions, particularly at 4,000 Hz. Young, noise-exposed subjects showed a flattening of the temporal integration curve similar to that seen in old subjects, suggesting that sensorineural pathology is responsible for the decrease in temporal integration of the older subjects.

Temporal integration was measured in subjects with acoustic trauma (Pedersen, 1973) or presbycusis (Pedersen and Elberling, 1973). Very similar decreases in temporal integration, vis a vis hearing loss, were observed in both hearing-impaired groups. Individuals showed normal temporal integration for some frequencies but not others. In subjects diagnosed as having presbycusis, temporal integration was closely correlated with the degree of hearing loss.

Chung (1982) measured hearing thresholds for 20 msec. and 500 msec. tones in normal (average age of 30.1 years) and generally older, noise-impaired listeners (average age of 60.2 years). The mean temporal integration function (hearing thresholds for long- and short-duration sounds as a function of frequency) was inversely related to peripheral hearing loss, as found by others. However, temporal integration for individuals was not predictable from the audiogram.

Thresholds were obtained by Goldstein and Kramer (1960) for tones of varying durations (20 msec. to 2000 msec.) in normal hearing adults (HLs no worse than 10 dB at 0.5, 1, and 2 kHz). They divided subjects into two groups, older or younger than 40 years. The older group had thresholds that were 2.5 to 3 dB higher than those of the younger group at all durations. However, there was no age-by-duration interaction; the curves were parallel as a function of duration. These findings indicate that older subjects with good hearing sensitivity had normal temporal integration. However, several older subjects required a loud sample of the shortest (20 msec.) tone in order to "orient" themselves, after which performance was, for the most part, normal.

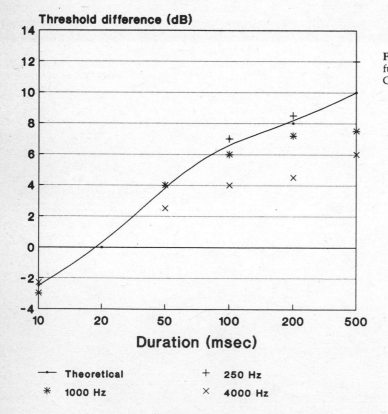

Figure 8-16. Threshold change as a function of tone duration (adapted from Corso et al., 1976).

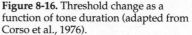

In summary, presbycusis appears to be associated with deficiencies in temporal integration that are correlated with the severity of hearing loss. There is little evidence that other age-related factors exacerbate the deficiency.

SPATIAL LOCALIZATION

When binaural cues are used to locate sounds, the CAS must make exquisitely precise computations of interaural time and intensity data provided by the ears. Thus, it would be expected that both central and peripheral processes must function well if localization is to be optimal.

It can be predicted that peripheral presbycusis would pose problems for sound localization because it has been shown that some young subjects with bilateral, symmetrical sensorineural impairment have deficits in the ability to discriminate a major cue in spatial localization, interaural time differences (Hawkins and Wightman, 1980; Rosenhall, 1985). Conductive impairment can also be associated with poor binaural hearing in some individuals, as indicated by MLD and time discrimination thresholds (Hall and Derlacki, 1986).

Several studies have provided evidence that older listeners can have diminished spatial localization. Konig (1969) cited two German articles that reported an age-related decline in directional hearing but differed with regard to the age of onset. Matzker and Springborn (1958) found an age-related decline in the ability to discern interaural time differences that began at a fairly young age. Preibisch-Effenberger (1966) observed a decline in directional hearing in the free field, but only after age 60. In a study by Baschek (1979), subjects aged 70 to 90 years had diminished ability to differentiate small directional changes in the location of a sound source. Colburn, Barker, and Milner (1982) tested free-field localization abilities in several hearing-impaired listeners, at least one of which was diagnosed as having presbycusis. Impaired subjects' vertical localization abilities were much worse than normal, and they made many front-back errors.

Hausler, Colburn, and Marr (1983) used pairwise discrimination tests to measure sound localization ability in subjects with various types of hearing impairments, including presbycusis. Included in their subject population were individuals diagnosed as having strial presbycusis and neural presbycusis. They measured both the minimal audible angle (MAA) in the free field and the ability to discriminate interaural time and intensity cues delivered from headphones. Subjects with good speech discrimination scores (strial presbycusis and others) had normal localization performance, whereas those with poor speech discrimination (neural presbycusis and others) performed poorly on localization tasks. In fact, vertical MAA could not even be measured in the subjects with neural presbycusis. Figure 8-17 presents examples of results from each type of subject. Hausler and colleagues also found that the results were not dependent upon sensation level; performance was similar at 85 dB SPL irrespective of the degree of hearing loss. Determination of the just noticeable difference (JND) for interaural time differences was also made for some subjects. In one individual with neural presbycusis, JNDs were modestly increased (30 µsec compared to 10–20 µsec in a subject with good speech discrimination) for broadband noise, 1000 Hz low pass noise, and 500 Hz tones; however, JNDs were grossly increased (greater than 500 µsec) for 3300 Hz tones.

The ability of patients to identify the location of a sound source in a free-field listening situation was assessed by Nordlund (1964). Individuals with (non-presbycusis) cochlear lesions had only slightly impaired performance. By contrast, patients with lesions of the auditory nerve or brainstem (pons) had great difficulty in locating sounds. Extrapolating these findings to presbycusis suggests that peripheral neural presbycusis or central presbycusis would be associated with difficulties in spatial localization.

A phenomenon associated with spatial localization is the precedence effect. The precedence effect can be observed by presenting identical sounds from opposite sides of a subject's head. With short delays to normal hearing subjects, the pair of sounds becomes fused and is perceived as originating in the leading sound source. This is presumed to involve suppression of the second sound by the CAS. Cranford, Boose, and Moore (1990) tested normal hearing young subjects and elderly subjects with a small degree of hearing loss. At inter-speaker delays of less than 0.7 msec., the older subjects performed more poorly in identifying the leading side. While there was some indication that high-frequency hearing loss may have contributed to the findings, subgroups of older subjects differing with respect to hearing loss did not differ in performance. The findings suggest that the precedence effect

Figure 8-17. Minimal audible angle in two cases of presbycusis (adapted from Hausler et al., 1983).

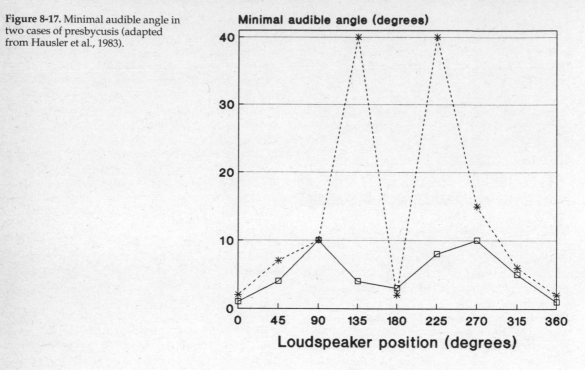

Minimal audible angle (degrees)

Loudspeaker position (degrees)

Sensorineural with:

Good speech discrim.   Poor speech discrim.

Note: Maximum values are greater than 40

is affected by age, although (as the authors point out), further work is needed to be sure that conservative response criteria did not influence the elderly subject's performance.

SUMMARY: SPATIAL LOCALIZATION

There is evidence that peripheral auditory dysfunction contributes to a decline in spatial localization performance in older people. However, as suggested by the findings of Hausler et al. (1983) and Nordlund (1964), it may be necessary that significant neural pathology is involved before spatial localization is greatly affected. There is also evidence that the use of localization cues may be deficient in some elderly listeners who do not have significant peripheral presbycusis. This was seen in research on the precedence effect (Cranford et al., 1990) and the use of binaural time cues discussed earlier. These changes are likely to involve central mechanisms that have been impaired by aging.

BEHAVIORAL STUDIES WITH ANIMALS

Little behavioral work has been done on the auditory capacities of animal models of presbycusis. A few behavioral studies have demonstrated age-related hearing loss in rodents and cats (Chapter 4). A behavioral study by Bennett, Davis, and Miller (1983) used both cross sectional and longitudinal approaches to demonstrate presbycusis in rhesus monkeys. Other auditory capacities that have been behaviorally examined are directional hearing, temporal processing, and the acoustic startle response.

Harrison (1981) employed a cross-sectional design to evaluate the ability of aging Sprague-Dawley rats to localize sounds. Stimuli were 300 msec. noise pulses at 70 dB SPL emitted from one of two loudspeakers. The rats, aged 12 and 30 months, were trained to press a lever (for food reward) close to the speaker emitting sound during a trial. Both old and young rats acquired the learned response quickly. Across trials, the percentage of correct responses reached an asymptotic level which was lower (i.e., fewer correct responses) for the older rats. However, the effect was small, since the old rats responded at a level of more than 90 percent correct. Harrison attributed the small decrease in performance level of the old rats to the modest age-related threshold elevation that occurs in this strain (see Chapter 4). In another study, Brown (1984) used a longitudinal design with Sprague-Dawley rats. They were trained to press one bar (on the left side of the testing apparatus) if a 200 msec. pink noise (75 dBA) was presented from the left side and to press a bar on the right when the sound was presented on that side. By 21 months of age, accuracy of localization had declined from greater than 90 percent to less than 69 percent correct. The age-related decline was greater in Brown's study than Harrison's, but results were otherwise similar. Brown attributed the quantitative differences to procedures that made his task more difficult (e.g., Harrison's stimuli had more high frequencies which are more easily localized by rats).

These studies, particularly that of Brown (1984), indicate that aging is accompanied by decreased directional hearing ability in Sprague-Dawley rats. Since the degree of hearing loss is not great at this age (Chapter 4), it seems unlikely that this would account for Brown's findings. However, the medial nucleus of the trapezoid body, a brain region important for the localization of sounds, exhibits a 34 percent loss of neurons by 2 years of age (see the work of Casey and Feldman, Chapter 4). One might speculate, therefore, that central changes are responsible for the localization deficits.

The phenomenon of reflex modification was used to evaluate auditory capacities in aging CBA mice by Ison and colleagues (Ison, O'Neill, and Walton, 1991). The acoustic startle response (ASR) can be inhibited by an audible sound preceding the startle-eliciting stimulus. The ability of sounds to affect the startle indicates that the auditory system responded to the modifying sound. Using this method, Ison and colleagues found a degree of hearing loss in the oldest mice (22 to 28 months) since more intense sounds were required to modify the startle. Despite a mild loss of sensitivity in old CBA mice, a good ASR could be elicited, allowing the reflex modification technique to be applied. Ison and colleagues used a gap of silence as the inhibiting stimulus and varied gap parameters to determine if gap detection was altered in the old mice. Gap detection was not significantly affected by aging. They did observe that, under certain conditions, there was an increase in the time required to modify the startle response in the old mice, suggesting a slowing of auditory processing.

The ASR was measured in aging C57 and CBA mice by Parham and Willott (1988). They were interested in the ASR as an auditory behavior in its own right, rather than as a test of modifiers. As shown in Figure 8-18, rather different patterns of age-related change are exhibited by the two strains. "Thresholds" of the ASR of aging CBA mice were modestly elevated at all frequencies across the actuarial life span of 18 months. By comparison, ASR thresholds of aging C57 mice became elevated by 6 months of age, but only at the higher frequencies. By 10 months the elevation of ASR thresholds progressed, and by 12 months (not shown), ASRs could not be elicited with tone pips. The differences between the strains is likely to be due to the progressive high-frequency hearing loss exhibited by C57 mice versus the less severe, "flat" loss exhibited by CBA mice (Chapter 4). However, the relationship between absolute sensory thresholds and ASR thresholds is not a simple one in C57 mice. Absolute sensory thresholds are only minimally elevated at 8 and 12 kHz in 10-month-old C57 mice, yet the ASR threshold elevations are pronounced at this age. This is an example, in an animal model, of a suprathreshold auditory behavior that declines more with age than would be predicted from the age-related decrease in pure-tone sensitivity.

One can speculate on possible mechanisms that might account for the exaggerated decrease in the ASR at middle frequencies, when the hearing loss occurs at high frequencies. For instance, at high sound levels an 8 kHz tone will activate regions of the basilar membrane basal to the "8 kHz region." When the cochlea is normal the central auditory system receives neural input from the basal cochlea in addition to the 8 kHz region when the ASR is evoked. When sensorineural pathology is present, the impaired basal region cannot provide its normal share of the neural activity in the auditory nerve; the net input to the brain is diminished with 8 kHz tones despite the fact that the 8 kHz region of the cochlea is normal.

Other explanations are also feasible. It was shown in Chapter 6 that the responsiveness of neurons in the ventral division of the cochlear nucleus (VCN) is reduced in middle-aged C57 mice compared to the dorsal cochlear nucleus (DCN). Davis and coworkers (Davis, 1984) have provided evidence that the VCN (not the DCN) is a component of the primary ASR circuit. Thus, impairment of the VCN might have exaggerated effects on the ASR. Alternatively, peripheral impairment might affect the normal balance of central excitatory and inhibitory circuits to affect the ASR in unpredictable ways. Yet another speculative hypothesis involves the efferent cochlear system. Evidence was provided in Chapter 3 to suggest that the efferent system is less vulnerable to age-related

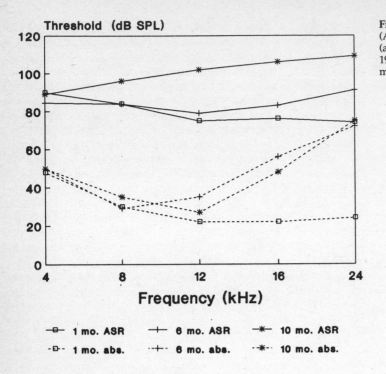

Figure 8-18a. Acoustic startle response (ASR) and absolute threshold in mice (adapted from Parham and Willott, 1988; Willott, 1986). a. CBA mice; b. C57 mice.

ASR data from Parham & Willott '88
Absolute threshold data extrapolated
from Willott '86

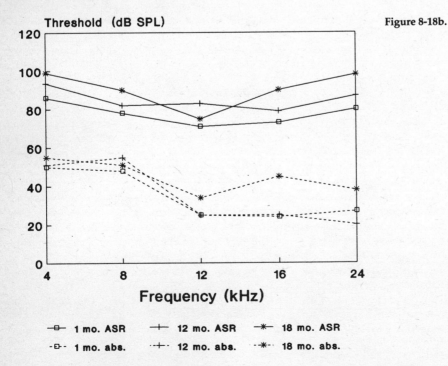

Figure 8-18b.

ASR data from Parham & Willott '88
Absolute threshold data extrapolated
from Willott, 1986

decline than the afferent system. Because the efferent system can suppress afferent activity, it might have exaggerated suppressive effects if the sensory cells of the cochlea are impaired.

The fact that a variety of hypotheses can be generated to account for these findings underscores the potential for complex interactions among aging, hearing loss, and auditory behaviors and the difficulty in trying to understand them.

prevalence data from the Framingham Heart Study in which audiograms of elderly subjects were characterized as rising, flat, gradually sloping high-frequency loss, and sharply sloping high-frequency loss (adapted from Lloyd and Kaplan, 1978). The results of this analysis are presented in Figure 8-29. Note that the distribution differed significantly as a function of gender, with women being most likely to exhibit flat or gradually sloping audiograms and men being most likely to exhibit sharply sloping audiograms.

CONCLUSIONS

Many elderly listeners manifest deficiencies in their ability to process information about frequency, intensity, time, and space. Most deficits can be largely accounted for by peripheral presbycusis, since similar deficits occur in young people with sensorineural impairment. Presumably, neural information provided by the impaired inner ear is distorted and/or incomplete, so that the CAS cannot use it effectively. However, peripheral dysfunction alone cannot adequately account for many of the performance deficiencies, and a number of studies have provided indications of central involvement, albeit less prominent. The central deficits could involve the effects of biological aging (CEBA) or the central effects of peripheral presbycusis (CEPP), described in Chapter 6. This topic is discussed in Chapter 10.

APPENDIX 8-1: AUDIO METRIC SURVEYS OF PURE TONE THRESHOLDS

Numerous surveys have been conducted from which the relationship of hearing and aging can be derived, as exemplified earlier in Figures 8-1 and 8-2. To provide a richer sense of the findings of various surveys, Figures 8-19 to 8-27 present further examples from a range of populations and time periods. Chapter 5 provides examples of hearing surveys from rural, nonindustrialized listeners including the Mabaans of the Sudan (Fig. 5-1) and natives of Easter Island (Figs. 5-2, 3).

Surveys, of course, mask the variability in audiograms that occurs among individual elderly listeners. Examples of the types of audiograms that can be associated with presbycusis were presented in Chapter 3 (Figs. 3-6, 9, 15, 18, 23, 24). Gates et al. (1990) presented

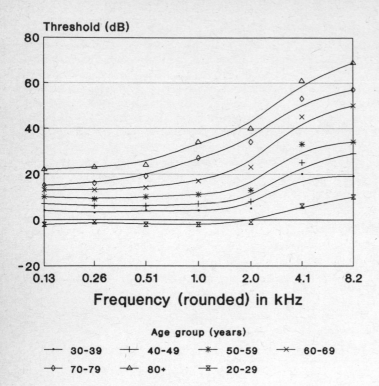

Figure 8-19a. Pure tone thresholds (adapted from Leisti, 1949). a. men; b. women. Subjects were patients in a Finnish clinic and other, healthy people screened to eliminate those with otological problems. Thresholds in dB re: audiometer settings.

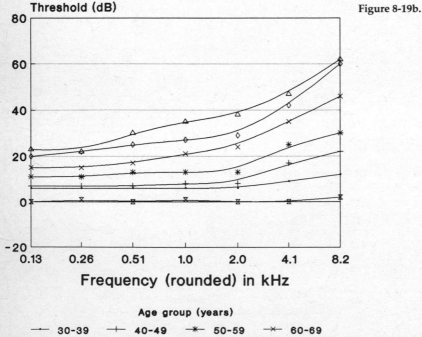

Figure 8-19b.

Figure 8-20a. Pure tone thresholds (adapted from Glorig, 1957). a. men; b. women. Subjects were from the Wisconsin State Fair Survey of 1954. Thresholds in dB re: ASA standards.

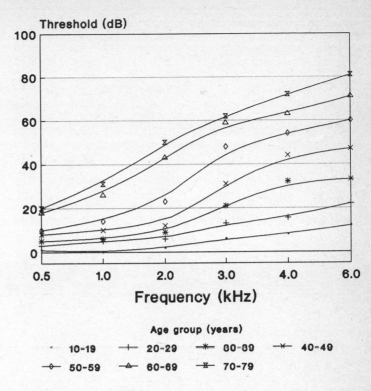

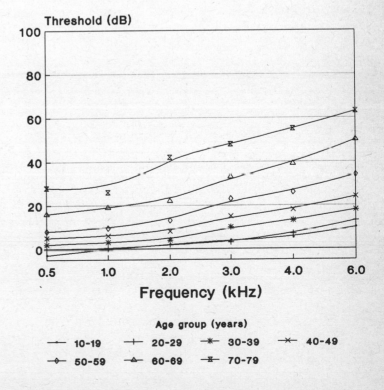

Figure 8-20b.

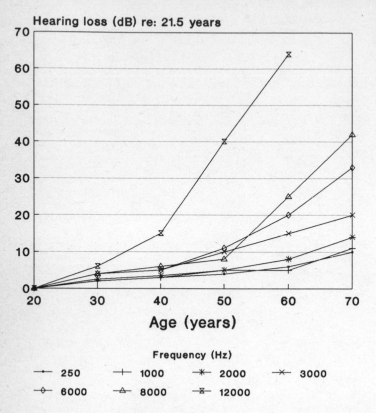

Figure 8-21. Pure tone hearing loss re: young listeners (adapted from Hinchcliffe, 1959). Subjects were otologically normal, selected in Scotland. Thresholds in dB re: young subjects' mean thresholds.

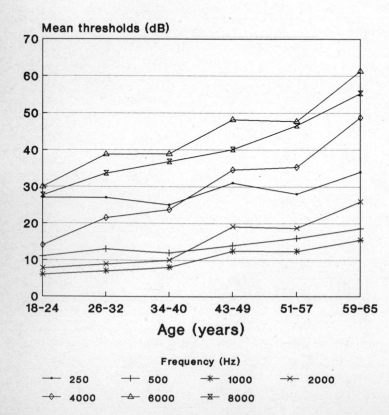

Figure 8-22. Pure tone thresholds (adapted from Corso, 1963). Subjects were college students (young group) and registered voters in rural Pennsylvania and were otologically screened. Thresholds in dB re: SPL.

Figure 8-23a. Pure tone thresholds (adapted from Hinchcliffe and Jones, 1968). a. men; b. women. Subjects were from suburban Jamaica. Thresholds in dB re: ISO, 1964 standards.

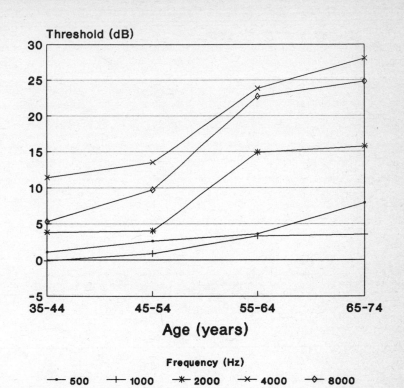

Right ears re: ISO '64

Figure 8-23b.

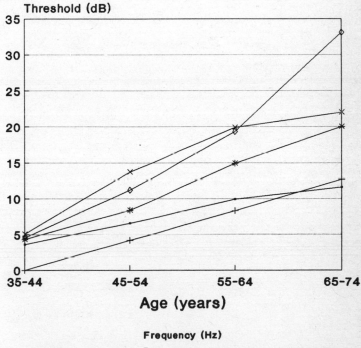

Right ears re: ISO '64

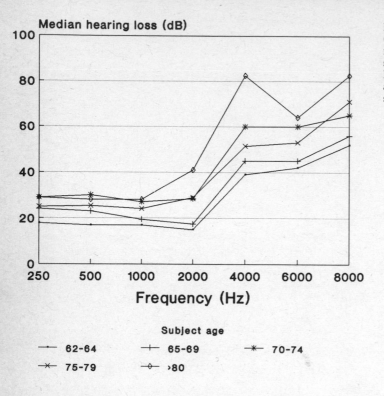

Figure 8-24a. Median hearing loss (adapted from Milne and Lauder, 1975). a. men; b. women. Subjects were randomly selected from doctors' patient lists in Edinburgh, Scotland. Thresholds in dB re: audiometer settings calibrated by British standards.

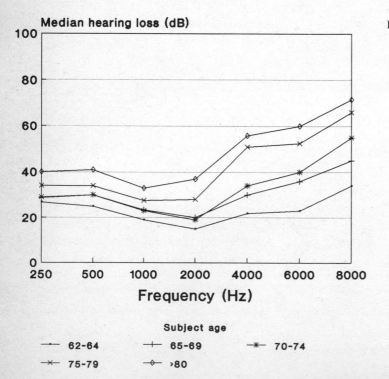

Figure 8-24b.

Figure 8-25. Pure tone hearing levels (adapted from Schow and Nerbonne, 1980). Subjects were obtained from nursing homes in Idaho and were not otologically or otherwise screened. Thresholds in dB re: ANSI standards.

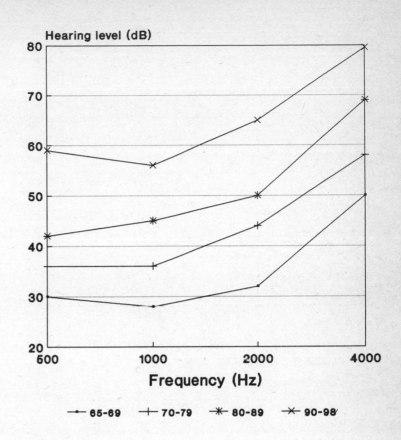

HL re: ANSI 1969

Figure 8-26. Pure tone thresholds (adapted from Waudby, 1984). Subjects were employees of a large food and drink manufacturing company throughout the United Kingdom undergoing routine audiological testing. Thresholds in dB re: ANSI standards.

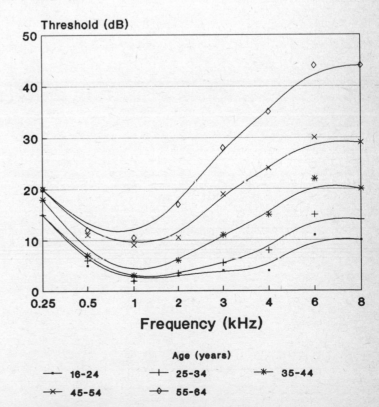

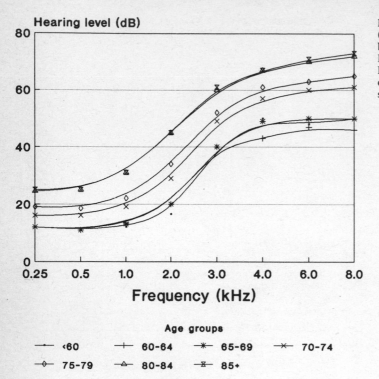

Figure 8-27a. Pure tone hearing level (adapted from Moscicki et al., 1985). a. men; b. women. Subjects were from the Framingham Heart Study, Framingham, Massachusetts and were not screened otologically. Thresholds in dB re: ANSI standards.

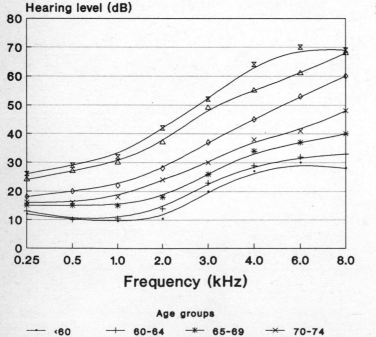

Figure 8-27b.

Figure 8-28. Fifteen-year threshold changes (right ear) as a function of age and frequency (adapted from Brant and Fozard, 1990). Subjects were men from the Baltimore Longitudinal Study of Aging.

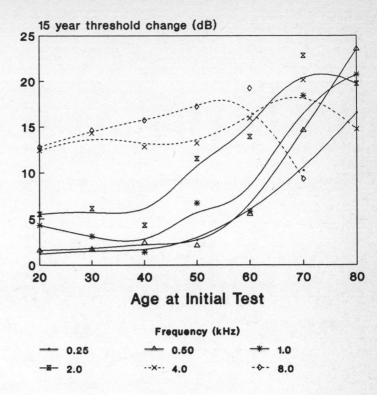

Figure 8-29. The percent of elderly men and women with various audiogram patterns, from the Framingham Heart Study (adapted from Gates et al., 1990). Almost all subjects were older than 65 years.

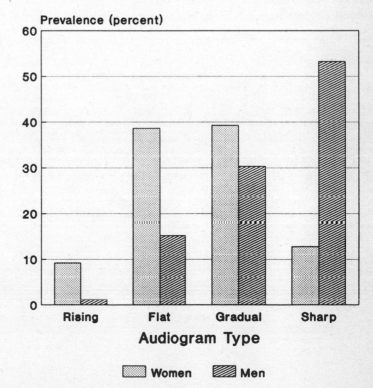

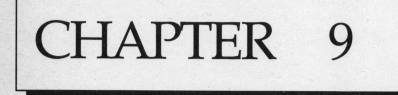

CHAPTER 9

Psychophysical Aspects of Aging and Presbycusis: Speech Perception

Understanding of speech is undoubtedly the most important of human auditory functions. It is also very complex, requiring the integration of auditory, cognitive, linguistic, and communicative skills. In keeping with the focus of this book, we shall emphasize research findings that are most relevant to the auditory system. Such research is primarily concerned with the ability of elderly people to detect, discriminate, and recognize words, phrases, and simple sentences—what we shall refer to as speech perception. Studies dealing with the understanding (comprehension) of speech material or complex sentences will not be reviewed, since they rely heavily on nonauditory regions of the brain and fall under the purview of cognitive psychology, communication science, and psycholinguistics. The reader is referred to other works for discussions of aging and comprehension, cognition, linguistics, or communicative skills (Beasley & Davis, 1981; Bergman, 1980; Gilad and Glorig, 1979a; Hayes, 1984; Marshall, 1981; Maurer & Rupp, 1979; Moller, 1983; Oyer and Oyer, 1976; Pickett, Bergman & Levitt, 1979; Salomon, 1991; Schow, Christensen, Hutchinson, and Nerbonne, 1978; Shadden, 1988; Spilich, 1985; Tamir, 1979; WGSUA, 1988).

Even after limiting the review, the literature on aging and speech recognition/discrimination is formidable. Consequently, many studies cannot be discussed in the text, but appear in Tables 9-1 through 9-4.

a tendency to withhold verbal responses or are slower in their verbal responses. In addition, the type of test material used is critical for demonstrating age effects. If tests are too easy or too hard, results tend to cluster, obscuring age differences. Finally, different ways of presenting material may influence age effects (e.g., fixed versus adjustable masking noise; Gordon-Salant, 1987b, Table 9-2).

(d) Cognitive factors such as attention, motivation, confidence, and inconsistent strategies during a test can influence performance on speech tests (see Chapter 10). However, this may not necessarily be true in all cases. Jerger, Johnson, and Jerger (1988) addressed an important issue involving aging and cognition, the possibility that conservative response criteria may influence the results of speech tests. If older individuals were less likely to respond positively to test material, speech testing could be affected. Jerger and colleagues used a signal detection task to divide elderly subjects into three response criteria groups: lax, intermediate, and strict. Response criteria groupings did not significantly affect performance on several conventional speech audiometry tests, suggesting that conservative response tendencies need not significantly affect test performance. It seems that the influences of cognitive factors should be determined on an empirical basis.

These and other factors can add to the variance of research findings, and have the potential to result in misleading conclusions about the role of the *auditory system* (central and peripheral) in age-related changes in speech perception.

RESEARCH CONSIDERATIONS

Several methodological issues that are particularly germane to speech perception research—in addition to those discussed in Chapter 1—have been noted by reviewers of the literature (Bergman, 1980; Marshall, 1981; WGSUA, 1988; Pickett, Bergman, and Levitt, 1979; and others).

(a) The listener's language and dialect history or linguistic skills may affect performance on speech tests and contribute to age differences.

(b) Practice effects can affect performance on speech perception tests. It is possible that the degree or rate of improvement from practice may differ as a function of age.

(c) Testing procedures may influence results. For instance, various speech testing procedures require subjects to respond verbally. Some older subjects have

PHONEMIC REGRESSION

Gaeth (1948) coined the term "phonemic regression" to describe his observation that, among other things, older subjects' speech perception was poorer than would be expected from their audiograms. Although the term is not widely used today, we shall employ it for the present discussion in deference to its historical significance. However, as Jerger (1973) has suggested, it is doubtful that either diminished ability to identify phonemes or regressive tendencies are major factors in the phenomenon.

The concept of phonemic regression in the elderly implies that some age-related change that is not revealed by pure tone threshold elevations (e.g., in the central auditory system or elsewhere) affects speech perception. This notion raises two related questions. First, are deficits in speech perception in older listeners

TABLE 9-1. AGING AND PERCEPTION OF SPEECH IN GOOD LISTENING CONDITIONS

Study	Test	Performance of older subjects
Kelley '39	word lists, 10–40 dB SL	poorer, especially for consonants ****
Gaeth '48	PB words	poorer in disproportion to audiogram in hl-OSs over 60 ***
Pestalozza & Shore '55	PB words	poorer in nm-OSs; hl and recognition correlated **** (Fig. 9-1)
Goetzinger et al. '61	PB words	progressively poorer from 60–90yrs; correlation of SRT and 5–2kHz thresholds; partial correlation with age ****
Klotz & Kilbane '62	PB words	recognition scores decreased with age from 51–80+, as did PTA and SRT ****
Harbert et al. '66	PB words	recognition more closely correlation with SRT than age ***
Feldman & Reger '67	monosyllabic words, 40 dB re:SRT	poorer (50–89yrs.); largest correlation 250, 1000 Hz thresholds and reaction time ****
Toyoda & Yoshisuke '69	PB words at various levels	performance-intensity functions less steep ***
Punch & McConnell '69	PB words, 10–40 dB re: spondee SRT	hl-OSs < nm-OSs; nm-OSs < YSs *,*** (Fig. 9-2)
Blumenfeld et al. '69	Fairbanks Rhyme test	poorer, especially over 60 yrs. *
Kasden '70	PB words 10–50 dB SL	maximum word recognition at 50 dB re: SRT; ns: hl-YSs & hl-OSs; both hl groups < nm-YSs ** (Fig. 9-3)
Bergman '71	sentences at telephone level	little change until 80-89 yrs. * (marginal hl)
Berkowitz & Hochberg '71	SRT, words and sentences	poorer SRT and word recognition paralleled PTA; sentence discrimination good ****
Hallerman & Plath '71	German syllables maximum score	upward shift, performance-intensity curve but no decline in max. score *(nonclinical population)
Kell et al. '71	PB words words 50% SRT	50% recognition poorer by more than 20 dB; minimal change in tone thresholds below 3kHz * (OSs not exposed to excessive noise)
Eisdorfer & Wilkie '72	spondee SRT, longitudinal	7-year decline less than that for pure tones ****
Jokinen '73	monosyllabic words	reduced by 12% between 20's and 70's at +22 S/N (Fig. 9-9)****
Jerger '73	PB words	PB max declined as an exponential function of age, but little decline in OSs with mild hl ****
Rintelmann & Schumaier '74	relatively difficult NU-6 words	poorer at 60+ yrs **
Stevenson '75	conventional & "adaptive" speech audiometry	correlation of speech and tone threshold; recognition poorer with hl ****
Bergman et al. '76	sentences	small decrement through 9th decade (Fig. 9-7) * ("relatively nm hearing")
Gang '76	PB words	Rollover (indicative of retrocochlear pathology) in oldest OSs, but normal tone decay (Fig. 9-21) *
Bess & Townsend '77	retrospective, word discrimination	no age effect for OSs with hl less than 50 dB PTA; age effect more pronounced with greater hl **** (Fig. 9-5)
Findlay & Denenberg '77	PB words	OSs recognized 94% in quiet *** (Fig. 9-11)
Surr '77	monosyllabic words, 40 dB SL re: SRT	no age effect, 30 –90 years ** (Fig. 9-4)

TABLE 9-1. CONTINUED

Study	Test	Performance of older subjects
Parnell & Amerman '79	syllables & subsyllables	poorer processing of coarticulatory cues, but better than 96% recognition in quiet *
Townsend & Bess '80	40 dBSL mono-syllabic words	OSs v. YSs: ns **
Moller '81	longitudinal, SRT and words	poorer, but recognition was in line with pure tone audiogram ****
Ginzel et al. '82	synthetic syllables	60–80 yr. hl-OSs poorer, especially when hl was severe *,***
Beattie & Warren '83	monosyllabic words	intelligibility slope not correlated with spondee threshold; slight decrease with high freq. hl. *,***
Dubno et al. '84	speech in quiet (see Table 9-2)	effect of hl, but not age *,**,***
Grady et al. '84	spondees (SRT) & PB words (SD)	when the effect of hl was taken into account, no age effect (21–83 yrs.) ****
Dorman et al.'85	phonemic identification tasks (words)	no age effect re: use of duration; OSs poorer in using dynamic spectral cues if other information is unavailable *,***
Gelfand et al. '85	nonsense syllables	recognition decreased with age *
Gelfand et al. '86	nonsense syllables	recognition decreased with age (see Table 9-2)*
Butts et al. '87	nonsense syllable test (NST)	correlation with hl at 250 and 2000 Hz, but not with age (5–90 yrs.) ****
Dubno et al. '87	consonant-vowel pairs	OSs with sloping hl had poor consonant recog. for short-duration stimuli***
Gordon-Salant '87a	consonant recognition & confusion tests	nm-OSs >hl-OSs (65 yrs.+); but confusions were not specific to hl or configuration of hl *,***
Gordon-Salant '87b	monosyl. words, open and closed sets in quiet (see Table 9-2)	ns: nm-OSs v. nm-YSs and hl-OSs v. hl-YSs *,**,***
Holmes et al. '88	closed & open set tests, California Consonant Test	no age effects *
Elliott et al. '89	single-formant frequency transitions	required larger acoustic differences between transitions
Gimsing '90	monosyllabic words	recognition decreased with hearing loss, but more so in very old hl-OSs ***
Holmes et al. '90	California Con-sonant Test	non age effect, closed or open set measures *
Rodriguez et al. '90	PB words	about 98% performance in OSs *
Plath '91	word recognition	nm-OSs: minimal losses; OSs with noise-induced hl: poor and became worse with age *,****

hl = hearing loss; nm = normal hearing for age; YSs = young subjects; OSs = older subjects; S/N = signal to noise ratio; ns = no significant difference
< = poorer relative performance; > = better relative performance
*hearing within normal limits, at least for age
** hl matched in YSs & OSs
*** OSs had hl for age
**** hl heterogeneous

TABLE 9-2. AGING AND PERCEPTION OF SPEECH IN THE PRESENCE OF NOISE, BABBLE, OR COMPETING SPEECH

Study	Test	Performance of older subjects
Blumenfeld et al. '69	Rhyme test in quiet or noise	tended to decrease, both conditions, especially after 60 yrs. (but OSs had some hl) ****
Smith '69	nonsense syllables in noise	poorer recognition but no age effect for noise level or S/N *
Tillman et al. '70	30 dB SL mono-syllabic words in competing sentences	ns: hl-OSs v. hl-YSs, but hl-OSs & hl-YSs < nm-YSs ***
Carhart & Nicholls '71	spondee thresh. in talkers &/or noise	poorer
Smith & Prather '71	nonsense syllables in noise	poorer, all S/Ns; dependence on S/N was parallel for YSs & OSs *
Jokinen '73	monosyllabic words in noise	increasingly poor at low S/Ns, 60–80 yrs. **** (many hl-OSs) (Fig. 9-9)
Garstecki & Mulac '74	monosyllables and sentences in competing speech	poorer ***
Mayer '75	sentences in traffic noise	poorer especially at low S/Ns *
Bergman et al. '76	sentences from competing talkers	poorer (Fig. 9-7) * ("relatively nm hearing")
Findlay & Denenberg '77	30 dB SL mono-syllabic words in -4 S/N babble	OSs poorer; hl-YSs < nm-YSs (Fig. 9-11) **,***
Jerger & Hayes '77	PB words (quiet) & SSI sentences with competing speech	SSI performance with age declined more than PB recognition ** (Fig. 9-22)
Kalikow et al. '77	SPIN	poorer at 80 dB SPL for PH & PL, low S/Ns PH > PL*
Orchik & Burgess '77	SSI, ipsilateral competition	poorer only at lower S/Ns * (Fig. 9-10)
Surr '77	monosyllables in multi-talker babble, 40 dB SL 6.4 S/N	no age effect, 30-90 years ** (hl-YSs and hl-OSs) (Fig. 9-4)
Punch '78	spondees, masked with interrupted noise	poorer ***
Hayes & Jerger '79	PB words & SSI	OSs varied re: PB v. SSI; OSs w/ poor SSI re: PB also had low freq. loss of CAS origin; some OSs performed very well ****
Leshowitz & Lindstrom '79	speech in noise	most (not all) OSs needed higher S/Ns ***
Plomp & Mimpen '79	SRT for sen-tences in noise	poorer in quiet & noise; smaller age effect with high noise levels ****
Bergman '80	Hebrew SPIN	PL and PH poorer in OSs, but PH > PL in OSs (age effect re: absolute but not relative scores)
Bergman '80	competing talkers	poorer with age even at age 40
Townsend & Bess '80	40 dB SL monosyllabic words in noise, 10 S/N	poorer by 5% **
Mayer '81	sentences in urban noise	poorer especially at low S/Ns *
Bosatra & Russolo '82	ipsilateral competition, PB words and SSI	poorer, some rollover *** ("a degree of presbycusis")
Dubno et al. '82	speech in babble (see Table 9-1 also)	poorer for hl-OSs, nm-OSs (required higher S/N) re: matched YSs *,**, ***

TABLE 9-2. CONTINUED

Study	Test	Performance of older subjects
Marks '82	speech in noise	poorer in quiet or noise, especially for female voice; correlated with high-frequency hl *
Nabelek & Robinson '82	Modified Rhyme, reverberation	poorer * (Fig. 9-12)
Otto & McCandless '82	PB words and SSI	30% of hl-OSs: SSI rollover; SSI > PB with increasing age; hl-YSs had normal SSI/PB ***
Shirinian & Arnst '82	PB words and SSI	SSI < PB at high levels ("rollover" phenomenon) in most OSs, especially R. ear **** (most had hl) (Figs. 9-23)
Duquesnoy '83a	SRT (sentences) in noise or babble	OSs: SRT in noise = SRT in babble; YSs: SRT in noise > SRT in babble; OSs benefited less from spatial separation of noise & speech ***
Duquesnoy '83b	SRT (sentences) in noise	PTA was a poor predictor of SRT; SRT in quiet v. noise often differed ***
Matthies et al. '83	several speech tests	poorer performance by OSs disappeared with practice
Kaplan & Pickett '84	PB and SSI	poorer, especially for "mild-moderate" hl-OSs (Fig. 9-24)***
Obler and Albert '85	SPIN	PH > PL OSs & YSs; no age effect
Era et al. '86	sentences in cafe noise	poorer and correlated with 4 kHz and .5-2 kHz thresholds ****
Gelfand et al. '86	nonsense syllables in babble	poorer but no interaction with S/N * strong correlation with 8000 Hz hl
Gordon-Salant '86	nonsense syll- ables in babble	poorer *
Gordon-Salant '87b	monosyllabic words, open and closed set for- mats in babble (see Table 9-1)	ns: nm-OSs v. nm-YSs and hl-OSs v. hl-YSs for fixed noise but significant age effect with adaptive noise paradigm *,**,***
Gelfand et al. '88	Sentence recept- ion and babble detection (BDT) thresholds; ratio of sentence to babble (S/B)	hl-OSs < nm-OSs < nm-YSs, sentence reception, BDT, & S/B ratio; hl-OSs had re- duced advantage from separation of speech and noise *,***
Nabelek '88	vowels in quiet and babble + reverberation	In quiet, no age effect; In noise + reverberation: age and hl effect ****
Debruyne & Tyberghein '89	PB and SSI	SSI <PB in OSs but ns correlation with ABR wave V latency *
Hutchinson '89	SPIN	PH & PL poorer, PH > PL *
van Rooij et al. '89	various tests with noise	poorer *
Nittrouer & Boothroyd '90	syllables, words, and sentences in noise	poorer at 0 and -3 S/N ****
Rodriguez et al. '90	SSI with ipsi- lateral competition	rollover at 0 S/N in more than half of OSs *
Schum & Matthews '90	SPIN	OSs who performed poorly on PH had hl ****

hl = hearing loss; nm = normal hearing for age; YSs = young subjects; OSs = older subjects; S/N = signal to noise ratio; ns = no significant difference
< = poorer relative performance; > = better relative performance
*hearing within normal limits, at least for age
** hl matched in YSs & OSs
*** OSs had hl for age
**** heterogeneous hl

really more severe than what the pure tone audiogram would predict? Second, if hearing level is accounted for, does the perception of speech by older subjects decline relative to young subjects?

SPEECH PERCEPTION: RELATIONSHIP TO THE PURE TONE AUDIOGRAM AND AGE OF THE LISTENER

Kryter (1988) reviewed the relationship between hearing level (HL) for pure tones and speech perception, noting the importance of 3000 and 4000 Hz sensitivity. He cited the study of French and Steinberg (1947) which introduced the articulation index (AI) as an estimation of the relative importance of tone frequencies to speech understanding. The percentage weights were 10 percent at 500 Hz, 20 percent at 1000Hz, 26 percent at 2000Hz, 21 percent at 3000Hz, and 15 percent at 4000Hz. Correlational studies (Chapter 10) have shown that 4000 Hz tone thresholds are more highly correlated with accuracy of speech perception than 500 Hz (although the lower frequency has a better correlation with speech reception threshold). The conclusion is that pure tone averages that do not include 3000 and 4000 Hz underestimate audiometric losses relevant to speech perception in individuals with sensorineural hearing loss (e.g., many older people).

An early study by Pestalozza and Shore (1955) is most often cited as supporting the concept of phonemic regression. They reviewed audiometric data for patients over 60, comparing pure tone audiograms at 500, 1000, and 2000 Hz with spondee thresholds and recognition of phonetically balanced (PB) words presented at 40 dB SL (*or lower* if the patient had a greatly elevated absolute threshold and could not tolerate such a level). The subjects were clinical patients with hearing problems, and some had substantial losses. Data from old subjects were also compared with young controls exhibiting sensorineural impairment of varied etiology, gradually sloping audiograms, and "an overall average hearing loss for pure tones in the same range as the group of old people." As seen in Figure 9-1, for the older subjects the relationship between word recognition and hearing loss was nearly linear: 10 dB HL was associated with 70 percent recognition (PB words); 50 dB HL was associated with 20 percent recognition. Recognition scores of the young subjects were 10 to 18 percent better, except at 40 dB HL, where the two age groups were virtually the same, and at 45–

50 dB HL, where old subjects performed much more poorly.

The evidence for phonemic regression in the Pestalozza and Shore study is inconclusive. The age group differences for word recognition were not especially large, except when hearing loss was pronounced, and statistical analyses were not performed, making it impossible to determine if the differences were reliable. Furthermore, the absence of threshold data for the important frequencies of 3000 Hz and 4000 Hz makes it impossible to adequately compare HLs of the groups or to assess the severity of pure tone losses in the old group.

Another study that is sometimes cited as an example of phonemic regression is that of Punch and McConnell (1969). They obtained word recognition scores for two groups of older subjects (mean age about 74 years) differing in the degree of hearing loss: an "old, impaired" group (mean PTA 500–2000 Hz: 45 dB) and a "minimal loss" group (mean PTA 500–2000 Hz: 13 dB). Word recognition was plotted as a function of sensation levels (re: SRT) of 10–40 dB (Fig. 9-2). Recognition scores of the "old, minimal loss" group were lower than those of young subjects from an earlier study by Hirsh et al. (1952), and "old, impaired" subjects' scores were even poorer. These findings may indicate that, when threshold is taken into account by plotting the results re: SL, older subjects' intelligibility curves achieve a lower maximum level. However, this assumes that a performance curve obtained 17 years earlier, undoubtedly under nonidentical conditions, is a valid standard for comparison. A less equivocal conclusion from this study is that aging plus hearing loss ("old, impaired" group) results in lower speech intelligibility than aging with minimal hearing loss. It is likely, however, that the differences in word recognition between the older groups would be predicted by the pure tone thresholds, which differed by more than 30 dB. In the Pestalozza and Shore study (Fig. 9-1), a difference in HL of 30 dB was associated with a 40 percent decrease in word recognition scores in young subjects. Thus, the Punch and McConnell (1969) study, like the study by Pestalozza and Shore (1955), does not provide convincing evidence that word recognition in the elderly is out of line with sensory thresholds, when PB words are presented in quiet conditions.

Kasden (1970) used testing procedures similar to those of Punch and McConnell (1969) but obtained different results. Young and old subjects with hearing loss (500–2000 Hz PTAs of 42 and 39 dB, respectively) had poorer word recognition than young, normal-hearing subjects (Fig. 9-3). However, young and old subjects with hearing loss performed similarly. Slopes of the functions with respect to SL were similar for all three groups. Thus, hearing loss was associated with

Figure 9-1. Recognition score as a function of average pure-tone hearing loss (adapted from Pestalozza and Shore, 1955).

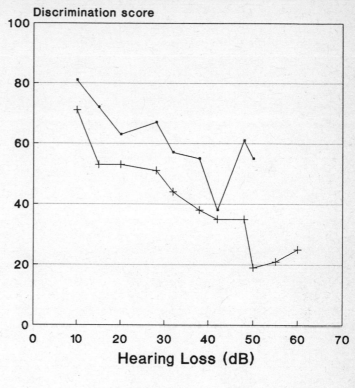

Figure 9-2. Percent intelligibility of PB words as sensation level (re: SRT) is varied (adapted from Punch and McConnell, 1969). Hirsh et al. (1952) data were obtained from young subjects.

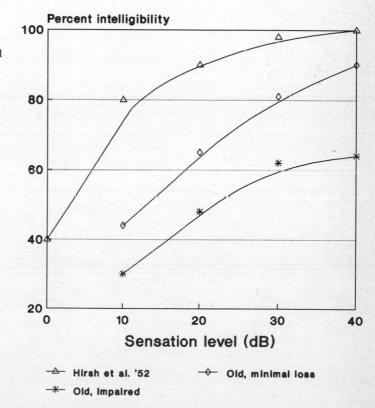

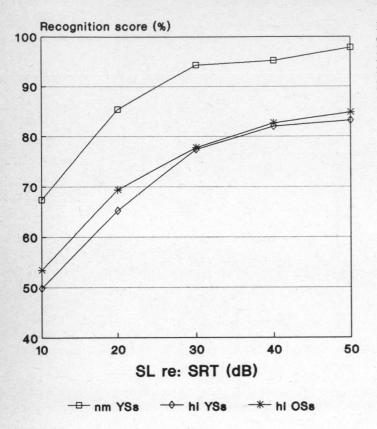

Figure 9-3. Recognition scores as a function of sensation level (re: SRT) (adapted from Kasden, 1970). nm YSs = normal-hearing young subjects; hl YSs = young subjects with hearing loss; hl OSs = old subjects with hearing loss.

poorer recognition, but age per se was not an important factor. In another study, Surr (1977) discerned only a slight decline in the identification of PB words in older subjects who had small increases in SRT (Fig. 9-4).

No age-related decline in recognition of words was observed by Bess and Townsend (1977) in subjects having flat cochlear hearing loss of less than 50 dB average (Fig. 9-5). When young and old subjects with more severe hearing losses were compared (dashed lines), word recognition dropped in older subjects. Unfortunately, their pure tone averages did not include 3 kHz and 4 kHz, so it is difficult to determine if the most severely impaired young and old subjects were truly comparable; they may very well have had more severe high-frequency losses than the "matched" young subjects (see Chapter 8). In any event, aging per se was not detrimental for subjects unless PTA was rather high.

The relationship among age, hearing level, and speech perception was addressed by Marshall and Bacon (1981). They used multiple regression techniques to assess the contributions of age and hearing loss at various frequencies to recognition of W-22 PB words. The most important predictor of word recognition

was pure tone threshold at high frequencies, with age accounting for a lesser amount of the variance. This relationship is shown in Figure 9-6, which plots PB recognition score as a function of age and threshold for 2000 Hz tones. When 2 kHz thresholds were good (e.g., 40 dB or better, little age-related decline in recognition was observed (less than 20 percent from ages 14 to 30 to ages 91 to 94). When hearing loss was more severe, recognition declined more steeply with age.

As seen in Table 9-1, a number of studies have found little evidence of age-related decline in speech perception when hearing loss was minimal. Other studies found that, when hearing loss was present, it appeared to account for deficits in perception in older listeners.

To summarize, the evidence leads one to conclude that older listeners who do not exhibit severe hearing loss typically perceive speech material effectively, if it is of good quality and presented in a relatively quiet environment. There does not appear to be a significant "age effect" under such conditions. When substantial hearing loss is present (e.g., on the order of 50 dB HL or more), the story may be different, as suggested by the data shown in Figures 9-5 and 9-6. The age-related decline in perception of speech may be more pronounced when individuals with substantial hearing

Figure 9-4. SRT and PB word recognition in quiet and noise (adapted from Surr, 1977).

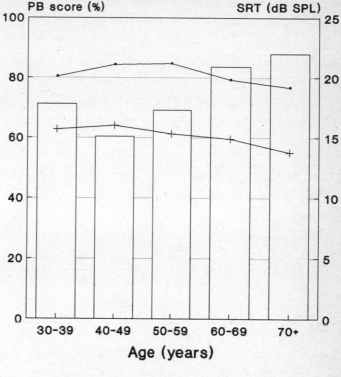

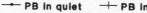 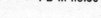

Figure 9-5. Word recognition as a function of pure tone average and age (adapted from Bess and Townsend, 1977). Each curve represents subjects with a range of PTAs, as noted.

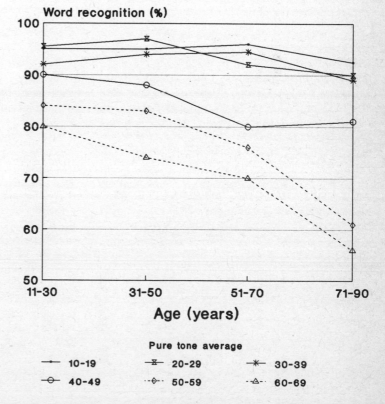

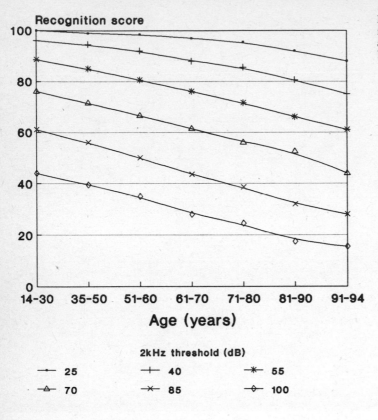

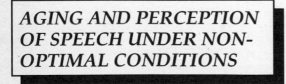

Figure 9-6. Word recognition as a function of threshold at 2 kHz (dB HL) and age (adapted from Marshall and Bacon, 1981).

impairment are compared. As Moller (1983) pointed out, Pestalozza and Shore (1955) and others who have found phonemic regression selected subjects with clinical hearing problems. With unselected older subjects (e.g., Moller, 1981) speech perception is more in line with the pure tone audiogram. Thus, the concept of phonemic regression may be useful in demonstrating that, when peripheral impairment is rather severe in the elderly, factors exist that are detrimental to speech perception but are not revealed by pure tone audiograms (although the absence of high frequency thresholds qualifies this statement). The possible identity of the factor(s) is discussed in Chapter 10.

AGING AND PERCEPTION OF SPEECH UNDER NON-OPTIMAL CONDITIONS

When speech must be perceived under less-than-optimal acoustic conditions, the capacities of the au-

ditory system may be seriously taxed, perhaps revealing age-related auditory deficits that would not be manifested under good listening conditions. Consequently, a number of investigators have evaluated speech perception in the presence of noise or competing speech, or when the message is degraded by altering time, continuity, or spectral properties of speech stimuli. Under such conditions older listeners often encounter difficulties. This point was well made by Bergman and colleagues (1976), who summarized the relationship between age and perception of speech under a variety of nonoptimal conditions (Fig. 9-7). With aging, performance declined on all speech tests, with the smallest decline occurring for speeded speech and the greatest decline occurring for interrupted speech. (These tests are discussed below.)

Poor performance on degraded speech tasks by young subjects with normal pure tone audiograms is typically interpreted as being diagnostic of problems within the central auditory system (CAS) (Noffsinger and Kurdziel, 1979; Musiek and Baran, 1987). For instance, temporal lobe lesions contralateral to the stimulated ear are associated with poor performance on lowpass filtered speech and accelerated speech;

Figure 9-7. Percent decrement of recognition under various conditions (adapted from Bergman et al. , 1976). Control = speech in quiet ; speeded = speeded rate of speech; bin. filt = binaurally filtered speech; select lstng = selective listening; reverb = reverberated speech; bin ovlpng = binaural overlapping of speech; interrupted = interrupted speech.

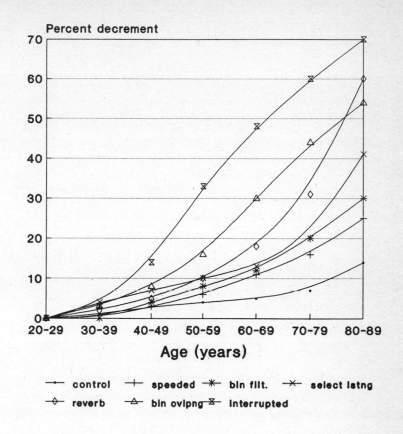

recognition of words presented in competing noise tends to be reduced with eighth nerve or brainstem lesions (Musiek and Baran, 1987). However, peripheral impairment also affects perception of degraded speech, as demonstrated in Figure 9-8 (Korsan-Bengtsen, 1973). In a patient with unilateral, sensorineural impairment caused by trauma, interrupted and time-compressed speech, in particular, were greatly affected by sensorineural impairment, with performance becoming worse as SL increased. Since most older individuals have at least some degree of peripheral dysfunction, caution must be exercised in attributing poorer performance of older subjects to CAS processes alone. One should always consider the possibility of peripheral and central involvement in speech perception deficits.

SPEECH PERCEPTION IN NOISE AND OTHER COMPETING SIGNALS

A number of studies have tested for the effects of noise or competing speech on speech perception in older listeners (Table 9-2). The interfering effects of noise are typically more extreme in elderly listeners.

Jokinen (1973) observed that the recognition of words in broadband noise decreased with age (Fig. 9-9). Lower signal-to-noise ratios (S/Ns) produced poorer recognition as expected, and there was a small interaction between age and S/N: the age difference in recognition between subjects in their 20's and those in their 70's was less than 15 percent when S/N was +22, but was almost 30 percent when S/N was +2. An interaction of age and S/N was also obtained by Orchik and Burgess (1977) when they measured recognition of synthetic sentences with ipsilateral competing speech (the "noise") in subjects with normal hearing for age (Fig. 9-10). At message-to-competition ratios (MCRs) of 0 and 20 (i.e., S/Ns), no age effect was found (dashed lines); at less favorable MCRs, recognition declined with age (dashed lines). In another study, Smith and Prather (1971) found older subjects to have poorer performance in noise at S/Ns of -5 to +10, but the magnitude of the age differences did not differ. These studies are in agreement in showing that perception of speech by older listeners is especially

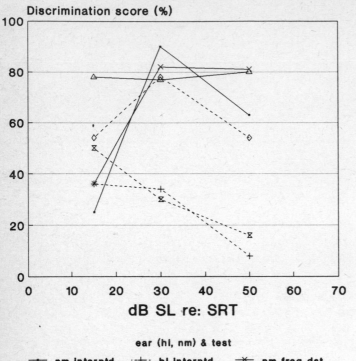

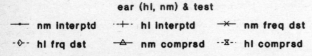

Figure 9-8. Recognition of speech as a function of hearing loss under various conditions in one subject (adapted from Korsan-Bengtsen, 1973). This subject had normal hearing in one ear and sensorineural loss in the other. nm = normal ear (solid lines); hl = ear with hearing loss (broken lines); interptd = interrupted speech; freq dst = frequency distortion of speech; comprsed = compressed speech.

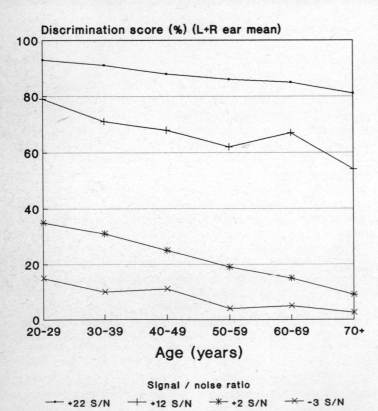

Figure 9-9. Recognition scores as a function of signal-to-noise ratio for monosyllabic words in broadband noise (adapted from Jokinen, 1973).

Figure 9-10. Recognition of SSI in ipsilateral competing babble as a function of message-to-competition ratio (adapted from Orchik and Burgess, 1977).

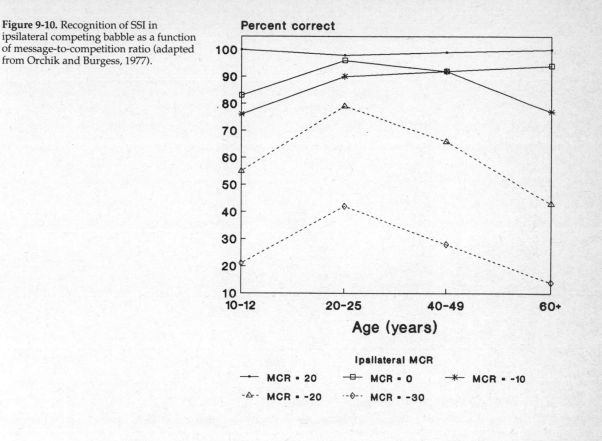

vulnerable to noise interference, but the S/N is an important variable in determining the magnitude of the age effect.

Findlay and Denenburg (1977) investigated the relationships among age, hearing loss, and competing babble. As shown in Figure 9-11, normal-hearing young subjects, young subjects with hearing loss, and old subjects performed similarly on recognition of PB words in quiet. In the presence of competing babble young subjects with hearing loss performed more poorly than normal-hearing subjects, suggesting that hearing loss exacerbates the effects of noise. Older subjects performed even more poorly, suggesting an additional age effect. However, the old subjects had more severe hearing loss than the young subjects with hearing loss (SRT about 8 DB higher), so it is possible that hearing loss, rather than age, was responsible for this finding.

The potential contribution of hearing loss to the masking or interfering effects of noise (Fig. 9-11) makes it difficult to interpret aging effects. For example, Bergman (1980) felt that hearing loss was not a necessary factor in his study of "selective listening" because a significant decline was seen by age 40, prior to the appearance of significant pure tone losses. It is possible, however, that significant hearing loss was present at untested, high frequencies (see Chapter 8).

Several ways in which noise masking experiments may be confounded by the presence of hearing loss in older subjects were outlined by the National Research Council Committee on Hearing, Bioacoustics, and Biomechanics (WGSUA, 1988). First, the spectrum of the noise versus the audiometric profile will influence the masking properties, making comparisons difficult (note, for instance, the "LP noise" versus "Noise" conditions in Fig. 9-11). Second, the presence of hearing loss produces significant differences in the masking level referenced to sensation level versus sound pressure level; if an experimenter chooses to equate SL, the SPL needed for impaired listeners may be rather high. Third, hearing-impaired listeners' performance can be sub-par even without noise, making it difficult to determine the extent of detrimental performance attributable to the noise. Whether or not peripherally impaired and normal-hearing individuals are affected similarly by noise remains an unanswered question.

Another variable that can affect the results of experiments on the effects of noise is the type of noise employed, as demonstrated by two recent European

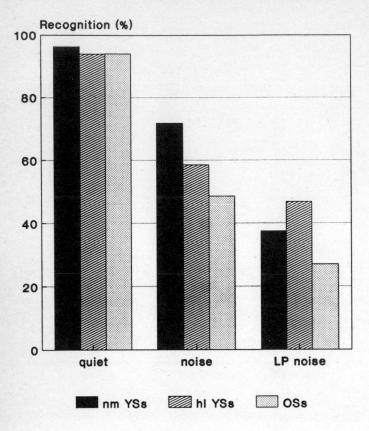

Figure 9-11. Recognition of monosyllabic words in competing babble (adapted from Findlay and Denenberg, 1977). nm YSs = normal-hearing young subjects; hl YSs = young subjects with hearing loss; OSs = old subjects. Noise was babble.

studies. A German study by von Wedel and Streppel (1991) showed that older subjects required higher signal-to-noise ratios than younger subjects, but this depended on the kind of masking noise used (e.g., competing speech or noise). An Italian study (Prosser, Turrini, and Arslan, 1991) reached similar conclusions. Traffic or "pink" noise maskers had similar effects on young and old hearing impaired listeners, whereas masking with continuous discourse was more problematic for the elderly listeners.

In this regard, the relationships among S/N and word recognition differed greatly between the Jokinen (1973) and Orchik and Burgess (1977) studies (Figs. 9-9 and 9-10). Performance was more deleteriously affected by comparable S/Ns in the former study. Furthermore, an age difference of more than 20 percent appeared in Jokinen's study when S/N (N = broadband noise) was +12, whereas in Orchik and Burgess' study, a S/N (N = babble) of -10 did not produce a comparable age effect.

While it is safe to conclude that the intelligibility of speech in noise decreases with age, the roles of peripheral hearing impairment and the nature of the competing noise are important.

AGING AND THE PERCEPTION OF ALTERED SPEECH

Performance of subjects on various listening tests involving altered speech has been used to diagnose central disorders of hearing and to uncover deficits that are not severe enough to be revealed by tests of speech perception under good conditions. Consequently, such tests may provide insight into changes in speech perception in the elderly.

REVERBERATED SPEECH

Reverberation produces exaggerated difficulties in the elderly (Table 9-3a). For example, Nabelek and Robinson (1982) obtained aging functions for reverberated speech delivered monaurally and binaurally at reverberation times (time taken for decay of sound) of 0, 0.4, and 1.2 seconds (Fig. 9-12). Longer reverberation times were more detrimental and binaural performance (dashed lines) was better than monaural. Performance of older listeners was more deleteriously affected by reverberation. For instance, when

TABLE 9-3. AGING AND PERCEPTION OF ALTERED OR LOW QUALITY SPEECH

(a) Reverberated speech

Study	Test	Performance of older subjects
Shubert '58 cited in Bergman '71	nonsense syllables with reverberation	poorer
Bergman et al. '76	sentences with reverberation	poorer (Fig. 9-7) * ("relatively nm hearing")
Harris & Reitz '85	word lists in quiet noise +/or reverberation	ns: YSs v. nm-OSs, except noise + reverberation; hl-OSs < other groups, all conditions *,*** (Fig. 9-13)

(b) Alteration of speed

Study	Test	Performance of older subjects
Calearo & Lazzaroni '57	sentences at increased rate	rates with little effect on YSs had drastic effect on OSs (prob. hl) (Fig. 9-14)
Luterman et al. '66	compressed & expanded PB words SRT+40 dB	hl-OSs < hl-YSs < YSs, all conditions, but no interaction of group and speed **,***
Hill '68	spondees, altered time & frequency	hl OSs < nm-OSs, nm-OSs < YSs ","""
Sticht & Gray '69	compressed PB words, SRT	hl-OSs < hl-YSs <nm-OSs < nm-YSs; OSs affected more by compression (Fig. 9-16) *,**
Schon '70	monosyllabic words compressed and expanded	compressed: ns: nm-OSs v. hl-OSs v. hl-YSs; all < nm-YSs. expanded: hl-OSs < nm-YSs; ns: nm-OSs v. nm-YSs. *,*** (Fig. 9-17)
Antonelli '70	time-compressed speech	normal speed: 80% compressed: 52% *
Korsan-Bengtsen '73	sentences spoken at 290 wpm	small decline for 50–60-year-olds *
Bergman et al. '76	sentences at 2.5 X nm rate	poorer (Fig. 9-7) * ("relatively nm hearing")
Konkle et al. '77	monosyllabic words	poorer as time compression & age increased (54–84) & as SL decreased; age effect accelerated * (Fig. 9-15)
Korabic et al. '78	expanded monosyllabic words	expanded: OSs poorer, especially at low SLs ****
Moller '81	accelerated low redundancy sentences	70 yr. OSs slightly poorer than YSs at 300 wpm ****
Schmitt & McCroskey '81	rate altered sentences	comprehension higher at compressed and expanded conditions in OSs
Bosatra & Russolo '82	"sensitized speech" (altered speed and filtering)	poorer in 60% of OSs; normal in 40% (no data provided); OSs with "a degree of presbycusis"
McCroskey & Kasten '82	rate altered sentences	Best comprehension at slow (125 wpm) & fast (291 wpm) rates in OSs ****
Schmitt '83	speech passages compressed and expanded	good at normal rate; OSs affected more by compression; at ages 65–74 yrs.: aided by expansion *
Schmitt & Carroll '85	comprehension of speaker generated alteration	poorer with 60% compression; not affected by expansion *

Continued over

TABLE 9-3. CONTINUED

(b) Alteration of speed (continued)

Study	Test	Performance of older subjects
Wingfield et al. '85	compression, sentences varying structural difficulty	increased age effect with increased rate, especially for difficult material *
Rastatter et al. '89	phonemic contrast discrimination at 50% compression	linear regression: significant age effect *
Paludetti et al. '91	bisyllabic PB words	poorer recognition by age and hl (60–80 yrs) *,***

(c) Interrupted speech

Study	Test	Performance of older subjects
Bocca & Calearo '56	interrupted low-redundancy speech	poorer over 75
Kirikae '69	interrupted, monaural speech	poorer, age 50–70 ***
Marston & Goetzinger '72	interrupted sentences, 50 dB re: SRT contralateral noise or competing messages	OSs (mean age 48.4) poorer * see Table 9-3d
Korsan-Bengtsen '73	interrupted sentences	poorer in 50–60-year-olds *
Bergman et al. '76	sentences interrupted 8 times/sec.	poorer (Fig. 9-7) * ("relatively nm hearing")
Moller '81	interrupted low-redundancy sentences	70 year OSs: 88% at 10 interruption/sec; 68% at 7 interruption/sec.; YSs near 100% ****
Era et al. '86	interrupted sentences	poorer and correlated with 4 kHz & .5–2 kHz thresholds ****

(d) Filtered speech

Study	Test	Performance of older subjects
Harbert et al. '66	bandpass filtered PB words, monaural & binaural	poorer than hl-YSs monaural & binaural ***
Kirikae '69	LP (1.2 kHz) filtered monosyllables	poorer
Palva & Jokinen '70	bandpass-filtered words see Table 9-4	monaural poorer as early as 30–39 yrs.; **** (Fig. 9-19)
Marston & Goetzinger '72	LP filtered monosyllabic words, 50 dB re: SRT contralateral noise or competing messages	ns age effect (OSs' mean age 48.4 yrs.) see Table 9-3c
Korsan-Bengtsen '73	band-filter distorted sentences	poorer in 50–60-year-olds *
Findlay & Denenberg '77	LP filtered monosyllabic words in babble	poorer than predicted from high-freq. hl (Fig. 9-11) ***
Bergman '80	LP filtered words	poorer
Grady et al. '84	LP filtered PB words	poorer, even when the effect of hl was taken into account ****

TABLE 9-3. CONTINUED

(e) Poor talker quality

Study	Test	Performance of older subjects
Goetzinger & Rousey '59	poor quality Rush-Hughes PB recordings vs. easier W-22 words	age effect greater than for good quality recordings *
Bergman '80	good, hoarse, or whisper voices	poorer, especially for whisper
Bergman '80	telephone	poorer, especially with competing babble
Clark '85	sentences, normal & alaryngeal speech in noise	poorer, especially for alaryngeal speech in noise *

hl = hearing loss; nm = normal hearing for age; YSs = young subjects; OSs = older subjects; S/N = signal to noise ratio; ns = no significant difference
< = poorer relative performance; > = better relative performance
*hearing within normal limits, at least for age
** hl matched in YSs & OSs
*** OSs had hl for age
**** heterogeneous hl

Figure 9-12. Effect of reverberation (seconds) on monaural and binaural speech recognition for the Modified Rhyme Test (adapted from Nabelek and Robinson, 1982). Solid lines = monaural; broken lines = binaural.

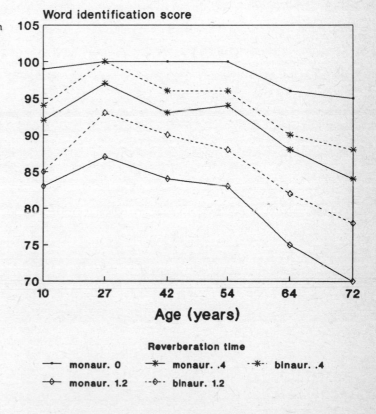

reverberation was increased from zero to 1.2, monaural scores decreased by about 13 percent in young subjects and by about 25 percent in the oldest subjects.

Harris and Swenson (1990) showed that the detrimental effects of reverberation on speech perception, especially with the addition of noise, were directly related to the degree of hearing impairment in young adults. This suggests that peripheral presbycusis would contribute to the difficulties older listeners have with reverberated speech. This conclusion can be reached from an earlier study by Harris and Reitz (1985). As seen in Figure 9-13, normal-hearing older subjects performed almost as well as young subjects on reverberated speech in quiet, while older subjects with hearing loss performed more poorly, especially with reverberation. When noise was added to reverberation (broken lines), the performance of all three groups declined, but the additive effects were somewhat more detrimental to older subjects.

ALTERATIONS OF SPEED

As shown in Table 9-3b, a number of studies have degraded speech by speeding it up (compression) or, in a few studies, by slowing it down (expansion).

Calearo and Lazzaroni (1957) pioneered the use of speech presented at high speed. As shown in Figure 9-14, performance-intensity functions of subjects older than 70 were a bit worse for normal speech, compared to young subjects. Speeding up the speech shifted the function by about 10 dB in young subjects. For older subjects, the function was shifted by about 20 dB at low intensities (referenced to hearing level) and "rolled over" at moderate intensities, after reaching a maximum of only about 50 percent correct (see also Fig. 9-8).

Recognition of words was measured by Konkle, Beasley, and Bess (1977) as a function of age and percent of time compression (Fig. 9-15). Recognition decreased with compression for all age groups, but the drop was greater for older subjects. For instance, recognition in young subjects decreased by about 8 percent when compression was increased from 0 to 60 percent; for older subjects, the same compression decreased performance by 25 to 30 percent.

Sticht and Gray (1969) showed that both age and hearing loss contributed to problems with compressed speech (Fig. 9-16). Normal-hearing, young subjects performed best (fewest errors), followed by older subjects with good hearing. Young subjects with hearing loss performed worse than old, normal-

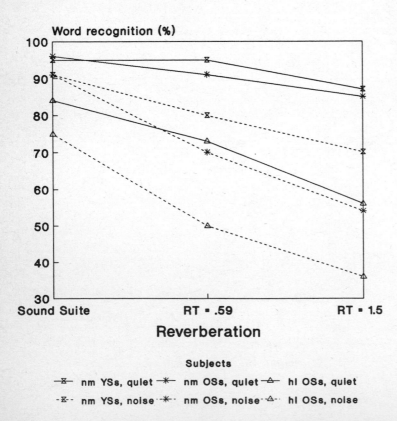

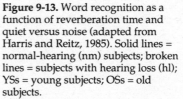

Figure 9-13. Word recognition as a function of reverberation time and quiet versus noise (adapted from Harris and Reitz, 1985). Solid lines = normal-hearing (nm) subjects; broken lines = subjects with hearing loss (hl); YSs = young subjects; OSs = old subjects.

Figure 9-14. Sentence recognition as a function of speed and intensity of presentation re: HL (adapted from Calearo and Lazzaroni, 1957). Old subjects were >70 years old.

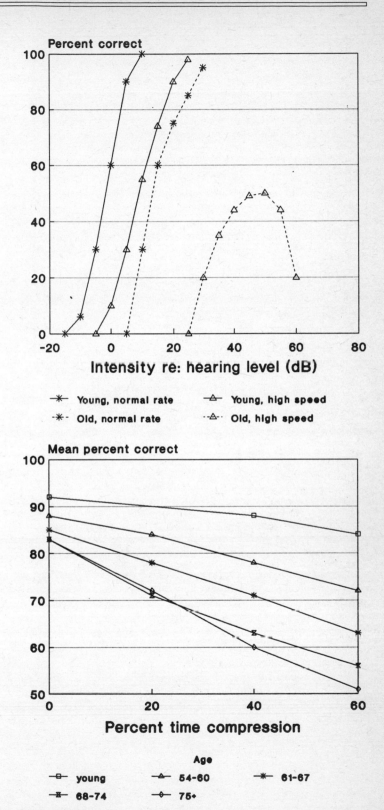

Figure 9-15. Recognition of monosyllabic words as a function of time compression (adapted from Konkle et al., 1977). NU-6 Words were presented at 24 dB SL.

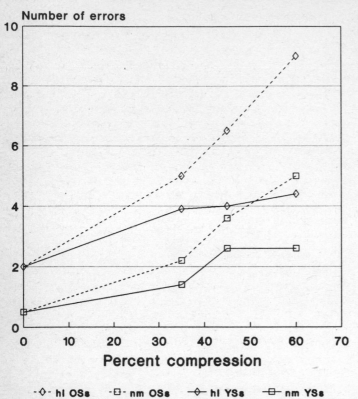

Number of errors

Percent compression

-◇- hl OSs   -□- nm OSs   -◆- hl YSs   -□- nm YSs

Figure 9-16. Number of errors in PB word recognition as a function of time compression (adapted from Sticht and Gray, 1969). hl = subjects with hearing loss; nm = normal-hearing subjects; YSs = young subjects; OSs = old subjects.

hearing subjects at lower degrees of compression, but these groups were similar at greater compression. Old subjects with hearing loss performed most poorly at all levels of compression. Both older groups (dashed lines) appeared to be more deleteriously affected at higher percent compression, as indicated by accelerating error functions.

Both compressed and expanded speech were employed by Schon (1970). All subjects, regardless of age or hearing loss, were more affected by compression than by expansion (Fig. 9-17). With expanded speech, normal-hearing young subjects missed the fewest words, followed by normal-hearing older subjects. Old and young subjects with hearing loss performed similarly to normal-hearing old subjects on compressed speech (but all performed worse than normal young subjects). Expansion had some detrimental effects on the subjects with hearing loss, particularly the older subjects.

Luterman, Welsh, and Melrose (1966) tested recognition of PB words across a range of compression/expansion times. Older subjects with hearing loss performed more poorly than young subjects with hearing loss. The young subjects with hearing loss, in turn, performed more poorly than normal-hearing young subjects. No interactions among compression,

expansion, and subject group were found. Thus, hearing loss and age were associated with reduced recognition, but greater degrees of expansion or compression did not alter the relative differences between groups.

Time expansion was studied in detail by Korabic, Freeman, and Church (1978). In this study, older subjects did more poorly at increased expansion times, particularly at lower sensation levels. For instance, at 32 dB SL, recognition of monosyllabic words by older subjects decreased by about 10 percent as speech was expanded by 100 percent. The same expansion produced no decline in young subjects. At 8 dB SL, expansion decreased performance by up to 40 percent in older subjects (again, no effect was seen in young subjects). Unfortunately, this study did not control for hearing loss in the older subjects.

In summary, there is general agreement that older subjects have difficulty with compressed speech when compared with young subjects (Table 9-3b). Hearing loss appears to pose additional difficulties, at least under certain experimental conditions (Luterman et al., 1966; Hill, 1968; Sticht & Gray, 1969). Testing for perception of expanded speech has produced mixed results. Older subjects have been hindered (Luterman et al., 1966; Korabic et al., 1978), unaffected (Schon,

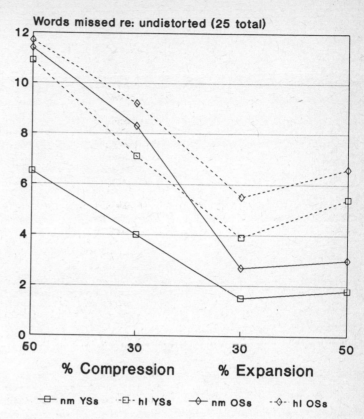

Figure 9-17. Number of monosyllabic words missed (re: undistorted words) as a function of time compression and expansion (adapted from Schon, 1970).

1970; Schmitt, 1983; Schmitt & Carroll, 1985), or helped (Schmitt, 1983). The reason for the inconsistent findings with expanded speech is unclear.

INTERRUPTION OF SPEECH

The studies summarized in Table 9-3c indicate that rapid interruption of speech is especially detrimental to perception by older listeners. There is some indication that the performance is affected by hearing loss as well (Era, 1986). Figure 9-7 provides an example of the relationship between aging and perception of interrupted speech (hour glass symbols), and Figure 9-8 demonstrates the effect of hearing loss. (Compare solid line with dot symbols, indicating the normal ear, and broken line with + symbols, indicating the hearing-impaired ear.)

FILTERED SPEECH

As seen in Table 9-3d, older listeners' perception of speech that has been degraded by lowpass or band pass filtering is generally poorer than that of young listeners.

Bergman (1980) investigated the relationship between lowpass cutoff and word recognition (Fig. 9-18). The age difference in recognition scores for unfiltered speech was about 4 percent. Filtering frequencies above 3000 Hz resulted in about the same age difference, whereas filtering frequencies above 2000 Hz increased the age difference to more than 20 percent.

Palva and Jokinen (1970) extracted two filtered bands (480–720 Hz and 1800–2400 Hz) from words and presented them to subjects ranging in age from 20 to 89. Either both bands were presented simultaneously to one ear (monaural presentation), or one band was presented to each ear (diotic binaural presentation). Binaural performance was similar to monaural, except in the oldest subjects, where it was superior (Fig. 9-19). However, performance in all conditions showed an age-related decline. This was becoming evident even in the 30- to 39-year group, despite normal tone thresholds in the filtered ranges. Two interesting aspects of this study should be noted. First, older listeners appeared to benefit from binaural presentation of speech material, but younger listeners did not (although poorer monaural performance in the older subjects allowed more room for improvement). Second, Palva and Jokinen found a greater decline in the older subjects' performance when stimuli were presented

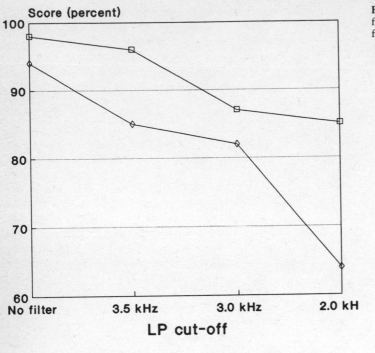

Figure 9-18. Recognition of words as a function of low-pass filter cut-off (adapted from Bergman, 1980).

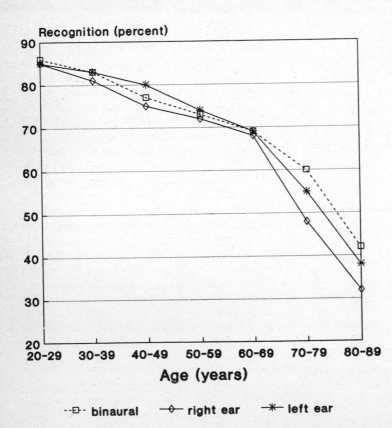

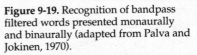

Figure 9-19. Recognition of bandpass filtered words presented monaurally and binaurally (adapted from Palva and Jokinen, 1970).

monaurally to the right ear. They interpreted this as having something to do with age-related changes in cerebral dominance. Whether this would impact on the superior binaural performance (e.g., better summation with reduced dominance?) is open to speculation.

CONCLUSIONS

Older listeners generally have exaggerated difficulties in perceiving speech that has been degraded or is of poor quality (Table 9-3a-e). Although elevation of hearing thresholds contributes significantly to the poor performance of elderly subjects, it is often not sufficient to account for the perceptual deficits. The problems appear to be influenced by other age-related factors that are not related to, or revealed by, pure-tone audiometry. In this context, the phenomenon of phonemic regression seems to apply, even when age-related hearing loss is not severe.

OTHER MONAURAL TESTS OF SPEECH PERCEPTION

THE SPEECH PERCEPTION IN NOISE (SPIN) TEST

The SPIN test was developed to provide information about the listener's ability to understand speech as a function of context and every-day conditions (e.g., babble in background) (Kalikow, Stevens, and Elliott, 1977). The listener hears a sentence in which the final word is obscured by noise and is asked to repeat the last word. Two types of sentence are used: those with high predictability with regard to context (PH) and those with low predictability (PL). Comparison of performance on PH and PL sentences provides an indication of the listener's ability to benefit from linguistic information (PH) versus phonemic information alone (PL).

In the initial development of the SPIN test (Kalikow et al., 1977), young subjects performed better with PH than with PL sentences when S/N was -5 and 0 dB. Similarly, old subjects whose hearing loss was within normal limits performed better on PH sentences at these S/Ns, but for both types of sentence, performance level was 10 to 15 percent below that of young subjects. At S/Ns of +5 and +10 dB, both groups performed near 100 percent. Thus, perception of older subjects was more deleteriously affected by background babble, but they benefited substantially from

contextual information. Bergman (1980) utilized a Hebrew version of the SPIN test with background babble presented at a level 4 dB below that of the sentences. The median performance of the young subjects was about 85 percent on the PL sentences, with a mean increase of about 10 percent on PH sentences. Median PL performance for old subjects was about 55 percent with highly variable, but similar mean improvement on material. While both groups benefited similarly from contextual cues (PH scores were higher than PL scores), older subjects performed more poorly on both types of material. Hutchinson (1989) presented the SPIN test at 0 dB S/N to young and old (mean age of 69 years) listeners who had normal hearing for their age. Scores on the PL sentences were about 10 percent lower in the older group whereas the PH scores were about 5 percent lower. Stated differently, older subjects were less effective in using acoustic-phonemic cues in the presence of background noise, but they were quite capable of improv-ing their performance by using contextual cues. Obler and Albert (1985) reported similar findings.

These studies are consistent in demonstrating that, under moderate-to-high S/Ns, recognition of both PL and PH material is somewhat depressed in older individuals compared to young, normal-hearing subjects. However, older listeners are capable of enhancing their performance with the addition of contextual information to a degree similar to that of young listeners. The ability to use acoustic-phonemic information (PL sentences) is more adversely affected by high levels of background babble in the older listeners. (This, of course, impacts on PH sentences as well.) The maximum performance levels of older listeners tend to be lower at high S/Ns, suggesting that an enhanced masking or interference effect is operating. One obvious possible cause of enhanced masking effects is peripheral presbycusis (see Chapter 8), and there is evidence to support this view. Elliott, Lyons, and Busse (1983) found that performance on PB word recognition in noise (but not in quiet) and sensitivity at 4 kHz (but not lower frequencies) were significantly related to performance on PH and PL SPIN sentences. This suggests that high-frequency hearing loss and increased susceptibility to masking are correlated with reduced performance on PL and PH material.

An important role of both hearing loss and other age-related factors was indicated by the work of Dubno, Dirks, and Morgan (1984). They used an adaptive method to determine the speech levels required for 50 percent performance on PH and PL sentences in young normal-hearing, young mildly-impaired, elderly normal-hearing, and elderly mildly-impaired subject groups. As seen in Figure 9-20, old and young normal-hearing subjects performed better on SPIN sentences

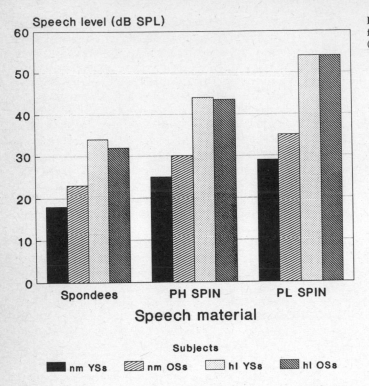

Figure 9-20. SPIN test performance as a function of age and hearing impairment (adapted from Dubno et al., 1984).

at lower SPLs than their hearing-impaired counterparts, indicating a role of hearing loss. Age was also a correlate of reduced performance, since young, normal-hearing subjects identified words at lower SPLs than old, normal-hearing subjects. Because age effects were not observed in quiet listening conditions, threshold sensitivity differences were not responsible. Rather, the findings suggest that older listeners were more vulnerable to the effects of noise. Whatever the reason may be for the poorer overall performance of older subjects, neither age nor hearing impairment was associated with a reduction in the ability to benefit from contextual information. Normal-hearing and hearing-impaired older listeners performed better on PH sentences than on PL sentences to a degree similar to that seen in young subjects.

Recently Schum and Matthews (1990) tested elderly hearing-impaired subjects using the SPIN test. Twenty percent of the subjects had depressed performance on the PH test items. However, in most cases, the poor performance on high predictable items occurred for presentation of items to one ear only and was correlated with threshold elevations. These findings indicate that in cases (albeit rare) when PH items are depressed in elderly listeners, peripheral impairment is largely responsible for the deficits.

In summary, there is little evidence from research using the SPIN test that older subjects are less able to make use of contextual cues. As the level of background babble increases, scores on PH and PL sentences are likely to decrease to a relatively greater degree in older subjects. The enhanced vulnerability to interference of both PL and PH sentences by background noise appears to be related, at least in large part, to peripheral presbycusis.

PERFORMANCE-INTENSITY FUNCTIONS FOR PB WORDS AND SSI

The synthetic sentence identification test (SSI) involves seven-word, grammatically correct but meaningless sentences presented with ipsilateral or contralateral competing continuous discourse (Jerger, 1973). The SSI and PB word recognition have been used diagnostically in several ways. According to Jerger and Hayes (1977), performance-intensity (PI) functions for PB words (PI-PB) and SSI (PI-SSI) are related to the type of hearing loss. When the audiometric pattern is flat, the two functions are similar. When the audiogram is sloping with high-frequency loss, the PB function falls below the SSI function; this indicates a peripheral, rather than central, deficit. When the audiometric contour slopes "up" (poorer low-frequency hearing), the SSI function is poorer than the PB function; this may indicate a central dysfunction;

In the case of an eighth nerve (retrocochlear) lesion, "rollover" of PB and/or SSI functions occur; in cases of central disorders, the SSI function falls well below the PB function despite normal sensitivity. The effects of ipsilateral versus contralateral masking are also diagnostic. Poor performance with ipsilateral competition is indicative of brainstem dysfunction, while poor performance with contralateral competition indicates temporal lobe pathology.

With regard to rollover of performance-intensity functions, Jerger and Jerger (1971) found 9 subjects, from a total of 741 ears in a general clinical population, that had rollover indices (PB max-PB min/PB max) of .50 or more. Seven of these 9 subjects were over age 60. The Jergers concluded that, when high rollover occurs in the general population, the individuals are likely to be elderly. Gang (1976) obtained performance-intensity functions for W-22 PB words in older listeners with varying degrees of hearing loss and observed an age-related increase in the rollover index (Fig. 9-21). Six of 32 subjects had pronounced rollover. Compared to the subjects with smaller rollover indexes, these six

were older (79 versus 61.8 years) but also had elevated SRTs (23.3 versus 10.9). Shirinian and Arnst (1982) also observed rollover of PI-PB in older subjects (see Fig. 9-23 below). In contrast to these studies, Punch and McConnell (1969) found no rollover to 40 dB SL (Fig. 9-2, above) in older subjects with or without hearing loss. However, many of the subjects in the studies by Gang (1976) and Shirinian and Arnst (1982) required intensities greater than 40 dB SL before rollover occurred. Thus, Punch and McConnell (1969) might have observed more rollover had they used higher SLs.

Jerger and Hayes (1977) and Hayes and Jerger (1979) compared performance on the SSI and PB word recognition. Older subjects performed more poorly on the SSI (Fig. 9-22). As shown previously in Figure 9-10, Orchik and Burgess (1977) observed poorer performance on the SSI with ipsilateral competition by older subjects with less than 25 dB hearing loss through 2000 Hz (30 dB loss at 4 kHz for some subjects). They did not test PB recognition. Otto and McCandless (1982a) found that the mean SSI maximum scores declined

Figure 9-21. Rollover index (adapted from Gang, 1976).

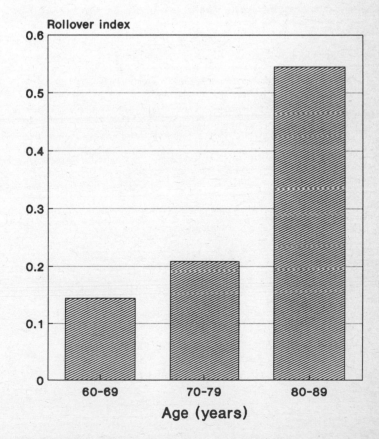

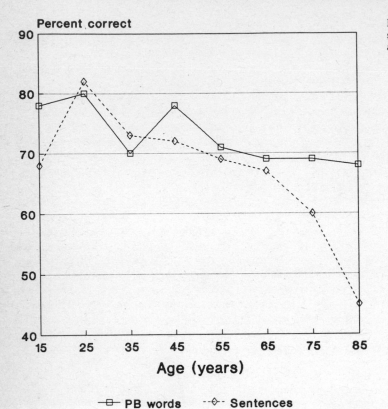

Figure 9-22. Recognition of PB words and synthetic sentences (adapted from Jerger and Hayes, 1977).

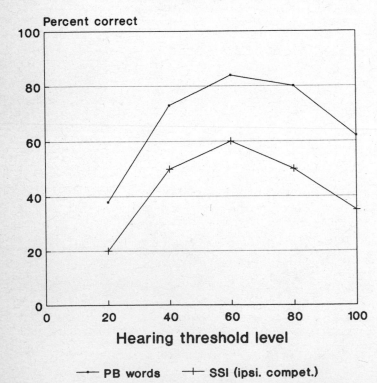

Figure 9-23. Performance-intensity functions for PB words and SSI for a subgroup of 60- to 89-year-olds exhibiting "central" patterns of performance (adapted from Shirinian and Arnst, 1982).

between 60 and 80+ years in presbycusis subjects, while PB max scores did not change systematically in this age range.

PI-SSI and PI-PB functions were obtained by Shirinian and Arnst (1982) in a group of subjects aged 60 to 89 years. The functions indicated that 37 of 62 subjects had central deficits. Most of the "central" patients displayed one of two patterns of performance: either PI-SSI performance fell below PI-PB by 14 percent or more at the highest intensity measured, or PI-PB and PI-SSI functions were interweaving until the final intensity level, where PI-SSI performance was depressed by 14 percent or more. Rollover of both SSI and PB functions was typical in this group of "central" patients, as suggested by the mean performance summarized in Figure 9-23.

Bosatra and Russolo (1982) used ipsilateral and contralateral competing messages with the SSI on 15 subjects aged 60 to 65. In the ipsilateral condition, performance decreased from 80 to 75 percent at zero message-to-competition ratio to 60 to 35 percent at -20 MCR. The contralateral competition had a lesser effect (100 percent at 0 MCR compared to 100 to 80 percent

at -30 MCR). Both PB and (unmasked) SSI scores were excellent in this group. Bosatra and Russolo also reported that subjects over 65 with presbycusis had reduced maximum performance on both SSI and PB performance, sometimes with rollover, and that the maximum SSI performance "usually falls below the PB function" (p.339).

Elderly subjects were divided by Kaplan and Pickett (1984) into two groups based on degree of hearing loss: a "borderline" group (thresholds of 20 dB or less at 500, 1000, and 2000 Hz but with greater losses at 4000 and 8000 Hz) and a "mild to moderate" group (thresholds of 25 dB or higher at two or more of the three lower frequencies as well as deficits at the two high frequencies). The mean ages of the two groups were 71.6 years and 78.5 years, respectively. The "mild to moderate" group did more poorly than the "borderline" group on PB max and SSI max (differences were statistically significant, computed from their raw data) (Fig. 9-24). This suggests an influence of peripheral hearing loss that is stronger for the PI-SSI than the PI-PB, which could contribute to the "central" PI profile. The mean percent rollover did not differ significantly.

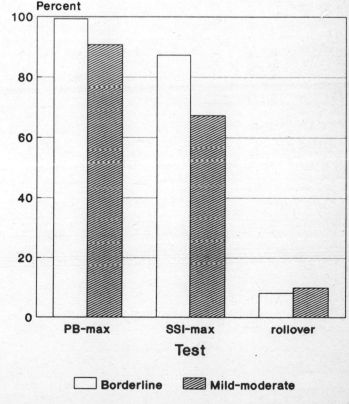

Figure 9-24. PB max, SSI max, and rollover as a function of degree of hearing impairment in older subjects (adapted from Kaplan and Pickett, 1984). Borderline = slight degree of hearing loss.

Irrespective of group, 4 of 7 subjects (57 percent) aged 80 or more had rollover of at least 10 percent, compared to 7 of 18 (39 percent) subjects less than 80 years old.

To summarize, PB max decreases in some elderly listeners, but the mean decrease in the general population is not impressive. Rollover of SSI-PB functions apparently occurs in many older individuals, but rather high intensities may be required to demonstrate the phenomenon. Rollover may be rather common in individuals over 80. The PI-SSI with ipsilateral competing message declines relative to the PI-PB in a good portion of elderly people. While performance of some elderly subjects in these studies may have been influenced by hearing loss, the patterns of PB and SSI performance imply central auditory dysfunction (assuming validity of the tests).

BINAURAL TESTS OF SPEECH PERCEPTION

Binaural hearing requires the integration and/or synthesis of input from the two ears by the central auditory system. Therefore, tests of speech perception in which the same stimuli are presented to both ears simultaneously (diotic presentation) or when different stimuli or portion of stimuli are presented to each ear (dichotic presentation) can be sensitive to CAS deficiencies. A number of such binaural tests have been applied to elderly subjects.

THE STAGGERED SPONDAIC WORD TEST (SSW)

Katz (1962) developed the SSW, in which one spondee word is presented to each ear in overlapping fashion. The first syllable is presented to one ear with no competing signal; the second syllable overlaps with the first syllable of the spondee to the opposite ear; the second syllable of the second word has no competition. The listener is asked to repeat both words. A low score is diagnostic of a central deficit on the side contralateral to the affected ear. Arnst (1982) obtained SSW and corrected SSW (CSSW, raw SSW adjusted for word recognition performance; the CSSW is thought to account for distortion due to peripheral hearing loss). A significant decline in performance was observed for subjects over 80 who were matched for hearing loss with young subjects (Fig. 9-25). Subjects

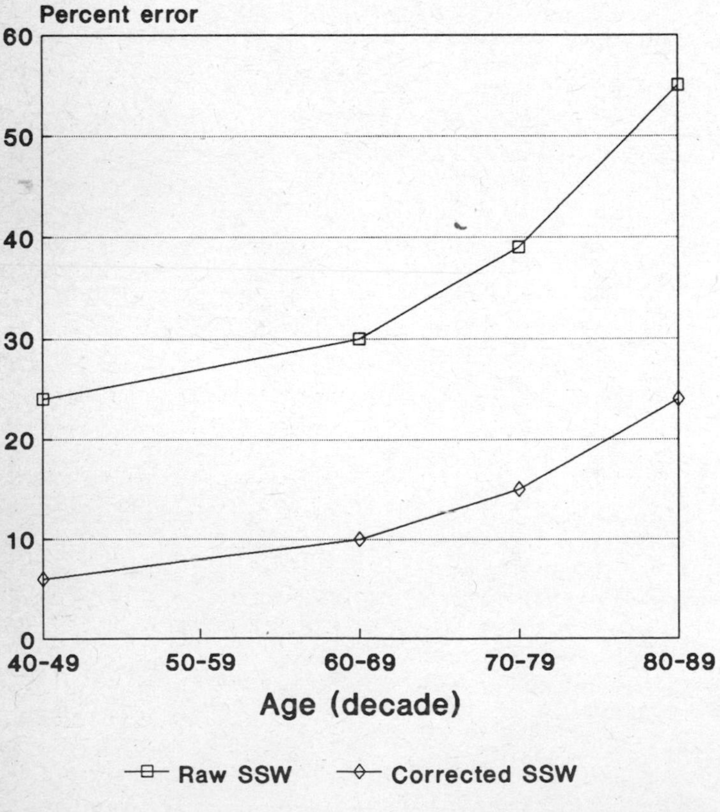

Figure 9-25. Staggered spondaic word (SSW) test performance (adapted from Arnst, 1982).

aged 70 to 79 years performed more poorly only if their loss exceeded 40 dB HL, while the remaining older subjects did not differ significantly from HL-matched young subjects. Because the CSSW score increased in the oldest subjects (relative to SSW), Arnst felt that central dysfunction was implicated.

Kaplan and Pickett (1984) also administered the SSW to their "borderline" and "mild to moderate" hearing loss groups, described previously. None of the borderline subjects had moderate or severe SSW deficits, whereas 9 of 15 subjects in the mild to moderate group did. The mean age of the subjects with moderate or severe SSW deficits was 81.1 years compared to 72.6 years for the subjects without a SSW deficit (irrespective of group).

These findings suggest that both hearing loss and age may be factors in SSW performance.

FILTERED SPEECH TESTS

One procedure used to assess CAS function employs speech material that has been subjected to two different complementary filtering conditions (e.g., two frequency bands); one of the filtered conditions is presented to each ear, and the CAS must fuse the two. The study by Palva and Jokinen (1970), discussed previously (Fig. 9-19), indicated that older subjects were able to fuse binaurally filtered speech material, as indicated by their good performance relative to monaural speech. Kaplan and Pickett (1981), Nabelek and Robinson (1982; Fig. 9-12), and Haas (1982) also found that diotic and dichotic speech was discriminated better than monotic speech by older subjects. Grady and colleagues (1984) detected no significant age effect on binaural fusion when the effects of hearing loss were taken into account. Thus, although filtering has deleterious effects on speech perception in the elderly, the ability to binaurally fuse the information appears to persist.

THE LAG EFFECT

Data from two research groups indicate that older subjects have an abnormal lag effect, a phenomenon observed when dichotic stimuli are presented with an interaural delay, and the lagging signal causes "backward masking" of the leading signal (Gelfand, Hoffman, Waltzman, and Piper, 1980; Martini et al., 1988). Martini and colleagues (Fig. 9-26) observed that young subjects' performance improved when the lag was increased from 0 to 90 msec.; the improvement from 180 to 500 msec. was not statistically significant and probably reflected a ceiling effect. Older subjects

(55 to 74 years) with normal hearing for age performed more poorly with no lag and had no significant improvement from 0 to 90 msec.; however, improvement did occur from 180 to 500 msec. Gelfand and colleagues compared performance on leading versus lagging scores. Perception of leading stimuli was actually better in older subjects (but not in young subjects) for the 30 msec. delay, indicating an aberrant lag effect. They interpreted a reduced overall dichotic performance (no lag, binaural input) in older subjects as suggesting a reduced capacity for processing binaural information. The reduced and/or aberrant lag effect was interpreted as poorer temporal processing by older subjects.

MASKING LEVEL DIFFERENCE (MLD)

The binaural masking level difference (MLD) refers to the improvement in masked thresholds as signals are made to differ between the two ears. For instance, a tone or spondee word is presented to one ear with a masker of intensity just sufficient to mask the tone. The same type of masker is presented 180 degrees out of phase to the opposite ear, making the stimulus sound audible. A number of variations with regard to the stimuli and maskers (some not involving phase manipulation) have been used with speech stimuli. Normal subjects typically enjoy an improvement in threshold (release from masking, or MLD). A reduced MLD appears to be diagnostic of brainstem dysfunction (Musiek and Baran, 1987).

Tillman, Carhart, and Nicholls (1973) used a variety of masking conditions to determine MLDs for spondees in young and elderly listeners. MLDs for the younger listeners were "usually somewhat larger" than those of older listeners. For 18 different masking conditions, only three t-tests were significant ($p < 0.05$); however, most mean MLDs were larger for young listeners. There was little age difference when the masker complex was given antiphasically (young subjects' mean 7.86, range 5.5–10.8; old subjects' mean 6.03, range 4.6–8.0). Similarly, time delay (0.8 msec.) of the masker between ears resulted in small differences (young subjects' mean 5.14, range 3.6–7.1; old subjects' mean 4.33, range 3.5–5.9). With opposed delay (one signal in the masker complex delayed in one ear and the remainder of the masker complex delivered to the other ear), the age effect was stronger (young subjects' mean 4.5, range 2.1–3.4; old subjects' mean 2.3, range 1.8–3.0).

As seen in Table 9-4, some studies (Bocca and Antonelli, 1976; Findlay and Schuchman, 1976; Olsen et al., 1976) have found that older listeners have smaller MLDs than young listeners. However, the magnitude

TABLE 9-4. AGING AND PERCEPTION OF SPEECH: BINAURAL EXPERIMENTS

Study	Test	Performance of older subjects
Balas '62	SSW	poorer, especially for competing conditions*
Berruecos '70	time compressed sentences	binaural recognition much better than monaural in OSs *
Palva & Jokinen '70	bandpass-filtered words monaural & binaural	monaural poorer by 30–39 yrs.; after 60, binaural > left ear > right ear **** (Fig. 9-19)
Tillman et al. '73	spondees in noise	MLDs slightly smaller in OSs; greatest age effect for opposed delay *
Bergman et al. '76	sentences binaurally HP, LP, filtered	poorer (Fig. 9-7) * ("relatively nm hearing")
Bocca & Antonelli '76	sentences in speech noise	MLD, OSs = 6.0 dB; MLD, YSs = 7.2 dB (prob. ns) * (high-frequency hl)
Findlay & Schuchman '76	monosyllabic words, cocktail party conditions	smaller MLDs in OSs, but age effect not strong; high variability ***
Olsen et al. '76	MLD for spondees	25% of OSs had smaller MLDs than 96% of normals ***
McCoy et al. '77	SSW	poorer, especially males, but when hl accounted for, little age effect ****
Warren et al. '78	voice in 4 spatially separate background voices	no improvement in dichotic v. diotic; smaller MLDs*
Amerman & Parnell '80	SSW	poorer in 60–79-year OSs, despite nm word recognition but ns age effect ****
Gelfand et al. '80	CV stimuli with interaural delay	poorer recognition; abnormal lag effect; no "right ear advantage" *
Kaplan & Pickett '81	Rhyme test in cafeteria noise & babble, LP-HP filtered; SPIN	diotic & dichotic > monotic for hl-OSs ***
Arnst '82	corrected SSW	ns: hl-YSs v. hl-OSs to age 70; 70–79 hl-OSs poorer; OSs over 80 poorer (Fig. 9-25) **,****
Haas '82	PB words,LP, HP filtered (780 Hz) split signal	hl-OSs: nsage effect re: unfiltered diotic & HP diotic in quiet ***
Nabelek & Robinson '82	Modified Rhyme words with reverberation	binaural scores 5% better than monaural * (Fig. 9-12)
Kelly-Ballweber & Dobie '84	speech & non-speech	ns age effect on binaural interactions tasks **
Grady et al. '84	binaural fusion, LP/HP filtered spondees	when the effect of hl was taken into account, ns age effect (23–83 yrs.) ****
Kaplan & Pickett '84	first-formant masking, synthetic vowels; SSW	dichotic > monotic presentation; SSW decline correlated with hl & age ***
Martini et al. '88	CV stimulus with interaural delay	poorer dichotic performance; abnormal lag effect; no "right ear advantage" * (Fig. 9-26)
Rodriguez et al. '90	SSW	about 98% performance in OSs *

hl = hearing loss; nm = normal hearing for age; YSs = young
subjects; OSs = older subjects; S/N = signal to noise ratio; ns =
no significant difference
< = poorer relative performance; > = better relative performance
*hearing within normal limits, at least for age
** hl matched in YSs & OSs
*** OSs had hl for age
****heterogeneous hl

Figure 9-26. The lag effect: recognition as a function of interaural lag (adapted from Martini et al., 1988).

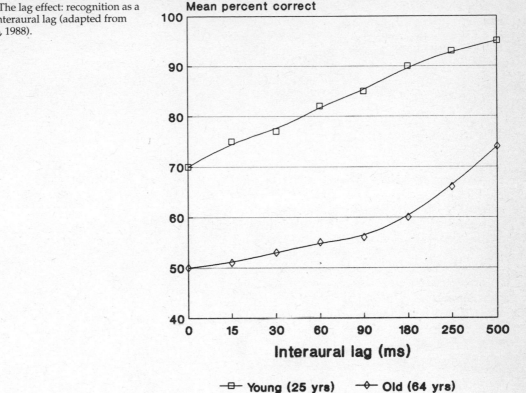

COCKTAIL PARTY PROBLEM

Warren, Wagener, and Herman (1978) had subjects listen to a target voice in four background voices originating from adjacent locations in space. The material was presented both dichotically (preserving normal interaural cues) or diotically (same input to either ear). Older subjects showed less improvement than young subjects for the dichotic condition, suggesting that older listeners have reduced ability to perform the binaural analysis needed to separate the target speech from the competing speech.

and incidence of MLD change is not impressive (a conclusion also reached for MLDs to tones; Chapter 8). Furthermore, hearing loss per se may result in a decrease in MLD (see Olsen et al., 1976, for references). Thus, the small differences in MLD that have been observed do not provide strong evidence of a central defect.

FIRST-FORMANT MASKING

Kaplan and Pickett (1981; 1984) investigated the observation that, in hearing-impaired listeners, the first formant (F1) of some speech sounds may mask second formant (F2) transitions. They found that the upward spread of masking was reduced in older listeners with some degree of hearing loss if F2 was presented to one ear and F1 was presented to the other ear; performance was better with dichotic presentation than when the formants were presented monotically. Scores on the Modified Rhyme Test and SPIN Test sentences against competing noise were also significantly better with dichotic (and diotic) presentation versus monotic. Peripheral hearing loss was not a factor, as subject subgroups with "borderline" and "mild to moderate" pure tone hearing loss did not differ significantly. Some of the subjects had "central" patterns in SSI max, rollover, or SSW tests (see Fig. 9-24). Correlations among the performance of individuals on these tests and formant masking experiments were not reported. Nevertheless, because the elderly subjects, as a group, had indications of suboptimal retrocochlear performance, the authors felt that their data suggested that binaural listening may not be impaired even with a degree of central dysfunction.

SUMMARY: BINAURAL TESTS

Performance of older listeners on binaural tasks appears to vary depending on the task and on hearing loss. For instance, older subjects tend to perform more poorly on the SSW, but it is affected by hearing loss as well. Binaural fusion is not greatly diminished if hearing loss is taken into account. The MLD tends to be smaller in older subjects, but the age effect is not consistent or large. Thus, while age-related declines in binaural processing may occur, they are not especially pronounced in many cases.

GENERAL CONCLUSIONS

For most people, aging in the absence of audiometrically significant hearing loss has little effect on the perception of relatively easy speech material. For masked or degraded speech, perceptual deficits associated with moderate peripheral presbycusis and/or other correlates of aging are manifested. Some speech perception deficits can be largely accounted for by peripheral hearing loss; in other cases, hearing loss is not a sufficient explanation. Some binaural speech perception tasks are often performed well by older listeners, suggesting little central dysfunction, whereas poor performance on other tasks suggests a deficit in central mechanisms. Perhaps the greatest challenge to understanding the empirical findings reviewed here is to understand the roles of hearing loss and other age-related factors and their interactions. This question requires integration of information presented throughout this book and is discussed in the following chapter.

CHAPTER 10

Etiology and Mechanisms of
Speech Perception Deficits
in the Elderly

We saw in Chapter 9 that elderly people encounter various difficulties in discriminating speech under unfavorable listening conditions. These difficulties could result from peripheral presbycusis, dysfunction of the central auditory system, impaired cognitive-linguistic processing, or from an interaction among two or all three of these variables. In this chapter we examine the contributions of cognitive-linguistic, central auditory, and peripheral auditory processes to age-related perceptual deficits.

CONTRIBUTIONS OF COGNITIVE AND LINGUISTIC PROCESSES TO SPEECH PERCEPTION: THEORETICAL AND OTHER CONSIDERATIONS

Age-related changes in cognitive processes have the potential to impact perception of both speech and non-speech material. Presumably, certain general abilities must remain intact if the auditory system is to function effectively. Important factors might include speed of central processing, attention, arousal level, and motivation. In addition, information-processing and linguistic abilities are required to make use of the acoustic and phonemic information extracted by the auditory system. Two issues must be addressed: the changes in relevant cognitive and linguistic skills that may accompany aging and the effect of such changes on the ability to perceive speech and other sounds.

AGING AND GENERAL COGNITIVE SKILLS

Jerger and co-workers have argued against a necessary role of cognitive deficits in contributing to the decline in speech perception in the elderly. Jerger, Jerger, Oliver, and Pirrozzolo (1989a) determined the auditory and cognitive status in subjects aged 51 to 91. The subjects had similar hearing for both ears; for the right ear, pure tone losses ranged from 2 to 48 dB HL (mean 23 dB) at 500 to 2000 Hz and from 5–70 dB HL for 1 to 4 kHz (mean 31 dB HL). The PB word test, SSI, SPIN, and dichotic sentence identification test (DSI)

were used for speech audiometry. Subjects were also given a battery of psychological tests including the Minnesota Multiphasic Personality Inventory, Wechsler intelligence scales, tests of visual and auditory reaction times, and other tests of cognitive ability. The prevalence of central auditory "processing disorders" (defined as abnormality on one or more of the three speech measures) was 50 percent. Forty-one percent of the subjects had cognitive deficits (evidence of mild or moderate cerebral dysfunction in one or both hemispheres as judged by an evaluation of the neuropsychological test battery by a neuropsychologist who was "blind" to the audiological or medical data).

Central processing disorders and cognitive function were congruent in 63 percent of the individuals (i.e., they were normal or abnormal on both). Central processing was abnormal despite normal cognitive functioning in 23 percent of the sample, while 14 percent had normal central processing but abnormal cognitive performance. Jerger et al. (1989a) argued that, since 37 percent of the subjects performed differently on cognitive versus central audiometric tests, speech understanding deficits cannot be explained by cognitive deficits in many cases. In addition, when subjects with and without central processing disorders were matched for age, hearing loss, and intellectual ability, they did not differ significantly on most measures of cognitive performance.

Jerger, Stach, Pruitt, Harper, and Kirby (1989b) evaluated the role of cognitive competence in speech understanding by testing patients suffering from dementia. Performance was "consistent with normal central functioning" in about half of the demented patients. Because these patients exhibited a number of cognitive deficits, Jerger and colleagues argued against a critical role of general cognitive incompetence in the decline of speech perception in the elderly.

One possible criticism of the above studies is that the tests used by Jerger and colleagues were not sensitive to all cognitive skills relevant to speech understanding. The psychological measures they used may be well suited for identifying clinically relevant changes in cognitive performance such as intellectual decline, senility, memory deficits, and increased sensorimotor reaction time. While their data indicate that these skills need not be closely linked to speech perception in some individuals, other (unmeasured) cognitive or linguistic skills might be involved. It should also be noted that poor cognitive performance was associated with poor performance on speech tests in a good proportion of their subjects. For instance, the majority of the subjects in the Jerger et al. (1989a) study had congruent cognitive and central processing status, and about half of the demented subjects in the Jerger et al. (1989b) study had abnormal central processing. In these cases, the role of cognitive deficits cannot be ruled out.

Nevertheless, the work of Jerger and colleagues indicates that considerable cognitive impairment can exist in some individuals without concomitant deficits in performance on SSI, PB word, and SPIN tests. Conversely, poor performance on these tasks can occur without general cognitive impairment.

AGING AND THE SPEED OF CENTRAL PROCESSING

There is little question that the speed of many mental processes is slowed in the elderly (Salthouse, 1985). Whether such slowing would have an impact on the perception of speech, however, is unclear. Interestingly, one likely exception to the slowing of functions in the aged is vocal reaction time, which, in some studies, has been found to fare well with aging (Salthouse, 1985). This suggests that slowing of the ability to deal with words may not be substantial. The notion of an "un-slowed" rate of speech processing in the elderly is supported by the fact that speech material presented under good listening conditions is not affected very much as a function of age (Chapter 9). On the other hand, the perceptual "fusion" of rapidly presented stimuli is poorer in the elderly (Chapter 8), and compressed speech presents particular problems (Chapter 9). While these findings could be a function of peripheral hearing loss (see below), they could also be interpreted as resulting from a slowing of auditory processing.

Feldman and Reger (1967) assessed reaction time and recognition of W-22 PB words under good listening conditions. They found a significant age-related increase in auditory reaction time, suggesting slower central processing of information. However, multiple regression analysis indicated that 72 percent of the variance in PB word recognition scores was accounted for by pure-tone thresholds at two frequencies, with relatively little variance being accounted for by reaction time. It may be the case that whatever "slowing" occurs in the aging auditory system is only significant when words are presented at an unusually fast rate or under poor listening conditions. Under good listening conditions the aging auditory system functions fast enough to provide for accurate speech perception.

MOTIVATION, AROUSAL, AND ATTENTION

Reduced levels of motivation, arousal, and/or attention can affect the performance of elderly subjects in a laboratory setting. For instance, McCroskey and Kasten (1980) described a study by their research group in which older, hearing impaired individuals with poor speech perception were presented with words in the context of a learning/conditioning experiment. Seventeen of 18 subjects improved their performance significantly when they were reinforced appropriately for correct responses. Apparently, the testing environment and its effects on motivation, attention, and reinforcement of performance had a good deal to do with poorer performance of the elderly listeners. In a real-life (non-laboratory) setting, this may not be a serious problem for the healthy elderly, who would presumably be motivated to hear what is important to them.

SUMMARY

There is little evidence that age-related declines in general cognitive ability, cognitive speed, or motivation pose serious problems in the ability of the auditory system to process speech and other sounds when the individuals are healthy, and listening and motivational conditions are favorable. However, it is under unfavorable listening conditions that elderly listeners exhibit perceptual deficits, and it is difficult to rule out a role of diminished cognitive processes under such conditions. It would seem valuable to gain a better understanding of extra-auditory cognitive influences on auditory perception in the elderly under non-optimal circumstances.

INFORMATION PROCESSING

The processing of speech may be viewed from information processing and psycholinguistic perspectives.[1] The information processing perspective is often set in the framework of memory processes. Two stages of memory are *primary, or working memory* (the "workspace" for phrases and sentences for which meaning is being construed) and *secondary, or long-term memory* (the storehouse of learned knowledge). Both memory processes are important to the functioning of the auditory system. Acoustic-phonemic infor-

---

[1] The present discussion draws from recent reviews by Davis and Ball (1989), Poon (1985), and by the National Research Council's Committee on Hearing, Bioacoustics, and Biomechanics (WGSUA, 1988), to which the reader is referred for a more thorough treatment of these issues.

mation, once registered, must be maintained in working memory, where it is acted upon cognitively and linguistically via secondary memory processes. These processes can be viewed as "bottom-up" (incoming information working its way up the auditory system) and "top-down" (the application of knowledge of syntax, semantics, and the real world to understanding the ascending information). From a psycholinguistic perspective, top-down processing is related to language comprehension through the interaction of processing components, or "modules" (Davis and Ball, 1989). These include lexical access (i.e., word recognition), syntactic parsing (i.e., constituent boundary recognition), and semantic interpretation (e.g., inferencing). These processing components operate within the working memory using information stored in secondary memory.

The psychological literature is fairly consistent in showing that primary memory abilities are not substantially impaired in the elderly (Poon, 1985) at least for information that is not dynamically complex. That is, operations such as digit span tend to be unimpaired, whereas "dynamic" processes, in which information must be held in memory while other operations are performed, are more prone to age-related declines (WGSUA, 1988).[2] Because the understanding of sentences requires that some words be held in memory while subsequent words are incoming, it is possible that primary memory deficits could contribute to age-related declines in comprehension of more complex sentences. On the other hand, it seems much less likely that perception of single words or simple phrases would be seriously affected. The psycholinguistic literature (Davis and Ball, 1989) appears to support this view, since recognition and comprehension of words are not seriously impaired as people age. With regard to sentence comprehension, performance on aphasia batteries and comprehension tests and the ability to explain the meaning of ambiguous sentences are not compromised by aging. However, comprehension declines in the elderly when competing perceptual demands are made (e.g., competing babble) or when sentences are complex or implausible.

Age-related decrements in recall or recognition of information stored in secondary memory are well documented (Poon, 1985). From a bottom-up vantage point, secondary memory is concerned with the storage and evaluation of information in a time frame that would seem to follow, and have little relevance to, the *auditory system's* on-line perception of sound. As a top-down process, however, secondary memory can affect perception early on by making use of semantic or syntactic features of sentences or phrases. It seems likely that an age-related decline in secondary memory would make it more difficult for elderly subjects to follow extended discourse or stories, but recognition of phrases and simple sentences would probably be less affected. *Semantic memory* is particularly germane in this regard. This type of secondary memory contains knowledge about the meaning and rules of language that would be applied to words, phrases, and sentences. The WGSUA (1988) concluded that the research on semantic memory "suggests little if any change with age that might be a source of age differences in speech understanding" (p. 870). From a psycholinguistic perspective, a recent study by Davis and Ball (1989) concluded that the semantic component of language comprehension is unchanged through the lifespan. In this regard, Nittrouer and Boothroyd (1990) found that older listeners had unimpaired ability to use semantic (and syntactic) constraints in the perception of simple sentences. Thus, semantic memory and semantic processing appear to be robust in the face of aging and probably do not contribute greatly to speech perception deficits in the elderly.

The research on the SPIN test, presented in Chapter 9, is also relevant. Several studies showed that older subjects benefited to the same extent (re: improvement of scores) when contextual information was available (PH versus PL sentences). This suggests that this cognitive-linguistic ability remains intact. When deficits in PH sentences did occur in elderly listeners, peripheral hearing loss was implicated (Schum and Matthews, 1990).

In summary, age-related declines in working and/or secondary memory or in semantic language abilities are probably not major factors with respect to the types of psychophysical tests we have dealt with in this book—those focusing on perception of sounds or recognition of words or simple sentences. Speech understanding abilities that require the comprehension of speech content may be seriously compromised by primary and secondary memory deficits or by impairments in certain linguistic abilities (e.g., syntactic:

---

[2] The concept of "sensory memory" also appears in the cognitive psychology literature (Poon, 1985). Sensory memory precedes primary memory. It is a modality-specific buffer memory called "echoic" for the auditory modality—that provides a veridical representation and lasts for seconds at best. To the extent that the phenomenon of sensory memory is valid, the transfer of information from sensory to primary memory does not appear to be affected by aging (Poon, 1985). The point may be moot, however. Since primary memory of simple items is not affected by aging, it is evident that the input of information to primary memory is adequate.

Davis and Ball, 1989). However, these functions rely heavily on areas of the brain outside of the auditory system.

CONCLUSIONS

Any cognitive-linguistic declines that may occur in the elderly are typically not sufficient to interfere with the perception of words and sentences under favorable listening conditions. However, it cannot be concluded from such evidence that speech perception is unaffected by age-related deficits of a cognitive or linguistic nature when conditions are not good. It may be that cognitive or linguistic abilities are diminished, but the tasks used by psychological researchers have not been taxing enough to reveal a deficit. Thus, the exaggerated deficits in the elderly under difficult conditions (e.g., compressed or masked speech) might be due to over-taxing of weakened cognitive or linguistic abilities. The available evidence does not allow us to rule out this possibility.

CONTRIBUTIONS OF CENTRAL AUDITORY SYSTEM PROCESSES TO SPEECH PERCEPTION: THEORETICAL AND OTHER CONSIDERATIONS

If the processing of acoustic-phonemic information by the central auditory system were impaired in older people, perceptual problems would likely result. Compared to deficits associated with diminished linguistic abilities, the effects of CAS dysfunction should be more readily observed with words and phrases, as well as with non-speech material. However, this distinction is a fuzzy one because cognitive and/or linguistic competence is likely to be a factor in virtually any type of perceptual task (e.g., Hinchcliffe, 1962).

As noted in Chapter 6, age-related histopathological and physiological changes in the central auditory system may result from the central effects of biological aging (CEBA) and from the central effects of peripheral pathology (CEPP). At present, we are unable to adequately identify the role of each aspect of central presbycusis as contributors to perceptual dysfunction. Theoretically, either type of effect can influence the results of central tests of auditory function. Let us now examine the evidence for central presbycusis.

HISTOPATHOLOGICAL CHANGES

As demonstrated in Chapter 6, some central auditory neurons are lost or degenerate with aging (CEBA). It is feasible that a reduction in the number of functional neurons would be deleterious to CAS functioning, causing central presbycusis. Indeed, this is the assumption made by those who cite studies by Hansen and Reske-Nielsen (1965), Kirikae et al. (1964), and others as evidence of "central presbycusis." Unfortunately, this is not necessarily a valid assumption. Consider the following points. (a) Systems with few components may be more efficient than systems with many components. A committee of three is likely to reach a decision more quickly and efficiently than a committee of ten. Within certain limits, "simpler may be better." (b) There may be considerable redundancy in the nervous system with regard to the roles of individual neurons. Millions of cortical neurons are lost by healthy adults between young adulthood and middle age (e.g., Brody, 1955) without dire consequences. Even after considerable loss of neurons, an adequate number may remain to support normal functional capacities. (c) The brain is often adept at compensating for losses of neurons to injury, with functional recovery from minor strokes often occurring. The functions associated with lost neurons may be taken over by surviving neurons. In short, there is no reason to believe that a *modest loss* of CAS neurons will *necessarily* interfere with auditory perception.

The same caution regarding functional significance can be raised for other histopathological correlates of aging in the CAS, described in Chapter 6. The accumulation of lipofuscin, the loss of dendritic branches or spines, the loss of volume of CAS nuclei, and alterations in capillaries in the brain *may* impair the processing of auditory stimuli. However, there are no studies that demonstrate a relationship between age-related histopathological changes and deficits in auditory perception.

RESPONSES OF CAS NEURONS IN MOUSE MODELS

It was shown in Chapter 6 that changes occur in the response properties of CAS neurons of very old CBA mice that had minimal peripheral impairment (implying CEBA) and in middle-aged C57 mice that had substantial high-frequency losses (implying CEPP). The latter condition resulted in more serious disruptions of neural responses. The effects of aging and/or peripheral presbycusis include changes in the shape and sharpness of frequency tuning curves, diminution of differences in frequency responses across tonotopic maps, and an increased number of nonfunctional ("sluggish") neurons in the population. Two points are germane to the present discussion. First, these and other changes theoretically have the potential to disrupt auditory perception, if they were to occur in humans. Since most biological changes that occur in rodents also occur in humans, it is feasible that they do occur in the human CAS, at least in some respects. Second, in hearing-impaired C57 mice, none of these changes were predicted a priori from the "audiogram," or even from peripheral histopathology, yet the changes were undoubtedly caused by peripheral impairment. Even the most thorough of evaluations of the inner ear fail to reveal the types of changes that may occur in the central processing of sounds (CEPP). Unfortunately, the occurrence of the types of CAS changes found in mice has not yet been tested for in humans, and we have no knowledge of their significance.

NEURAL NOISE

The notion of an age-related decrease in the neural signal-to-noise ratio has been used by gerontologists to account for age-related cognitive and sensory changes (Cremer and Zeef, 1987; Gregory, 1974). Research findings discussed in Chapter 6 are interesting in this regard. First, enhanced spontaneous discharge rates are observed in neurons of the inferior colliculus of aged CBA and middle-aged C57 mice. Second, there is evidence that the inhibitory neurotransmitter, GABA, is diminished in the inferior colliculus of old rats (Caspary et al., 1990). Third, the utilization of glucose by CAS neurons is maintained at a high rate in old rodents, even when hearing impairment is severe. These findings suggest that high levels of "neural noise," the "base rate" of firing of action potentials in central auditory neurons, may occur in the elderly auditory system. Psychophysical evidence consistent with the notion of an increase in neural noise was provided in the study by Novak and Anderson (1982), described in Chapter 8 (Fig. 8-14). Their findings suggest that peripheral neural presbycusis is associated with enhanced neural noise that mimics the effects of external, acoustic noise in affecting the masking level difference.

The Novak and Anderson (1982) study obtained evidence of neural noise in subjects diagnosed as having neural presbycusis, but not in subjects with other types of presbycusis. The neural presbycusis diagnosis was made on the basis of poor word recognition, whereas other presbycusis patients had good word recognition. One way of viewing the selection of subjects and results of this study is that elderly subjects with hearing loss were grouped on the basis of word recognition ability. Only those subjects with poor word recognition showed evidence of neural noise. By this interpretation, when neural noise was present, word recognition was impaired; when neural noise was absent, word recognition was good. In other words, neural noise may have been responsible for poor speech perception.

It might prove valuable to subject this alternate interpretation of Novak and Anderson's findings to experimental evaluation. Certainly, future research should address the occurrence and functional significance of central neural noise in central presbycusis. The possibility that tinnitus can result from neural noise should also be investigated. At this time, however, the role of CAS neural noise role in age-related perceptual deficits is unknown.

EVOKED RESPONSES

Evoked responses provide some information about the physiological status of the human CAS, as reviewed in Chapter 7. Measurements of latencies of ABR waves indicate that the speed of transmission of information concerning simple acoustic stimuli is minimally affected by aging. On the other hand, in older listeners, the effect of increased stimulus rates on the ABR is exaggerated (Fig. 7-25). Observations on the amplitudes of ABR waves suggest that some changes at upper brainstem levels differ from those at peripheral or lower brainstem levels. Amplitudes of later ABR waves decrease only slightly with age, with or without peripheral presbycusis, but earlier waves are drastically affected if peripheral impairment is present. In addition, presbycusis can affect amplitude-intensity functions of early and late ABR waves differently. These types of observations suggest that central changes are occurring, but they provide little insight into how auditory perception may be affected. The utility of ABRs in detecting central presbycusis has yet to be demonstrated.

In fact, recent studies utilizing the ABR have provided little evidence of a relationship to clinical indices of central presbycusis. Debruyne and Tyberghein (1989) identified a number of patients who had reduced SSI versus PB performance-intensity functions and/or prolongation of ABR wave V latency at high stimulus rates. Both of these are clinical measures of central auditory dysfunction. No significant correlations were obtained between ABR latency and performance-intensity functions, suggesting that they represented different processes. Rawool (1989) computed correlations between ABR parameters and PB word recognition in noise for subjects aged 40 to 60 years who had hearing loss (high-frequency PTA of 50–60 dB HL). A significant correlation was obtained between the word recognition scores and the latencies of ABR waves I and II, but no significant correlations were found between word recognition and either the latency or amplitude of later waves. These findings suggest the presence of eighth nerve pathology, but they do not reveal central changes correlated with poor word recognition.

Other evoked responses reflect the activity of cortical or thalamic levels of the brain. As noted in Chapter 7, several studies have reported increased latencies of the middle-latency response (MLR), late (cortical) responses, and the P300. Enhanced MLR Pa amplitudes have also been seen in elderly people. The more robust changes in these measures suggests that they may be more useful in identifying central presbycusis. However, one report (Paludetti et al., 1991) found no correlation between abnormalities in MLR waves and performance on compressed speech.

EVIDENCE OF CENTRAL PRESBYCUSIS FROM AUDIOMETRIC TESTS

Of the various audiometric tests of central auditory function, those using binaural presentation of stimuli are the most compelling because binaural interactions must take place in the brain. Review of the studies summarized in Chapter 9 (Table 9-4) leads one to the conclusion that older subjects perform rather well on some binaural tasks. Several studies indicate either no age effect, no age effect when hearing loss is taken into account, or differences that are rather small. Thus, binaural tests do not provide much evidence that central presbycusis is widespread or has serious functional consequences. Performance of elderly listeners on monaural tests of "central" auditory function, such as degraded speech, is consistently diminished (Table 9-3). However, the interpretation of these tests is somewhat muddied by the potential influence of peripheral dysfunction and the rationale used to infer a central site of lesion (see below).

Also adding to the difficulty in interpreting the role of the CAS in performance on tests of central dysfunction are the potential influences of nonauditory variables such as practice effects, test conditions, response criteria, etc. (Chapter 9). Indeed, when the effects of such variables are minimized, tests of central function may be performed rather well by elderly listeners. A cogent example is the "Old Time Ears" project—a longitudinal study of well-known and respected hearing scientists aged 65 and up; a group of subjects that is highly sophisticated with respect to hearing tests (Hood, et al., 1991). A battery of peripheral and central tests was given to these subjects. Whereas a high incidence of peripheral dysfunction was observed (e.g., threshold elevations), little decline in performance has been seen on tests sensitive to central dysfunction (e.g., speech understanding in quiet and with competing noise, masking level difference, dichotic speech tests, ABRs, and MLRs).

The difficulties in using test results to determine the prevalence of central presbycusis in more typical subject populations is demonstrated in a recent study by Welsh, Welsh, and Healy (1985). They used a test battery to evaluate central deficits and found differences in test scores between young and elderly subjects (ninth decade) as follows, with respect to the better mean performance for left or right ear. For competing sentences, mean performance declined from near 100 percent to 90 percent. For lowpass filtered speech, the mean declined from about 65 percent to 40 percent Binaural fusion scores fell from about 85 percent to about 60 percent. Scores on the rapidly alternating speech test decreased by only about 10 percent. Finally, compressed speech decreased from about 75 percent to about 50 percent. For all tests, the range of scores was very large, and the upper range of scores, even for octogenarians, encompassed the mean for young subjects. This study suggests that there is a great deal of variance on central test performance both within and between subjects. While this could mean that individuals had different types of central disorders, no clear patterns were evident. Furthermore, high-frequency hearing loss was prevalent and could have affected performance in compressed speech, binaural fusion, and lowpass filtered speech tests (Chapter 9). In addition, cognitive tests were not given, so it is not clear if the total failure of some subjects on certain tests may have been related to cognitive or other nonauditory factors.

CONCLUSIONS

There is little direct evidence that age-related changes in the central auditory system are functionally significant with respect to hearing, let alone to the perception of speech. Central histopathological changes that might be associated with biological aging are well documented in humans, but we do not know if these changes affect perception. Central physiological changes that might arise from peripheral presbycusis are well documented in mice, but have not been evaluated in humans. Research on the ABR has found some age-related changes, but it is not clear that they are associated with altered perception. Performance of elderly subjects on certain tests of "central" dysfunction suggests the presence of central presbycusis when listening conditions are poor. However, interpretation of these tests is not without problems (see below). On the other hand, there is no evidence to indicate that CEBA or CEPP are *not* significant in many cases of perceptual impairment, and there are certainly theoretical reasons to believe that they are.

CONTRIBUTIONS OF PERIPHERAL PRESBYCUSIS TO SPEECH PERCEPTION: THEORETICAL AND OTHER CONSIDERATIONS

There is no question that peripheral presbycusis is highly prevalent and significantly affects auditory thresholds. The impact of peripheral presbycusis on speech perception is not well understood, however. There are several ways in which peripheral presbycusis might, in theory, affect the perception of speech.

THE NUMBER OF INPUT CHANNELS

Irrespective of absolute audiometric thresholds, the number of "channels" that are capable of carrying suprathreshold information is reduced in many older individuals as a consequence of cochlear neural pathology. In basal, high-frequency regions of the cochlea, there may be virtually no channels remaining in elderly listeners. Thus, the populations of neurons in the cochlear nucleus that receive the ganglion cells' input must operate with reduced amounts of information. A reduction in the number of efferent channels also accompanies peripheral presbycusis.

THE QUALITY OF NEURAL INFORMATION IN AUDITORY NERVE FIBERS

The quality of information carried by axons of surviving ganglion cells may be reduced as a function of

sensorineural or other pathology. The effects of cochlear pathology on the responses of eighth nerve fibers were outlined in Chapter 4 (Table 4-2). The alterations encompass frequency tuning curves, spontaneous firing rates, temporal discharge patterns, phase-locking to low-frequency tones, responses to tonal combinations, intensity functions, and more. Any of these would be expected to degrade the neural messages entering the brain.

If such changes in auditory nerve fibers occur in animals, it is likely that similar changes occur in humans with cochlear pathology. The result would be distortion of cochlear output. The notion of distortion was applied to presbycusis by Plomp and Mimpen (1979), using a model developed by Plomp to describe the intelligibility of speech in noise for impaired listeners. According to this model, problems result from the *attenuation* of sound by hearing loss and from *distortion* of the message. Attenuation can be overcome by increasing the intensity of speech, but distortion cannot. In the presence of noise, distortion is responsible for impairment of speech perception. According to this model, the effects of attenuation and distortion are described by comparison of the SRT in quiet (attenuation plus distortion) and in noise (distortion only). Pure tone thresholds are not good predictors of distortion or, therefore, of deficits in speech perception. This model has been successful in accounting for speech perception performance in elderly listeners in quiet and noise (Duquesnoy, 1983).

LOUDNESS FUNCTIONS

Evidence reviewed in Chapter 8 indicates that a percentage of older listeners exhibit loudness recruitment, a sign of sensory pathology. Hood (1968) has suggested that loudness recruitment (associated with cochlear pathology) or "loudness reversal" (shallower slopes of loudness, associated with auditory nerve lesions) may account for poorer speech perception by elderly listeners at higher intensities. He has shown that derangements of loudness are correlated with decreased speech discrimination and that these were not predicted by the pure tone audiograms in (nonpresbycusis) sensorineural listeners.

FREQUENCY RESOLUTION AND MASKING

Cochlear pathology is likely to interfere with frequency resolution and to result in exaggerated masking of signals by noise (see Chapter 8). For instance, behavioral data from animals suggest that intact inner hair cells (but perhaps not outer hair cells) are essential for frequency resolution (Dallos and Ryan, 1975; Dallos, et al., 1977; Nienhuys and Clark, 1978; 1979). Psychophysical experiments with humans have indicated that poor frequency resolution is likely to be deleterious to certain aspects of speech perception (Dreschler and Plomp, 1980; Festen and Plomp, 1983; Leshowitz, 1977; Pick et al., 1977; Rosen and Fourcin, 1986). For instance, Patterson et al. (1982) presented filtered speech in a notched noise. There was a decrease in speech recognition with age that appeared to be related to a loss in frequency selectivity (changes in the auditory filter) in the elderly subjects.[3]

It is well established that cochlear pathology results in enhanced masking effects (Tyler, 1986). A recent study by Klein, Mills, and Adkins (1990) found enhanced upward spread of masking that was related to hearing loss irrespective of age. There are several possible ways that peripheral presbycusis might affect the masking of signals by noise. Damage to outer hair cells is likely to affect masking, since the OHC system modulates cochlear mechanics and sensitivity of IHCs (Kim, 1984). Stimulation of the efferent olivocochlear bundle to the cochlea has been shown to reduce the masking of tones by noise in single auditory nerve fibers (Winslow and Sachs, 1987). Thus, loss of efferents or their targets within the cochlea could bring about enhanced masking. In addition, the responses of inner hair cells to tone stimuli are affected in complex ways by the presence of broadband noise. In the normal cochlea, enhancement, suppression, or no change in IHC receptor potentials can result, depending on spectral relationships between signal and noise and the sensitivity of the IHCs (Dolan and Nuttall, 1989). Consequently, age-related changes in the condition of IHCs (or OHC influences on IHCs) might alter the normal effects of masking noise on cochlear output.

TEMPORAL RESOLUTION

It was shown in Chapter 8 that temporal resolution is decreased in older listeners, and that this is probably in large part a function of peripheral presbycusis. Harris (1965) pointed out that deficits in binaural temporal resolution would also result in problems in discriminating speech in a noisy environment.

Price and Simon (1984) assessed the ability of young and old listeners to distinguish between the words "rabid" and rapid," since the voicing distinction that separates these words involves temporal

aspects of closure and vowel sounds. The older listeners (who had good hearing for their age, but had higher tone and speech reception thresholds than the young subjects) required longer silence durations to report hearing "rapid, " especially when vowel durations were short and intensity level was high. This was interpreted as indicating an age-related deficit in the processing of temporal information that could cause difficulties in speech perception. One possible explanation of these findings is that the responses of auditory nerve fibers may not recover as rapidly in older subjects. Another explanation is that the young and old listeners differed in inferring the presence of a voiced /b/ (i.e., a cognitive-linguistic factor).

CEPP

Peripheral sensorineural pathology causes changes in central neural activity in animal models that cannot be predicted from simple threshold elevations. Thus, in addition to degrading the neural message before it enters the brain (peripheral effects), peripheral pathology is likely to have various other effects on central processing and perception. CEPP is yet to be evaluated in humans because the tools have not been available to do so. Assuming that CEPP is valid in humans, it is interesting to speculate that high-frequency losses, which are nearly ubiquitous in the elderly, could have significant effects on hearing. Animal research has suggested several consequences of removing high-frequency input to the CAS. These include the induction of increased levels of central spontaneous activity (neural noise), alterations of tonotopic maps (diminution of tonotopic variance and sensitization of low-frequency responses), or elimination of tonic synaptic input (excitatory or inhibitory) to the central auditory neurons.

CONCLUSIONS

Peripheral presbycusis is likely to degrade neural input to the brain in many ways. The number of information-carrying channels (i.e., auditory nerve fibers) is reduced, the responses of the surviving channels are distorted with respect to their frequency, intensity, and temporal aspects, the frequency resolution of the overall cochlear output is reduced, and interference by background noise may be exacerbated. In addition, CEPP may occur.

---

[3] It has been suggested that threshold elevations are responsible for both poor word recognition and poor frequency resolution, leading to a faulty conclusion that poor frequency resolution per se hinders speech perception (Dubno and Dirks, 1989).

THE INTERACTION OF COGNITIVE-LINGUISTIC PROCESSES, CENTRAL PRESBYCUSIS, AND PERIPHERAL PRESBYCUSIS

Evaluation of the empirical and theoretical evidence indicates that peripheral hearing impairment affects not only thresholds, but also suprathreshold perceptual abilities such as temporal and frequency resolution and recognition of speech in noise. Such deficits would pose problems in discriminating speech under unfavorable listening conditions. Research on cognitive-linguistic processes in the elderly has not dealt adequately with speech perception under non-optimal conditions. However, there is reason to expect, on theoretical grounds discussed earlier, that diminished cognitive processing abilities would contribute to perceptual deficits when listening conditions are poor. The evidence for a role of impaired central processes, independent of peripheral hearing loss, is not strong at this time but is attractive theoretically.

On the basis of the evidence presented, it would be expected that peripheral presbycusis plays a major role in speech perception deficits, with age-related changes in cognitive-linguistic processes contributing, as well. Recent work has supported these expectations.

van Rooij and Plomp (1990, 1991) assessed the contributions of auditory and cognitive factors to speech perception in the elderly. They developed a test battery to evaluate basic auditory (sensitivity, frequency selectivity, temporal resolution), speech perception (phonemes, spondees, and sentences), and cognitive (memory, processing speed, intellectual abilities) performance. The battery was given to subjects aged 60 to 93 years. A canonical correlation analysis revealed two independent components that accounted for deterioration of speech perception: a large component related to progressive high-frequency hearing loss and a smaller component related to diminished cognitive performance. Both components were correlated with age, and the balance between their contributions to the variance did not change with age. An earlier study from the same group (van Rooij, Plomp, and Orlebeke, 1989) employed a smaller number of subjects. These consisted of young, normal-hearing subjects and older subjects within the ninetieth percentile of hearing

levels for their age group (re: Robinson and Sutton, 1979). This study also found that high frequency tone thresholds are the factor most predictive of perceptual impairment. Poorer frequency selectivity was related to reduced vowel perception in noise, but temporal resolution was not correlated with speech perception. The most important cognitive correlates of speech perception were processing speed and sensorimotor speed, whereas the contributions of verbal efficiency and short-term memory were negligible.

Glasberg and Moore (1989) employed a number of psychophysical tests on subjects (many of whom were over 60 but were not diagnosed as having presbycusis) that had either bilateral or unilateral sensorineural hearing loss. The subjects were well trained and well practiced. Subjects with moderate to severe cochlear hearing loss performed poorly on suprathreshold tasks including detection of gaps in noise bands, frequency discrimination of pure and complex tones, and frequency selectivity as determined from masking experiments. Intensity discrimination of pulsed tones, detection of amplitude modulation in tones, and detection of gaps in tones were unaffected by peripheral hearing loss and could actually be performed better at low SLs. SRTs in quiet were primarily determined by absolute thresholds, whereas SRTs in noise were largely determined by absolute threshold and suprathreshold discrimination abilities, especially frequency DLs and gap detection for noise bands. When the effects of absolute threshold were statistically controlled for, age was significantly correlated with SRT, particularly in noise. This was interpreted as being indicative of a cognitive effect that was independent of hearing loss per se.

These studies suggest that peripheral hearing loss can account for most of the perceptual deficits in the elderly, with cognitive processes (especially slowing) contributing a lesser amount. The following studies (and others reviewed in Chapter 9) suggest that peripheral presbycusis can account for many of the difficulties older listeners have with degraded or masked speech material.

McCoy and colleagues (1977) found an age effect for the Staggered Spondaic Word Test (SSW). However, when hearing level was accounted for, age did not affect dichotic performance. They concluded that SSW scores were related to hearing loss rather than age. In this regard, the original description of the SSW by Katz (1962) presented a case study of a young person with sensorineural hearing impairment who showed poor performance on the test.

Korsan-Bengtsen (1973) presented a battery of central tests to young people with acquired sensorineural hearing loss. They performed quite poorly on all of the tests: interrupted speech, frequency-distorted speech, and time-compressed speech (Fig. 9-8). Presumably, older individuals with peripheral presbycusis would also have difficulty because of their hearing loss.

Schon (1970) tested young and old normal and impaired listeners on time-compressed monosyllables (Fig. 9-17). Performance decrements were largely accounted for by hearing impairment, rather than age. Luterman et al. (1966) matched young and old listeners for pure tone hearing levels and observed no age difference in the effects of time-alteration on recognition of monosyllables. Hearing impairment affected performance of young and old listeners.

Sensorineural hearing loss was associated with poor performance on monosyllable recognition with competing sentences in the background irrespective of the subjects' age (Tillman, Carhart, and Olsen, 1970). In a study by Ross et al. (1965), the only factor related to speech perception in noise was hearing level.

Even the relationship between PI-SSI and PI-PB may be affected by peripheral hearing loss. The "mild to moderate" hearing loss group in the study by Kaplan and Pickett (1984) did more poorly than the "borderline" group on the SSImax compared to PBmax (Fig. 9-24), suggesting an influence of peripheral hearing loss on the "central" pattern of performance-intensity functions.

Gelfand et al. (1988) assessed the contributions of peripheral hearing loss and aging in their findings on sentence reception in babble. In quiet, sentence reception thresholds were accounted for by hearing loss, irrespective of age. With competing babble, older, normal-hearing subjects required a more favorable S/N, and presbycusis subjects required an even more favorable ratio. This suggests that both aging and hearing impairment contributed to elevated sentence-reception thresholds. More telling may be the finding that normal-hearing, older subjects benefited from spatial separation of babble and sentences to the same extent as young subjects, whereas presbycusis subjects did not benefit as much from spatial separation. This observation suggests that the ability of the CAS to process such spatially separated material is affected by peripheral presbycusis.

In summary, the occurrence of peripheral impairment plays a key role in the diminished ability of older listeners to accurately perceive speech under unfavorable listening conditions. Most older listeners have fewer cochlear neurons than young people, and the loss is often not revealed by threshold audiometry (Chapter 3). Threshold audiometry also does not reflect distortion or other changes in the quality of peripheral information. Thus, the conclusion that the results of various "central" tests in the elderly are due to central

disorders *rather than* peripheral hearing impairment is dubious in many cases.

AN INTERACTIVE MODEL

Resolution of the question of the contributions of cognitive-linguistic, peripheral, and central processes to speech perception may be reached by implicating all three in an interactive mechanism. For example, peripheral presbycusis must certainly stress the information processing capacity of a healthy CAS by distorting the neural message. The degraded information, in turn, must place extra demands upon cognitive and linguistic abilities, even if they are not greatly diminished with age. If, on the other hand, cognitive functioning was impaired, it could result in reduced levels of attention (to take one example), and the effectiveness of the auditory system in processing sounds might be reduced.

The notion that different alterations in auditory processes exert potentiating effects on each other was suggested some years ago by J.D. Harris (Harris, 1960). Normal listeners performed more poorly when different types of acoustic distortions were combined than the additive effects of either alone would predict (Harris, 1960). Similarly, subjects with severe high-frequency hearing loss performed more poorly than what would be predicted by either filtering or distortion of speech alone (LaCroix and Harris, 1979).

The combined effects of distortion in the work by Harris and colleagues appeared to be multiplicative. The term "interactive" is preferred in the present context because of its generality. An interaction can be multiplicative, but it can also be occlusive, additive, or even subtractive. It seems likely that such instances may often apply to presbycusis.

From the interactive model viewpoint, attempting to discern the peripheral versus central contributions to speech perception deficits is a frustrating endeavor. Age-related changes in the two parts of the auditory system cannot be divorced for two reasons.

First, in order to function effectively, the CAS must have high-quality information from the periphery. If the information is distorted or incomplete due to peripheral presbycusis, central problems are likely to result. This could account for the influence of peripheral hearing loss on "central" test scores. Consider the rationale used to interpret central tests in the elderly. Evidence for central presbycusis is often derived from the results of audiometric tests that have been used on young patients with brain injury. Certain profiles of performance on a particular audiometric test have been shown to be correlated with lesions of specific central auditory structures. The occurrence of a tell-tale test profile in old, noninjured brains has been interpreted as evidence that the implicated central structure is, therefore, damaged. The line of reasoning goes as follows: A lesion in central auditory structure "A" is associated with abnormal performance on test "B." Therefore, abnormal performance on test "B" in an old person indicates that structure "A" is defective. Consider an alternative interpretation: Central auditory structure "A" does in fact mediate performance on test "B." However, to do so, it requires high-quality, usable information from the ear. Because of peripheral dysfunction, structure "A" does not receive high-quality information, and cannot mediate test "B" effectively; The result is abnormal performance on test "B." In this scenario, the deficit *is* a central one, but the *cause* of the central deficit can be found in the inner ear. If one is unaware of existing inner ear neural pathology (as is often the case due to the inadequacy of audiometric thresholds in revealing such pathology), the interpretation might be that the brain was pathological.

Second, CEPP may result from the removal or attenuation of peripheral input, as discussed above and in Chapter 6. If CEPP exists in humans, response properties of central auditory neurons and neural circuits may become altered in individuals with peripheral presbycusis. It may be impossible to have peripheral presbycusis without concomitant changes in the CAS. Thus, when peripheral presbycusis occurs, CAS neural responses may be abnormal, *and* information from the ear may be distorted.

This is not to say that elderly individuals never have central disorders independent of peripheral presbycusis. Given the histopathological and physiological evidence for CEBA presented in Chapter 6, such cases are extremely feasible, and it is important to develop the tools to assess CEBA more effectively.

Interactions between cognitive-linguistic processes and presbycusis may also be important to understanding age-related deficits in speech perception. The work of Rabbitt (1991) provides an example of how hearing loss and cognitive processes may interact. When young subjects were required to correctly repeat (shadow) words in the presence of noise, they exhibited deficits in remembering what they heard. This was the case even though the noise was not sufficiently intense to interfere with their ability to shadow accurately. This is presumably due to the increased effort necessary to recognize the words in noise: rehearsal or encoding of the material is hampered. To extrapolate this finding to hearing-impaired older subjects, Rabbitt divided subjects aged 50 to 80 into normal-hearing (<35 dB)

and mildly-impaired (35–50 dB) groups. Word lists were presented both visually and auditorily under conditions that permitted correct recognition and repetition of all words. The subjects with mild hearing loss recalled visually presented words as well as the normal-hearing group; however, auditorily presented words were less successfully recalled by the mildly impaired subjects. Recall was reduced with age in both groups, but in the hearing-loss group, the relative advantage of visually presented material became greater with age. Subsequent work indicated that subjects with higher IQ test scores were able to overcome the negative effects of hearing loss better than those with lower IQ scores. Those with higher IQ scores also performed better on the more difficult task of recalling words presented at higher rates of speed. Measures of individual differences in information processing speed (e.g., maximum reading speed, choice reaction time) were better predictors than chronological age with regard to recall of auditorily presented words in elderly listeners with mild hearing loss.

This work suggests that both the degree of peripheral presbycusis and the level of cognitive skill interact to determine how effectively speech is processed. Peripheral distortion of the message leads to impaired processing of the material. Conversely, effective cognitive skills can mitigate the problems caused by peripheral distortion.

CONCLUSIONS

From an interactive perspective, the most important questions do not involve "which" age-related change is responsible for deficiencies in speech. The questions center on the contribution of each and the manner in which they interact. This may be a more productive approach to understanding presbycusis than trying to rule out the effects of age-related cognitive, central, or peripheral changes. It is hoped that future research on presbycusis will move in this direction.

BIBLIOGRAPHY

Abel, S.M., Krever, E.M., and Alberti, P.W. (1990) Auditory detection, discrimination and speech processing in ageing, noise-sensitive and hearing-impaired listeners. *Scandinavian Audiology, 19*, 43-54.

Adams, J.C., Tarnowski, B.I., Heaple, S., Hellstrom, L.I., and Schmiedt, R.A. (1989) Cochlear histopathology and hearing loss in quiet reared aged gerbils. *Association for Research in Otolaryngology Abstracts, 12*, 46-47.

Adams, J.C., Tarnowski, B.I., Schmiedt, R.A., Hellstrom, L.I., and Schulte, B.A. (1989) Age related changes in the cochlea. *Anatomical Record, 223*, 6A.

Alberti, P.W. and Kristensen, R. (1972) The compliance of the middle ear: Its accuracy in routine clinical practice. In D. Rose and L. Keating (Eds.), *Impedance symposium.* Mayo Clinic, Rochester, Minnesota, pp. 159-167 (cited in Thompson, et al., 1979).

Allam, A. (1970) Pathology of the human spiral ligament. *Journal of Laryngology and Otology, 84*, 765-779.

Allison, T., Hume, A.L., Wood, C.C. and Goff, W.R. (1984) Developmental and aging changes in somatosensory, auditory and visual evoked potentials. *Electroencephalography and Clinical Neurophysiology, 58*, 14-24.

Allison, T., Wood, C.C. and Goff, W.R. (1983) Brain stem auditory, pattern-reversal visual, and short-latency somatosensory evoked potentials: Latencies in relation to age, sex, and brain and body size. *Electroencephalography and Clinical Neurophysiology, 55*, 619-636.

Almadori, G., Ottaviani, F., Paludetti, G., Rosignoli, M., Gallucci, L., D'Alatri, L. and Vergoni, G. (1988) Auditory brainstem responses in noise-induced permanent hearing loss. *Audiology, 27*, 36-41.

Altman, P.L. and Dittmer, D.S. (1972) *Biology data book* (Vol. 1). Federation of the American Society for Experimental Biology. Bethesda, pp. 230.

Altmann, F. (1955) Entizundliche und degenerative erberkrankungen des peripheren cochlear-und vestibular-neurons. *Fortschritte der Hals -Nasen-Ohrenheilkunde, 2*, 80 (cited by Rosen, et al., 1964).

Altmann, F., Kornfeld, M., and Shea, J.J. (1966) Inner ear changes in otosclerosis. Histopathological studies. *Annals of Otology Rhinology and Laryngology, 75*, 5-32.

Altmann, F. (1966) Sensorineural deafness in otosclerosis. *Annals of Otology Rhinology and Laryngology, 75*, 469-480.

Altschuler, R.A., Bobbin, R.P., and Hoffman, D.W. (Eds.), (1986) *Neurobiology of hearing: The cochlea.* Raven Press, New York.

Altschuler, R.A., Miller, J.M., Zappia, J.J., Niparko, J.K., and Hawkins, J.E. (1989) Is inner hair cell survival necessary for spiral ganglion cell survival in primates? Disparate findings in simian and human ears. *Association for Research in Otolaryngology Abstracts, 12*, 134.

Amerman, J.D. and Parnell, M.M. (1980) The staggered spondaic word test: A normative investigation of older adults. *Ear and Hearing, 1*, 42-45.

Anderson, H., Barr, B., and Wedenberg, E. (1969) Intra-aural reflexes in retrocochlear lesions. In C. Hamberger and J. Wersall (Eds.), Nobel Symposium, 10. *Disorders of the skull base region.* Almquist and Wiksell, Stockholm, pp. 49-55.

Anderson, R.G. and Meyerhoff, W.L. (1982) Otologic manifestations of aging. In C.F. Koopmann (Ed.), *The Otolaryngologic Clinics of North America* (Vol., 15.) W.B. Saunders, Philadelphia, pp. 353-370.

Antonelli, A.R. (1970) Sensitized speech tests in aged people. *Speech Audiometry Second Danavox Symposium,* Odense, pp. 66-79 (cited in Antonelli, A.R., Auditory processing disorders and problems with hearing-aid

fitting in old age. *Audiology, 17*, 27-31, 1978).

Antonelli, A.R. (1978) Auditory processing disorders and problems with hearing-aid fitting in old age. *Audiology, 17*, 27-31.

Arnesen, A.R. (1982) Presbycusic loss of neurons in the human cochlear nuclei. *Journal of Laryngology and Otology, 96*, 503-511.

Arnold, W. (1987) Myelination of the human spiral ganglion. *Acta Oto-Laryngologica, 436*, 76-84.

Arnst, D.J. (1982) Staggered spondaic word test performance in a group of older adults: A preliminary report. *Ear and Hearing, 3*, 118-123.

Attias, J. and Pratt, H. (1984) Auditory evoked potentials and audiological follow-up of subjects developing noise-induced permanent threshold shift. *Audiology, 23*, 498-508.

Axelsson, A. (1971) The cochlear blood vessels in guinea pigs of different ages. *Acta Oto-Laryngologica, 72*, 172-181.

Axelsson, A. (1974) The blood supply of the inner ear of mammals. In W.D. Keidel and W.D. Neff (Eds.), *Handbook of sensory physiology* (Vol. 5) Auditory System. Springer-Verlag, New York, pp. 213-260.

Axelsson, A. (1991) Epidemiology of tinnitus in a general population. *Association for Research in Otolaryngology Abstracts, 14*, 2.

Babbitt, J.A. (1947) The endaural surgery of chronic suppourations. In S.J. Kopetzky (Ed.) *Nelson's loose-leaf surgery of the ear.* Thomas Nelsons and Sons, New York (cited in Covell, 1952).

Bagger-Sjoback, D. and Engstrom, B. (1985) Preservation of the human cochlea. *Annals of Otology Rhinology and Laryngology, 94*, 284-292.

Balas, R.F. (1962) *Results of the staggered spondaic word test with an old age population.* Master's thesis, Northern Illinois University.

Balle, V. and Linthicum, F.H. (1984) Histologically proven cochlear otosclerosis with pure sensorineural hearing loss. *Annals of Otology Rhinology and Laryngology, 93*, 105-111.

Barnes, C.A. (1979) Memory deficits associated with senescence: a neurophysiological and behavioral study in the rat. *Journal of Comparative and Physiological Psychology, 93*, 74-104.

Barnes, C.A. and McNaughton, B.L. (1979) Neurophysiological comparison of dendritic cable properties in adolescent, middle-aged and senescent rats. *Experimental Aging Research, 5*, 195-206.

Baschek, V. (1979) Die abhangigkeit des richtungshorens vom zerebralen alterungsprozess und die indikation zur applikation einer stereophonen horgerateversorgung. *Laryngologie, Rhinologie, Otology, 58*, 827-831, (Medline abstract).

Bauch, C.D., Rose, D.E., and Harner, S.G. (1982) Auditory brain stem response results from 255 patients with suspected retrocochlear involvement. *Ear and Hearing, 3*, 83-86.

Beagley, H.A. and Sheldrake, J.B. (1978) Differences in brainstem response latency with age and sex. *British Journal of Audiology, 12*, 69-77.

Beasley, D.S. and Davis, G.A. (Eds.), (1981) *Aging: Communication processes and disorders.* Grune & Stratton, New York, pp. 63-85.

Beattie, R.C. and Warren, V. (1983) Slope characteristics of CID W-22 word functions in elderly hearing-impaired listeners. *Journal of Speech and Hearing Disorders, 48*, 119-127.

Beattie, R.C. and Warren, V.G. (1982) Relationships among speech threshold, loudness discomfort, comfortable loudness, and PB max in the elderly hearing impaired. *American Journal of Otology, 3,* 353-, 358.

Beedle, R.K. and Harford, E.R. (1973) A comparison of acoustic reflex and loudness growth in normal and pathological ears. *Journal of Speech and Hearing Research, 16,* 271-281.

Bekesy, G. von (1960) *Experiments in hearing.* McGraw-Hill, New York.

Belal, A. (1975) Presbycusis: physiological or pathological. *Journal of Laryngology and Otology, 89,* 1011-1025.

Belal, A. (1980) Pathology of vascular sensorineural hearing impairments. *Laryngoscope, 90,* 1831-1839.

Bennett, C.L., Davis, R.T., and Miller, J.M. (1983) Demonstration of presbycusis across repeated measures in a nonhuman primate species. *Behavioral Neuroscience, 97,* 602-607.

Bergholtz, L.M., Hooper, R.E., and Mehta, D.C. (1977) Electrocochleographic response patterns in a group of patients mainly with presbycusis. *Scandinavian Audiology, 6,* 3-11.

Bergman, M. (1971) Changes in hearing with age. *Gerontologist, 11,* 148-, 151, 1971,

Bergman, M. (1980) *Aging and the perception of speech.* University Park Press, Baltimore.

Bergman, M. (1983) Central disorders of hearing in the elderly. In R. Hinchcliffe (Ed.) *Hearing and balance in the elderly.* Churchill Livingstone, Edinburgh, pp. 145-158.

Bergman, M., Blumenfeld, V.G., Cascardo, D., Dash, B., Levitt, H., and Margulies, M.K. (1976) Age-related decrement in hearing for speech. Sampling and longitudinal studies. *Journal of Gerontology, 31,* 533-, 538.

Bergman, M. (1966) Hearing in the Mabaans. *Archives of Otolaryngology, 84,* 411-415.

Bergstrom, L., Thompson, P., Sando, I., and Wood, R.P. (1980) Renal disease: Its pathology, treatment, and effects on the ear. *Archives of Otolaryngology, 106,* 567-572.

Berkowitz, A.O. and Hochberg, I. (1971) Self-assessment of hearing handicap in the aged. *Archives of Otolaryngology, 93,* 25-28.

Berruecos, P. (1970) Binaural temporal integration in presbyacusis. *International Audiology, 9,* 309-313.

Bess, F.H., and Townsend, T.H. (1977) Word discrimination for listeners with flat sensorineural hearing losses. *Journal of Speech and Hearing Disorders, 42,* 232-237.

Bhattacharyya, T.K. and Dayal, V.S. (1985) Age-related cochlear hair cell loss in the chinchilla. *Annals of Otology Rhinology and Laryngology, 94,* 75-80.

Bhattacharyya, T.K. and Dayal, V.S. (1989) Influence of age on hair cell loss in the rabbit cochlea. *Hearing Research, 40,* 179-183.

Bierman, E.L. (1985) Arteriosclerosis and aging. In C.E. Finch and E.L. Schneider (Eds.), *Handbook of the biology of aging.* Van Nostrand, New York, pp. 842-858.

Bilger, R.C. and Hirsh, I.J. (1956) Masking of tones by bands of noise. *Journal of the Acoustical Society of America, 28,* 623-630.

Billett, T.E., Thorne, P.R., and Gavin, J.B. (1989) The nature and progression of injury in the organ of Corti during ischemia. *Hearing Research, 41,* 189-198.

Blood, I. and Greenberg, H.J. (1977) Acoustic admittance of the ear in the geriatric person. *Journal of the American Audiological Society, 2,* 185-187.

Blood, I.M. and Greenberg, H.J. (1976) Acoustic impedance in the geriatric individual. *American Speech and Hearing Association, 18,* 600.

Blumenfeld, V.G., Bergman, M., and Millner, E. (1969) Speech discrimination in an aging population. *Journal of* *Speech and Hearing Research, 12,* 210-217.

Bocca, E. and Antonelli, A.R. (1976) Masking level difference: another tool for the evaluation of peripheral and cortical defects. *Audiology, 15,* 480-487.

Bocca, E. and Calearo, C. (1956) Aspects of auditory pathology of central origin in aged subjects. *Annali di Laryngologia, Otologia, Rinologia, Faringologia, 55,* 365-369.

Bochenek, Z. and Jachowska, A. (1969) Atherosclerosis, accelerated presbyacusis, and acoustic trauma. *International Audiology, 8,* 312-316.

Boettcher, F.A. and Salvi, R.J. (1991) Effects of acoustic trauma on response properties of single neurons in the anteroventral cochlear nucleus. *Association for Research in Otolaryngology, 14,* 43.

Bohme, G. (1989) [Hearing disorders in obliteration of the carotid artery. 2. Contribution to hearing loss in the aged] *Laryngorhinootologie, 68,* 367-371, 1989 (Medline abstract).

Bohne, B.A. (1976) Mechanisms of noise damage to the inner ear. In D. Henderson, R.P. Hamernik, D.S. Dosanjh, and J.H. Mills (Eds.), *Effects of noise on hearing.* Raven Press, New York, pp. 41-68.

Bohne, B.A., Gruner, M.M., and Harding, G.W. (1990) Morphological correlates of aging in the chinchilla cochlea. *Hearing Research, 48,* 79-92.

Bohne, B.A. and Rabbitt, K.D. (1983) Holes in the reticular lamina after noise exposure: Implication for continuing damage in the organ of Corti. *Hearing Research, 11,* 41-53.

Bonding, P. (1979) Critical bandwidth in presbycusis. *Scandinavian Audiology, 8,* 43-50, 1979.

Bonfils, P. (1988) Les alterations de l'audiometrie vocale dans la presbyacousie apport des emissions acoustiques cochleares. *Journal Otolaryngology, 17,* 207-210.

Bonfils, P., Bertrand, Y., and Uziel, A. (1988) Evoked otoacoustic emissions: Normative data and presbycusis. *Audiology, 27,* 27-35.

Borod, J., Obler, L., Albert, M., and Stiefel, S. (1983) Lateralization for pure tone perception as a function of age and sex. *Cortex, 19,* 281-285.

Bosatra, A. and Russolo, M. (1982) Comparison between central tonal tests and central speech tests in elderly subjects. *Audiology, 21,* 334-341.

Brant, L.J. and Fozard, J.L. (1990) Age changes in pure-tone hearing thresholds in a longitudinal study of normal human hearing. *Journal of the Acoustical Society of America, 88,* 813-820.

Bredberg, G. (1968) Cellular pattern and nerve supply of the human organ of Corti. *Acta Oto Laryngologica Supplement, 236,* 1-135.

Briner, W.B. and Willott, J.F. (1989) Ultrastructural features of neurons in the C57BL/6J mouse anteroventral cochlear nucleus: Young mice versus old mice with chronic presbycusis. *Neurobiology of Aging, 10,* 295-303.

Brody, H. (1955) Organization of the cerebral cortex: III. A study of aging in the human cerebral cortex. *Journal of Comparative Neurology, 102,* 511-556.

Brody, J.A. and Brock, D.B. (1985) Epidemiologic and statistical characteristics of the United States elderly population. In C.E. Finch and E.L. Schneider (Eds.), *Handbook of the biology of aging.* Van Nostrand, New York, pp. 3-26.

Brown, C.H. (1984) Directional hearing in aging rats. *Experimental Aging Research, 10,* 35-38.

Brown, M.C., Nuttall, A.L., Masta, R.I., and Lawrence, M. (1983) Cochlear inner hair cells: Effects of transient asphyxia on intracellular potentials. *Hearing Research, 9,* 131-144.

Brown, W., Marsh, J., and LaRue, A. (1983) Exponential

electrophysiological aging: P300 latency. *Electroencephalography and Clinical Neurophysiology, 55*, 277-285.

Browner, R.H. and Baruch, A. (1982) The cytoarchitecture of the dorsal cochlear nucleus in the 3-month and 26-month-old C57BL/6 mouse: A Golgi impregnation study. *Journal of Comparative Neurology, 211*, 115-138.

Browner, R.H. and Riedel, E.R. (1988) Individual neuronal area changes in the developing and aged medial nucleus of the trapezoid body of hearing impaired C57BL/6 mice. *Society for Neuroscience Abstracts, 14*, 1098.

Bruhl, G. (1905) Beitrage zur pathologischen anatomie des gehororgans, II. *Zeitschrift fuer Ohrenheilkunde, 50*, 5 (cited in Bredberg, 1968).

Buchanan, L.H. (1990) Early onset of presbyacusis in Down syndrome. *Scandinavian Audiology, 19*, 103-110.

Bunch, C.C. (1929) Age Variations in auditory acuity. *Archives of Otolaryngology, 9*, 625-636.

Burns, W. and Robinson, D.W. (1970) *Hearing and noise in industry.* Her Majesty's Stationary Office, London (cited in Erlandsson et al., 1982).

Butts, F.M., Ruth, R.R., and Schoeny, Z.G. (1987) Nonsense syllable test (NST) results and hearing loss. *Ear and Hearing, 8*, 44-48.

Calearo, C. and Lazzaroni, A. (1957) Speech intelligibility in relation to the speed of the message. *Laryngoscope, 67*, 410-419.

Canlon, B, and Schacht, J. (1983) Acoustic stimulation alters deoxyglucose uptake in the mouse cochlea and inferior colliculus. *Hearing Research, 10*, 217-226.

Carhart, C. (1957) Clinical determination of abnormal auditory adaptation. *Archives of Otolaryngology, 65*, 32-39.

Carhart, R. (1966) Cochlear otosclerosis: Audiological considerations. *Annals of Otology Rhinology and Laryngology, 75*, 559-571.

Carhart, R. and Nicholls, S. (1971) Perceptual masking in elderly women. *American Speech and Hearing Association, 13*, 535.

Casey, M.A. (1990) *The effects of aging on neuron number in the rat superior olivary complex.* Unpublished manuscript.

Casey, M.A. and Feldman, M.L. (1982) Aging in the rat medial nucleus of the trapezoid body. I. Light Microscopy. *Neurobiology of Aging, 3*, 187-195.

Casey, M.A. and Feldman, M.L. (1985a) Aging in the rat medial nucleus of the trapezoid body. II. Electron microscopy. *Journal of Comparative Neurology, 232*, 401-413.

Casey, M.A. and Feldman, M.L. (1985b) Aging in the rat medial nucleus of the trapezoid body. III. Alterations in capillaries. *Neurobiology of Aging, 6*, 39-46.

Casey, M.A. and Feldman, M.L. (1988) Age-related loss of synaptic terminals in the rat medial nucleus of the trapezoid body. *Neuroscience, 24*, 189-194.

Caspary, D.M., Raza, A., Lawhorn Armour, B.A., Pippin, J., and Arneric, S.P. (1990) Immunocytochemical and neurochemical evidence for age-related loss of GABA in the inferior colliculus: Implications for neural presbycusis. *Journal of Neuroscience, 10*, 2363-2372.

Chambers, R.D. and Griffiths, S.K. (1991) Effects of age on the adult auditory middle latency response. *Hearing Research, 51*, 1-10.

Chandler, J.R. (1964) Partial occlusion of the external auditory meatus: Its effect upon air and bone conduction hearing acuity. *Laryngoscope, 74*, 22-45.

Chase, M.H., Morales, F.R., Boxer, P.A. and Fung, S.J. (1985) Aging of motorneurons and synaptic processes in the cat. *Experimental Neurology, 90*, 471-478.

Chermak, G.D. and Moore, M.K. (1981) Eustachian tube function in the older adult. *Ear and Hearing, 2*, 143-147.

Chole, R.A. and Henry, K.R. (1983) Disparity in the cytocochleogram and the electrocochleogram in aging LP/J and A/J inbred mice. *Audiology, 22*, 384-392.

Chu, N.-S. (1985) Age-related latency changes in the brainstem auditory evoked potentials. *Electroencephalography and Clinical Neurophysiology, 62*, 431-436.

Chung, D.Y. (1982) Temporal integration: its relationship with noise-induced hearing loss. *Scandinavian Audiology, 11*, 153-157.

Chung, D.Y., Mason, K., Gannon, R.P. and Wilson, G.N. (1983) The ear effect as a function of age and hearing loss. *Journal of the Acoustical Society of America, 73*, 1277-1282.

Chung, D.Y. and Smith, F. (1980) Quiet and masked brief-tone audiometry in subjects with normal hearing and with noise-induced hearing loss. *Scandinavian Audiology, 9*, 43-47.

Church, M.W. and Shucard, D.W. (1986) Age-related hearing loss in BDF1 mice as evidenced by the brainstem auditory evoked potential. *Audiology, 25*, 363-372.

Citron, L., Dix, M.R., Hallpike, C.S., and Hood, J.D. (1963) A recent clinico-pathological study of cochlear nerve degeneration resulting from tumor pressure and disseminated sclerosis, etc. *Acta Oto-Laryngologica, 56*, 330-337.

Clark, J.C. (1985) Alaryngeal speech intelligibility and the older listener. *Journal of Speech and Hearing Disorders, 50*, 60-65.

Clemis, J.D. and McGee, T. (1979) Brain stem electrical response audiometry in the differential diagnosis of acoustic tumors. *Laryngoscope, 89*, 31-42.

Clerici, W.J. and Coleman, J.R. (1987) Resting and pure tone evoked metabolic responses in the inferior colliculus of young adult and senescent rats. *Neurobiology of Aging, 8*, 171-178.

Coats, A.C. and Martin, J.L. (1977) Human auditory nerve action potentials and brain stem evoked responses. Effects of audiogram shape and lesion location. *Archives of Otolaryngology, 103*, 605.

Cody, A.R., Robertson, D., Bredberg, G., and Johnstone, B.M. (1980) Electrophysiological and morphological changes in the guinea pig cochlea following mechanical trauma to the organ of corti. *Acta Oto-Laryngologica, 89*, 440-452.

Cohen, G.M. and Bullers, S. (1989) Age-and condition-related changes in levels of neuron specific enolase in spiral ganglion neurons of C57BL/6 mice. *Association for Research in Otolaryngology Abstracts, 12*, 357.

Cohen, G.M., Bullers, S.R., and Kronman, B.S. (1990) Myelin basic protein and glial fibrillary acidic protein as markers for Schwann cells in spiral ganglia of C57BL/6 mice. *Association for Research in Otolaryngology Abstracts, 13*, 151.

Cohen, G.M. and Grasso, J.S. (1987) Further observations on the degeneration of spiral ganglia in aging C57BL/6 mice. *Association for Research in Otolaryngology Abstracts, 10*, 120.

Cohen, G.M. and Lawrence, K.O. (1989) Age-related changes in acid phosphatase and carbonic anhydrase levels in spiral ganglion neurons of C57BL/6 mice. *Association for Research in Otolaryngology Abstracts, 12*, 356-357.

Cohen, G.M., Park, J.C., and Grasso, J.S. (1990) Comparison of demyelination and neural degeneration in spiral and Scarpa's ganglia of C57BL/6 mice. *Journal of Electron Microscopy Technique, 15*, 165-172.

Colburn, H.S., Barker, M.A., and Milner, P. (1982) Free-field tests of hearing-impaired listeners. In O.J. Pedersen and T. Poulsen (Eds.), *Binaural effects in normal and impaired hearing. Scandinavian Audiology Supplement, 15*, pp. 123-133.

Coleman, J.W. (1976a) Age dependent changes and acoustic trauma in the spiral organ of the guinea pig. *Scandinavian Audiology, 5*, 63-68.

Coleman, J.W. (1976b) Hair cell loss as a function of age in the normal cochlea of the guinea pig. *Acta Oto-Laryngologica, 82*, 33-40.

Conlee, J.W., Abdul-Baqi, K.J. McCandless, G.A., and Creel, D.J. (1988) Effects of aging on normal hearing loss and noise-induced threshold shift in albino and pigmented guinea pigs. *Acta Oto-Laryngologica, 106*, 64-70.

Conlee, J.W., Gill, S.S., McCandless, P.T., and Creel, D.J. (1989) Differential susceptibility to gentamicin ototoxicity between albino and pigmented guinea pigs. *Hearing Research, 41*, 43-52.

Conlee, J.W., Parks, T.N., Schwartz, I.R., and Creel, D.J. (1989) Comparative anatomy of melanin pigment in the stria vascularis. Evidence for a distinction between melanocytes and intermediate cells in the cat. *Acta Oto-Laryngologica, 107*, 48-58.

Cooper, W.A., Coleman, J.R., and Newton, E.H. (1990) Auditory brainstem responses to tonal stimuli in young and aging rats. *Hearing Research, 43*, 171-180.

Cooper, W.A., Coleman, J.R., Newton, E.H., and Youatt, A.E. (1986) ABR changes to tonal stimuli in the senescent Fischer, 344 rat. *Society for Neuroscience Abstracts, 12*, 1280.

Corcoran, J.G. and Axline, S.G. (1982) Infectious diseases in the geriatric patient. In C.F. Koopmann (Ed.), *The otolaryngologic clinics of north america.* (Vol. 15). W.B. Saunders, Philadelphia, pp. 421-438.

Corso, J.F. (1963) Age and sex differences in pure-tone thresholds. *Archives of Otolaryngology, 77*, 385-405.

Corso, J.F. (1976) Presbycusis as a complicating factor in evaluating noise-induced hearing loss. In D. Henderson, R.P. Hamernik, D.S. Dosanjh, and J.H. Mills (Eds.), *Effects of noise on hearing.* Raven Press, New York, pp. 497-524.

Corso, J.F., Wright, H.N., and Valerio, M. (1976) Auditory temporal summation in presbycusis and noise exposure. *Journal of Gerontology, 31*, 58-63.

Covell, W.P. (1952) The ear. In V. Cowdry (Ed.), *Problems of ageing: Biological and medical aspects.* Williams and Wilkins, Baltimore, pp. 268-276.

Covell, W.P. and Rogers, J.B. (1957) Pathological changes in the inner ears of senile guinea pigs. *Laryngoscope, 67*, 118-129.

Crace, R. (1970) *Morphologic alterations with age in the human cochlear nuclear complex.* PhD dissertation, Ohio Univ.

Cranford, J.L., Boose, M., and Moore, C.A. (1990) Effects of aging on the precedence effect in sound localization. *Journal of Speech and Hearing Research, 33*, 654-659.

Cremer, R. and Zeef, E.J. (1987) What kind of noise increases with age? *Journal of Gerontology, 42*, 515-518.

Crossman, E.R. and Szafram, J. (1956) Changes with age in the speed of information intake and discrimination. *Experientia Supplement, 4.*

Crowe, S.J., Guild, S.R., and Polvogt, L.M. (1934) Observations on the pathology of high-tone deafness. *Johns Hopkins Hospital Bulletin, 54*, 315-380.

Crowley, D.E. (1975) Conference on animal models of aging in the auditory system. *Annals of Otology Rhinology and Laryngology, 84*, 560-561.

Crowley, D.E., Schramm, V.L., Swain, R.E., and Swanson, S.N. (1972a) Analysis of age-related changes in electric responses from the inner ear of rats. *Annals of Otology Rhinology and Laryngology, 81*, 739-746.

Crowley, D.E., Schramm, V.L., Swain, R.E., Maisel, R.H., Rauchback, E., and Swanson, S.N. (1972b) An animal model for presbycusis. *Laryngoscope, 82*, 2079-2091.

Cutler, W.M., Lonsbury-Martin, B.L., and Martin, G.K. (1990) Effects of aging on acoustic-distortion product generation in humans. *Association for Research in Otolaryngology Abstracts, 13*, 234-235.

Dallos, P. and Harris, D. (1978) Properties of auditory nerve responses in absence of outer hair cells. *Journal of Neurophysiology, 41*, 365-383.

Dallos, P. and Ryan, A. (1975) Frequency selectivity mediated by inner hair cells alone. *Journal of the Acoustical Society of America, 57, Supplement, 1*, S40.

Dallos, P., Ryan, A., Harris, D., McGee, T., and Ozdamar, O. (1977) Cochlear frequency selectivity in the presence of hair cell damage. In E.F. Evans and J.P. Wilson (Eds.), *Psychophysics and physiology of hearing.* Academic Press, New York.

Davis, A. (1983) The epidemiology of hearing disorders. In R. Hinchcliffe (Ed.), *Hearing and balance in the elderly.* Churchill Livingstone, Edinburgh, pp. 1-43.

Davis, A.C. (1989) The prevalence of hearing impairment and reported hearing disability among adults in Great Britain. *International Journal of Epidemiology, 18*, 901-907.

Davis, G.A. and Ball, H.E. (1989) Effects of age on comprehension of complex sentences in adulthood. *Journal of Speech and Hearing Research, 32*, 143-150.

Davis, H. (1957) Biophysics and physiology of the inner ear. *Physiological Reviews, 37*, 1-49.

Davis, H. (1970) Abnormal hearing and deafness. In H. Davis and R. Silverman, *Hearing and deafness.* Harvard Univ. Press, Cambridge, pp. 87-143.

Davis, M. (1984) The mammalian startle response. In R.C. Eaton (Ed.), *Neural mechanisms of startle behavior.* Plenum Press, New York, pp. 287-351.

Dayal, V.S. and Barek, W.G. (1975) Cochlear changes from noise, kanamycin, and ageing. *Laryngoscope, 85*, 1-18.

Dayal, V.S. and Bhattacharyya, T.K. (1986) Comparative study of age-related cochlear hair cell loss. *Annals of Otology Rhinology and Laryngology, 95*, 510-513.

DeBoer, E. and Bouwmeester, J. (1974) Critical bands and sensorineural hearing loss. *Audiology, 13*, 236-259.

Debruyne, F. and Tyberghein, J. (1989) Age effects in speech audiometry and in brainstem electric response audiometry. *Audiology, 28*, 258-261.

Dickson, R.C. (1968) The normal hearing of Bantu and Bushmen. *Journal of Laryngology and Otology, 82*, 505-522.

Divenyi, P.L., Jerger, J., and Jerger, S. (1991) Factor structure of speech understanding and cognitive abilities in the elderly. *Association for Research in Otolaryngology Abstracts, 14*, 34.

Dolan, D.F. and Nuttall, A.L. (1989) Inner hair cell responses to tonal stimulation in the presence of broadband noise. *Journal of the Acoustical Society of America, 86*, 1007-1012.

Dorman, M.F., Marton, K., and Hannley, M.T. (1985) Phonetic identification by elderly normal and hearing-impaired listeners. *Journal of the Acoustical Society of America, 77*, 664-670.

Drescher, D.G. (Ed.) (1985) *Auditory biochemistry.* Charles C. Thomas, Springfield, Illinois.

Dreschler, W.A. and Plomp, R. (1980) Relation between

psychophysical data and speech perception for hearing-impaired subjects. I. *Journal of the Acoustical Society of America, 68,* 1608-1615.

Duara, R., London, E.D., and Rapoport, S.I. (1985) Changes in structure and energy metabolism of the aging brain. In C.E. Finch and E.L. Schneider (Eds.), *Handbook of the biology of aging.* Van Nostrand, New York, pp. 595-616.

Dublin, W.B. (1976) *Fundamentals of sensorineural auditory pathology.* Charles C. Thomas, Springfield, IL.

Dubno, J.R. and Dirks, D.D. (1989) Auditory filter characteristics and consonant recognition for hearing-impaired listeners. *Journal of the Acoustical Society of America, 85,* 1666-1975.

Dubno, J.R., Dirks, D.D., and Morgan, D.E. (1984) Effects of age and mild hearing loss on speech recognition in noise. *Journal of the Acoustical Society of America, 76,* 87-96.

Dubno, J.R., Dirks, D.D., and Schaefer, A.B. (1987) Effects of hearing loss on utilization of short-duration spectral cues in stop consonant recognition. *Journal of the Acoustical Society of America, 81,* 1940-1947.

Dum, N. (1983) Age-dependence of the auditory threshold-difference between albino and pigmented guinea pigs. (Cavia porcellus) *Zeitschrift Saugetierkunde, 48,* 95-99.

Dum, N., Schmidt, U., and von Wedel, H. (1980) Age-related changes in the auditory evoked brainstem potentials of albino and pigmented guinea pigs. *Archives of Oto-Rhino-Laryngology, 228,* 249-254.

Dum, N. and von Wedel, H. (1983) Langzeituntersuchung altersbedingter veranderungen der hirnstammpotentiale beim meerschweinchen. *Laryngologie, Rhinologie, Otologie, 62,* 378-381.

Duquesnoy, A.J. (1983a) Effect of a single interfering noise or speech source upon the binaural sentence intelligibility of aged persons. *Journal of the Acoustical Society of America, 74,* 739-749.

Duquesnoy, A.J. (1983b) The intelligibility of sentences in quiet and in noise in aged listeners. *Journal of the Acoustical Society of America, 74,* 1136-1144.

Duvall, A.J. (1968) Ultrastructure of the lateral cochlear wall following intermixing of fluids. *Annals of Otology Rhinology and Laryngology, 77,* 317-331.

Duvall, A.J., Ward, W.D., and Lauhala, K.E. (1974) Stria ultrastructure and vessel transport in acoustic trauma. *Annals of Otology Rhinology and Laryngology, 83,* 498-515.

Ehret, G. (1974) Age-dependent hearing loss in normal hearing mice. *Die Naturwissenschaften, 61,* 506-507.

Eisdorfer, C. and Wilkie, F. (1972) Auditory changes in the aged: a follow-up study. *American Geriatrics Society Journal, 20,* 377-382.

Elliott, L.L., Hammer, M.A., Scholl, M.E., and Wasowicz, J.M. (1989) Age differences in discrimination of simulated single-formant frequency transitions. *Perception and Psychophysics, 46,* 181-186.

Elliott, L.L., Lyons, L., and Busse, L.A. (1983) Speech understanding of older adults: a preliminary report. *Journal of the Acoustical Society of America, 74,* S66.

Engstrom, B. (1983) Stereocilia of sensory cells in normal and hearing impaired ears. *Scandinavian Audiology Supplement 19,* 1-35.

Engstrom, B., Hillerdal, M., and Laurell, G. (1987) Selected pathological findings in the human cochlea. *Acta Oto-Laryngologica Supplement, 436,* 110-116.

Era, P., Jokela, J., Qvarnberg, Y., and Heikkinen, E. (1986) Pure-tone thresholds, speech understanding, and their correlates in samples of men of different ages. *Audiology, 25,* 338-352.

Erlandsson, B., Hakanson, H., Ivarsson, A., and Nilsson, P. (1982) Hearing impairment caused by noise or age. *Acta Oto-Laryngologica, 386,* 40-42.

Etholm, B. and Belal, A. (1974) Senile changes in the middle ear joints. *Annals of Otology Rhinology and Laryngology, 83,* 49-54.

Evans, E.F. and Klinke, R. (1982) The effects of intracochlear and systemic furosemide on the properties of single cochlear nerve fibres in the cat. *Journal of Physiology, 331,* 409-427.

Fabinyi, G. (1931) Regarding morphological and functional changes of the internal ear in arteriosclerosis. *Laryngoscope, 41,* 663-670.

Feldman, M.L. (1982) Synaptic loss with advanced age in the cochlear nucleus. *Neuroscience, 7,* S67.

Feldman, M.L. (1984) Morphological observations on the cochleas of very old rats. *Association for Research in Otolaryngology Abstracts, 7,* 14.

Feldman, M.L. (1990) Reissner's membrane in aged rats. *Association for Research in Otolaryngology Abstracts, 13,* 421-422.

Feldman, M.L. and Burkard, R. (1991) Brainstem auditory evoked responses in aged rats. *Association for Research in Otolaryngology Abstracts, 14,* 27.

Feldman, M.L., Craig, C., and Keithley, E. (1981) *Differential age pigment accumulation in type I and type II ganglion cells of rat cochlea.* American Aging Association, New York.

Feldman, M.L. and Dowd, C. (1975) Loss of dendritic spines in aging Cerebral cortex. *Anatomy and Embriology, 148,* 279-301.

Feldman, M.L. and Peters, A. (1972) Intracellular rods and sheets in rat cochlear nucleus. *Journal of Neurocytology, 1,* 109-127.

Feldman, M.L. and Vaughan, D.W. (1979) Changes in the auditory pathway with age. In S.S. Han and D.H. Coons (Eds.), *Special senses in aging.* Institute of Gerontology, Ann Arbor, pp. 143-162.

Feldman, R.M. and Reger, S.N. (1967) Relations among hearing, reaction time, and age. *Journal of Speech and Hearing Research, 10,* 479-495.

Felix, H., Johnsson, L.-G., Gleeson, M., and Pollak, A. (1990) Quantitative analysis of cochlear sensory cells and neuronal elements in man. *Acta Oto-Laryngologica Supplement, 470,* 71-79.

Fernandez, C. (1958) Postmortem changes and artifacts in human temporal bones. *Laryngoscope, 68,* 1583-1615.

Ferraro, J.A. and Minckler, J. (1977a) The brachium of the inferior colliculus. *Brain and Language, 4,* 156-164.

Ferraro, J.A. and Minckler, J. (1977b) The human lateral lemniscus and its nuclei. *Brain and Language, 4,* 277-294.

Festen, J.M. and Plomp, R. (1983) Relations between auditory functions in impaired hearing. *Journal of the Acoustical Society of America, 73,* 652-662.

Fialkowska, M.D., Janczewski, G., Kochanek, K., and Dawidowicz, J. (1983) Studies on the temporary effect of noise on the auditory function in man. *Scandinavian Audiology, 12,* 295-298.

Fieandt, H. von and Saxen, A. (1937) Pathologie und klinik der altersschwerhorigkeit. *Acta Oto-Laryngologica Supplement, 23.*

Filling, S. (1958) *Difference limen for frequency.* Andelsbogtrykkeriet, Adense (cited in Marshall, 1981).

Findlay, R.C. and Denenburg, L.J. (1977) Effects of subtle mid-frequency auditory dysfunction upon speech discrimination in noise. *Audiology, 16,* 252-259, 1977.

Findlay, R.C. and Schuchman, G.I. (1976) Masking level

difference for speech: Effects of ear dominance and age. *Audiology, 15,* 232-241.

Fisch, L. (1970) The selective and differential vulnerability of the auditory system. In G.E.W. Wolstenenholme and J. Knight (Eds.), *Sensorineural hearing hearing loss.* Churchill, London, pp. 101-116.

Fisch, U., Dobozi, M., and Greig, D. (1972) Degenerative changes of the arterial vessels of the internal auditory meatus during the process of aging. *Acta Oto-Laryngologica, 73,* 259-266.

Fleischer, K. (1956) Atrophy of ganglionic cells in the inner ear in aging. *Experientia Supplement IV,* 122-127 (cited in Proctor, 1960).

Florentine, M., Buus, S., Scharf, B., and Zwicker, E. (1980) Frequency selectivity in normally-hearing and hearing-impaired observers. *Journal of Speech and Hearing Research, 23,* 646-669.

Ford, J.M., Hink, R.F., Hopkins, W.F., Roth, W.T., Pfefferbaum, A., and Kopell, B.S. (1979a) Age effects on event-related potentials in a selective attention task. *Journal of Gerontology, 34,* 388-395.

Ford, J.M., Roth, W.T., Mohs, R.C., Hopkins, W.F., and Kopell, B.S. (1979b) Event-related potentials recorded from young and old adults during a memory retrieval task. *Electroencephalography and Clinical Neurophysiology, 47,* 450-459.

Fowler, E.P. (1937) The diagnosis of diseases of the neural mechanism of hearing by the aid of sounds well above threshold. *Laryngoscope, 47,* 289-300.

Fowler, E.P. (1944) The aging ear. *Archives of Otolaryngology, 40,* 475-480.

Fowler, E.P. (1959) Presbycusis: The aging ear. *Annals of Otology Rhinology and Laryngology, 68,* 764-776.

Freeman, J. (1979) Progressive sensorineural hearing loss and cochlear otosclerosis: A prospective study. *Laryngoscope, 89,* 1487-1521.

French, N.R. and Steinberg, J.C. (1947) Factors governing the intelligibility of speech sounds. *Journal of the Acoustical Society of America, 19,* 90-119.

Fujikawa, S.M. and Weber, B.A. (1977) Effects of increased stimulus rate on brainstem electric response (BER) audiometry as a function of age. *Journal of the American Audiological Society, 3,* 147-150.

Gacek, R.R. and Schuknecht, H.F. (1969) Pathology of Presbycusis. *International Audiology, 8,* 199-207.

Gaeth, J. (1948) *A study of phonemic regression in relation to hearing loss.* Doctoral Dissertation, Northwestern University.

Gallo, R. and Glorig, A. (1964) Permanent threshold shift changes produced by noise exposure and aging. *Industrial Hygene Association Journal, 25,* 237-245 (cited in Schmidt, 1969).

Gang, R.P. (1976) The effects of age on the diagnostic utility of the rollover phenomenon. *Journal of Speech and Hearing Disorders, 41,* 63-69.

Garstecki, D.C. and Mulac, A. (1974) Effects of test material and competing message on speech discrimination. *Journal of Auditory Research, 3,* 171-178.

Gates, G.A., Cooper, J.C., Kannel, W.B., and Miller, N.J. (1990) Hearing in the elderly: the Framingham cohort, 1983-1985. *Ear and Hearing, 11,* 247-256.

Gatti, A. (1956) Considerations of the functional mechanisms of the tympanic cavity in the causation of presbycusis. *Annali di Laryngologia, Otologia, Rinologia, Faringologia, 55,* 415-418 (cited in Proctor, 1960).

Gelfand, S.A., Hoffman, S., Waltzman, S.B., and Piper, N.

(1980) Dichotic CV recognition at various interaural temporal onset asynchronies: effect of age. *Journal of the Acoustical Society of America, 68,* 1258-1261.

Gelfand, S.A. and Piper, N. (1981) Acoustic reflex thresholds in young and elderly subjects with normal hearing. *Journal of the Acoustical Society of America, 69,* 295-297.

Gelfand, S.A., Piper, N., and Silman, S. (1985) Consonant recognition in quiet as a function of aging among normal hearing subjects. *Journal of the Acoustical Society of America, 78,* 1198-1206.

Gelfand, S.A., Piper, N., and Silman, S. (1986) Consonant recognition in quiet and in noise with aging among normal hearing listeners. *Journal of the Acoustical Society of America, 80,* 1589-1598.

Gelfand, S.A., Ross, L., and Miller, S. (1988) Sentence reception in noise from one versus two sources: Effects of aging and hearing loss. *Journal of the Acoustical Society of America, 83,* 248-256.

Gentschev, T. and Sotelo, C. (1973) Degenerative patterns in the ventral cochlear nucleus of the rat after primary deafferentation: An ultrastructural study. *Brain Research, 62,* 37-60.

Gerken, G.M. (1979) Central denervation hypersensitivity in the auditory system of the cat. *Journal of the Acoustical Society of America, 66,* 721-727.

Gersdorff, M.C. (1978) Modifications du reflexe acoustico-facial chez l'homme en fonction de l'age. *Audiology, 17,* 260-270.

Gilad, O. and Glorig, A. (1979a) Presbycusis: The aging ear. Part I. *Journal of the American Audiological Society, 4,* 195-206.

Gilad, O. and Glorig, A. (1979b) Presbycusis: The aging ear. Part II. *Journal of the American Audiological Society, 4,* 207-217.

Gimsing, S. (1990) Word recognition in presbycusis. *Scandinavian Audiology, 19,* 207-211.

Ginzel, A., Pederson, C.B., Spliid, P.E., and Andersen, E. (1982) The effect of age and hearing loss on the identification of synthetic /b,d,g/-stimuli. *Scandinavian Audiology, 11,* 103-112.

Gjaevenes, K. and Sohoel, T. (1969) The tone decay test. *Acta Oto-Laryngologica, 68,* 33-42.

Glasberg, B.R. and Moore, B.J. (1989) Psychoacoustic abilities of subjects with unilateral and bilateral cochlear hearing impairments and their relationship to the ability to understand speech. *Scandinavian Audiology Supplement, 32.*

Glasberg, B.R., Moore, B.C.J., and Bacon, S.P. (1987) Gap detection and masking in hearing-impaired and normal-hearing subjects. *Journal of the Acoustical Society of America, 81,* 1546-1556.

Glasberg, B.R., Moore, B.J., Patterson, R.D., and Nimmo-Smith, I. (1984) Dynamic range and asymmetry of the auditory filter. *Journal of the Acoustical Society of America, 76,* 419-427.

Gleeson, M. and Felix, H. (1987) A comparative study of the effect of age on the human cochlear and vestibular neuroepithelia. *Acta Oto-Laryngologica Supplement, 436,* 103-109.

Glorig, A. (1957) *Wisconsin state fair hearing survey,* American Academy of Opthalmology and Otolaryngology.

Glorig, A. and Davis, H. (1961) Age, noise and hearing loss. *Annals of Otology Rhinology and Laryngology, 70,* 556-571.

Glorig, A. and Gallo, R. (1962) *Comments on sensorineural hearing loss in otosclerosis.* Little, Brown, and Co., Boston.

Glorig, A. and Nixon, J. (1962) Hearing loss as a function of age. *Laryngoscope, 72,* 1596-1610.

Goetzinger, C.P. and Rousey, C. (1959) Hearing problems in later life. *Medical Times, 87,* 771-780.

Goetzinger, C.P., Proud, G.O., Dirks, D., and Embrey, J. (1961) A study of hearing in advanced age. *Archives of Otolaryngology, 73,* 662-674.

Goldstein, R. and Kramer, J.C. (1960) Factors affecting thresholds for short tones. *Journal of Speech and Hearing Research, 3,* 249-256.

Goodhill, V. (1969) Bilateral malleal fixation and conductive presbycusis. *Archives of Otolaryngology, 90,* 107-112.

Goodin, D.S., Squires, K.C. and Henderson, B.H., and Starr, A. (1978) Age-related variations in evoked potentials to auditory stimuli in normal human subjects. *Electroencephalography and Clinical Neurophysiology, 44,* 447-458.

Gordon-Salant, S. (1986) Recognition of natural and time/intensity altered CVs by young and elderly subjects with normal hearing. *Journal of the Acoustical Society of America, 80,* 1599-1607.

Gordon-Salant, S. (1987a) Consonant recognition and confusion patterns among elderly hearing-impaired subjects. *Ear and Hearing, 8,* 270-276.

Gordon-Salant, S. (1987b) Age-related differences in speech recognition performance as a function of test format and paradigm. *Ear and Hearing, 8,* 277-282.

Goycoolea, M.V., Goycoolea, H.G., Farfan, C.R., Rodriguez, L.G., Martinez, G.C., and Vidal, R. (1986) Effect of life in industrialized societies on hearing in natives of Easter Island. *Laryngoscope, 96,* 1391-1396.

Grady, C.L., Grimes, A.M., Pikus, A., Schwartz, M., Rapoport, S., and Cutler, N.R. (1984) Alterations in auditory processing of speech stimuli during aging in healthy subjects. *Cortex, 20,* 101-110.

Gregory, R.I. (1974) Increase in neurological noise as a factor in aging. In R.I. Gregory (Ed.), *Concepts and mechanisms of perception.* Duckworth & Co., London.

Grigor, R.R., Spitz, P.W., and Furst, D.E. (1987) Salicylate toxicity in elderly patients with rheumatoid arthritis. *Journal of Rheumatology, 14,* 60-66.

Gross, C.W. (1969) Sensori-neural hearing loss in clinical and histologic otosclerosis. *Laryngoscope, 79,* 104-112.

Guild, S.R. (1936) Hearing by bone conduction: The pathways of transmission by sound. *Annals of Otology Rhinology and Laryngology, 45,* 736-755, (cited in Covell, 1952).

Guild, S. (1944) Histologic otosclerosis. *Annals of Otology Rhinology and Laryngology, 53,* 246-267.

Guild, S.R., Crowe, S.J., Bunch, C.C., and Polvogt, L.M. (1931) Correlations of differences in the density of innervation of the organ of Corti with difference in acuity of hearing, including evidence as to location in the cochlea of receptors for certain tones. *Acta Oto-Laryngologica, 15,* 269-308.

Gussen, R. (1968) Articular and internal remodeling in the human otic capsule. *American Journal of Anatomy, 122,* 397-418.

Gussen, R. (1969) Plugging of vascular canals in the otic capsule. *Annals of Otology Rhinology and Laryngology, 78,* 1305-1315.

Haas, G.F. (1982) Impaired listeners' recognition of speech presented dichotically through high and low-pass filters. *Audiology, 21,* 433-453.

Habener, S.A. and Snyder, J. M. (1974) Stapedius reflex amplitude and decay in normal hearing ears. *Archives of Otolaryngology, 100,* 294-297.

Habermann, J. (1891) Uber nervenatrophie in inneren ohre. *Zeitschrift Heilkunde, 12,* 357 (cited in Bredberg, 1968).

Hall, J. G. (1976) The Cochlear nuclei in monkeys after dihydrostreptomycin or noise exposure. *Acta Oto-Laryngologica, 81,* 344-352.

Hall, J.W. (1982a) Acoustic reflex amplitude. I. Effect of age and sex. *Audiology, 21,* 294-309.

Hall, J.W. (1982b) Acoustic reflex amplitude. II. Effect of age-related auditory dysfunction. *Audiology, 21,* 386-399.

Hall, J.W., III and Derlacki, E.L. (1986) Effect of conductive hearing loss and middle ear surgery on binaural hearing. *Annals of Otology Rhinology and Laryngology, 95,* 525-530.

Hall, J.W. and Harvey, A.D.G. (1985) The binaural masking level difference as a function of frequency, masker level and masking bandwidth in normal-hearing and hearing-impaired listeners *Audiology, 24,* 25-31.

Hall, R.D. (1990) Estimation of surviving spiral ganglion cells in the deaf rat using the electrically evoked auditory brainstem response. *Hearing Research, 49,* 155-168.

Hallerman, W. and Plath, P. (1971) Effect of age on the discrimination ability of the ear. *Hals Nasen Ohren, 19,* 26-32.

Hallpike, C.S. (1976) Sensori-neural deafness and derangements of the loudness function: Their nature and clinical investigation. In W.D. Keidel and W.D. Neff (Eds.), *Handbook of sensory physiology.* (Vol. 3). Springer-Verlag, Berlin, pp. 1-36.

Handler, S.D. and Margolis, R.H. (1977) Predicting hearing loss from stapedial reflex thresholds in patients with sensori-neural impairment. *American Academy of Ophthalmology and Otolaryngology Transactions, 84,* 425-431.

Hansen, C.C. (1967) *Vascular anatomy of the human temporal bone.* American Medical Society, Chicago (cited in Hansen, 1973).

Hansen, C.C. (1968) Perceptive hearing loss and arterial hypertension. *Archives of Otolaryngology, 87,* 119-122.

Hansen, C.C. (1973) The aetiology of perceptive deafness. *Acta Oto-Laryngologica, Supplement 309,* 1-92.

Hansen, C.C. and Reske-Nielsen, E. (1965) Pathological studies in presbycusis. *Archives of Otolaryngology, 82,* 115-132.

Harbert, F. and Young, I.K. (1965) Spread of masking in ears showing abnormal adaptation and conductive deafness. *Acta Oto-Laryngologica 60,* 49-58.

Harbert, F., Young, I.M. and Menduke, H. (1966) Audiologic findings in presbycusis. *Journal of Auditory Research, 6,* 297-312.

Harkins, S.W. (1981) Effects of age and interstimulus interval on the brainstem auditory evoked potential. *International Journal of Neuroscience, 15,* 107-118.

Harman, D. (1972) The biologic clock: The mitochondria? *American Geriatrics Society Journal, 20,* 145-147.

Harman, D. (1986) Free radical theory of aging: role of free radicals in the origination and evolution of life, aging, and disease processes. In J.E. Johnson, Jr., R. Walford, D. Harman, and J. Miquel (Eds.), *Free radicals, aging, and degenerative diseases.* Liss, New York, pp. 3-50.

Harris, J.D. (1965) Monaural and binaural speech intelligibility and the stereophonic effect based on temporal cues. Laryngoscope, 75, 428-446.

Harris, J.D. (1960) Combinations of distortions in speech. *Archives of Otolaryngology, 72,* 227-232.

Harris, R.W. and Reitz, M.L. (1985) Effects of room reverberation and noise on speech discrimination by the elderly. *Audiology, 24,* 319-324.

Harris, R.W. and Swenson, D.W. (1990) Effects of reverberation and noise on speech recognition by adults with various amounts of sensorineural hearing impairment. *Audiology, 29,* 314-321.

Harrison, J. and Buchwald, J. (1982) Auditory brainstem responses in the aged cat. *Neurobiology of Aging, 3,* 163-171.

Harrison, J.M. (1981) Effects of age on acquisition and maintenance of a location discrimination in rats. *Experimental Aging Research, 7,* 467-476.

Harrison, J.M. and Turnock, M. (1975) Animal psychophysics: Improvements in tracking method. *Journal of the Experimental Analysis of Behavior, 23,* 141-147.

Harty, M. (1953) Elastic tissue in the middle-ear cavity. *Journal of Laryngology and Otology, 67,* 723-729.

Hausler, R., Colburn, S. and Marr, E. (1983) Sound localization in subjects with impaired hearing. Spatial discrimination and discrimination tests. *Acta Oto-Laryngologica Supplement, 400,* 6-62.

Hausman, P.B. and Weksler, M.E. (1985) Changes in the immune response with age. In C.E. Finch and E.L. Schneider (Eds.), *Handbook of the biology of aging.* Van Nostrand, New York, pp. 414-432.

Hawkins, D.B. and Wightman, F.L. (1980) Interaural time discrimination ability of listeners with sensorineural hearing loss. *Audiology, 19,* 495-507.

Hawkins, J.E. (1976) Drug ototoxicity. In W.D. Keidel and W.D. Neff (Eds.), *Handbook of sensory physiology,* (Vol. 3). Springer-Verlag, Berlin, pp. 707-748.

Hawkins, J.E. and Johnsson, L.-G. (1985) Otopathological changes associated with presbycusis. *Seminars in Hearing, 6,* 115-133.

Hawkins, J.E., Miller, J.M., Rouse, R.C., Davis, J.A., and Rarey, K. (1985) Inner ear histopathology in aging rhesus monkeys (Macaca mulatta). In *Behavior and pathology of aging rhesus monkeys.* Liss, New York, pp. 137-154.

Hayes, D. (1984) Hearing problems of aging. In J. Jerger (Ed.), *Hearing disorders in adults.* College-Hill, San Diego, pp. 311-338.

Hayes, D. and Jerger, J. (1979) Low-frequency hearing loss in presbycusis: A central interpretation. *Archives of Otolaryngology, 105,* 9-12.

Hayes, D. and Jerger, J. (1979) Aging and the use of hearing aids. *Scandinavian Audiology, 8,* 33-40.

Hazell, J.W.P. (1979) Tinnitus. *British Journal of Hospital Medicine, 22,* 468-471.

Helmholtz, H. von (1863) *On the sensations of tone.* Dover Publications, New York (reprinted, 1954).

Hellbrook, J. (1988) Strukturelle veranderungen des horfeldes in abhangigkoit vom lebensalter. *Zeitschrift fur Gerontologie, 21,* 146-149.

Hellman, R.P. and Meiselman, C.H. (1990) Loudness relations for individuals and groups in normal and hearing. *Journal of the Acoustical Society of America, 88,* 2596-2606.

Hellstrom, L.I. and Schmiedt, R.A. (1989) A comparison of whole nerve potential input/output functions in aged and young gerbils. *Association for Research in Otolaryngology Abstracts, 12,* 43.

Hellstrom, L.I. and Schmiedt, R.A. (1990) Comparisons of compound action potential and single-fiber characteristics in young and quiet-aged gerbils. *Association for Research in Otolaryngology Abstracts, 13,* 149.

Hellstrom, L.I. and Schmiedt, R.A. (1991) Frequency selectivity and thresholds in auditory-nerve fibers in young and quiet-aged gerbils. *Association for Research in Otolaryngology Abstracts, 14,* 133.

Henry, K.R. (1983a) Lifelong susceptibility to acoustic trauma: Changing patterns of cochlear damage over the life span of the mouse. *Audiology, 22,* 372-383.

Henry, K.R. (1983b) Ageing and audition. In J.F. Willott (Ed.), *Auditory psychobiology of the mouse.* Charles C. Thomas, Springfield, Illinois, pp. 470-493.

Henry, K.R. (1984) Cochlear microphonics and action potentials mature and decline at different rates in the normal and pathologic mouse cochlea. *Developmental Psychobiology, 17,* 493-504.

Henry, K.R. (1986) Effects of dietary restriction on presbyacusis in the mouse. *Audiology, 25,* 329-337.

Henry, K.R. and Chole, R.A. (1980) Genotypic differences in behavioral, physiological and anatomical expressions of age-related hearing loss on the laboratory mouse. *Audiology, 19,* 369-383.

Henry, K.R., Chole, R.A., McGinn, M.D. and Frush, D.P. (1981) Increased ototoxicity in both young and old mice. *Archives of Otolaryngology, 107,* 92-95.

Henry, K.R. and Lepkowski, C. (1978) Evoked potential correlates of genetic progressive hearing loss: Age-related changes from the ear to inferior colliculus of C57BL/6 and CBA/J mice. *Acta Oto-Laryngologica, 86,* 366-374.

Henry, K.R., McGinn, M.D. and Chole, R.A. (1980) Age-related auditory loss in the Mongolian gerbil. *Archives of Oto-Rhino-Laryngology, 228,* 233-238.

Henson, M.M., Henson, O.W., and Jenkins, D.B. (1984) The attachment of the spiral ligament to the cochlear wall: Anchoring cells and the creation of tension. *Hearing Research, 16,* 231-242.

Herman, G.E., Warren, L.R., and Wagener, J.W. (1977) Auditory lateralization: Age differences in sensitivity to dichotic time and amplitude cues. *Journal of Gerontology, 32,* 187-191.

Hesse, G. and Hesch, R.D. (1986) [Evaluation of risk factors in various forms of inner ear hearing loss.] *Hals Nasen Ohren, 34,* 503-507, 1986 (Medline abstract).

Hildyard, V.H. and Valentine, M.A. (1962) Collapse of the ear canal during audiometry: A further report. *Archives of Otolaryngology, 75,* 422-423.

Hill, M.J. (1968) Speech intelligibility in presbycusis under conditions of simultaneous time and frequency distortion. *Dissertation Abstracts International, 28,* 4738-4739.

Hillerdal, M., Jansson, B., Engstrom, B., Hultcrantz, E., and Borg, E. (1987) Cochlear blood flow in noise-damaged ears. *Acta Oto-Laryngologica 104,* 270-278.

Hinchcliffe, R. (1959) The threshold of hearing as a function of age. *Acustica, 9,* 303-308.

Hinchcliffe, R (1961) Prevalence of the commoner ear nose and throat conditions in the adult rural populations of Great Britain. *British Journal of Preventive and Social Medicine, 15,* 128-134.

Hinchcliffe, R. (1962) The anatomical locus of presbycusis. *Journal of Speech and Hearing Disorders, 4,* 301-310.

Hinchcliffe, R. and Jones, W.I. (1968) Hearing levels of a suburban Jamaican population. *International Audiology, 7,* 239-258.

Hinojosa, R. and Marion, M. (1987) Otosclerosis and sensorineural hearing loss: A histopathologic study. *American Journal of Otolaryngology, 8,* 296-307.

Hinojosa, R., Seligsohn, R., and Lerner, S.A. (1985) Ganglion cell counts in the cochlea of patients with normal audiograms. *Acta Oto-Laryngologica, 99,* 8-13.

Hirsh, I.J. (1948) The influence of interaural phase on interaural summation and inhibition. *Journal of the Acoustical Society of America, 20,* 536-544.

Hirsh, I.J., Davis, H., Silverman, S., Reynolds, E.G., Eldert,

E., and Benson, R.W. (1952) Development of materials for speech audiometry. *Journal of Speech and Hearing Disorders, 17*, 321-337.

Hobson, W. and Pemberton, J. (1955) *The health of the elderly at home.* Butterworth, London.

Hoeffding, V. and Feldman, M.L. (1988) Changes with age in the morphology of the cochlear nerve in rats: Light microscopy. *Journal of Comparative Neurology, 276*, 537-546.

Hoeffding, V. and Feldman, M.L. (1989) The morphology of the inferior colliculus in young adult and aging macaques (M. mulatta). *Association for Research in Otolaryngology Abstracts, 12*, 93.

Hoffman, D.W., Jones-King, K.L., and Altschuler, R.A. (1988) Putative neurotransmitters in the rat cochlea at several ages. *Brain Research, 460*, 366-368.

Holmes, A.E., Kricos, P.B., and Kessler, R.A. (1988) A closed-versus open-set measure of speech discrimination in normally hearing young and elderly adults. *British Journal of Audiology, 22*, 29-33.

Hood, J. D. (1968) Speech discrimination and its relationship to disorders of the loudness function. *International Audiology, 7*, 232-258, l968.

Hood, L.J., Berlin, C.I., Collins, M.J., and Cullen, J.K. (1991) Peripheral and central components of aging in the auditory system: "Old Time Ears." *Association for Research in Otolaryngology Abstracts, 14*, 102.

Hotaling, A.J., Hillstrom, R.P., and Bazell, C. (1989) Sickle cell crisis and sensorineural hearing loss: Case report and discussion. *International Journal of Pediatric Otolaryngology, 17*, 207-211.

Hoyer, S. (1988) Glucose and related brain metabolism in normal aging. *Age, 11*, 150-156.

Humes, L.E. (1978) The aural-overload test: Twenty years later. *Journal of Speech and Hearing Disorders, 43*, 34-46.

Humes, L.E. (1984) Noise-induced hearing loss as influenced by other agents and by some physical characteristics of the individual. *Journal of the Acoustical Society of America, 76*, 1318-1329.

Hunter, K.P. and Willott, J.F. (1987) Aging and the auditory brainstem response in mice with severe or minimal presbycusis. *Hearing Research, 30*, 207-218.

Hutchinson, K.M. (1989) Influence of sentence context on speech perception in young and older adults. *Journal of Gerontology, 44*, 36-44.

Inglis, J. and Tansey, C.L. (1967) Age differences and scoring differences in dichotic listening performance. *Journal of Psychology, 66*, 325-332.

Irvine, D.R.F. (1986) The auditory brainstem. *Progress in sensory physiology* (Vol. 7). Springer-Verlag, Berlin.

Ishii, T., Murakami, Y., and Balogh, K. (1967a) Acetylcholinesterase activity in the efferent nerve fibers of the human inner ear. *Annals of Otology Rhinology and Laryngology, 76*, 69-82.

Ishii, T., Murakami, Y., Kimura, R.S., and Balogh, K. (1967b) Electron microscopic and histochemical identification of lipofuscin in the human inner ear. *Acta Oto-Laryngologica, 64*, 17-29.

Ison, J.R., O'Neill, W.E., and Walton, J.P. (1991) Reflex inhibition by acoustic transients in aged CBA mice. *Association for Research in Otolaryngology Abstracts, 14*, 157.

Jaehne, A. (1914) Die anatomischen veranderungen bei der alters-schwerhorigkeit. *Archiv fuer Ohrenheilkunde, 95*, 247-298 (cited in Johnsson and Hawkins, 1972b).

Jakimetz, J.J., Silman, S., Miller, M.H., and Silverman, C.A. (1989) Some effects of signal bandwidth and spectral density on the acoustic-reflex threshold in the elderly. *Journal of the Acoustical Society of America, 86*, 1783-1789.

Jastreboff, P.J. (1990) Phantom auditory perception (tinnitus): Mechanisms of generation and perception. *Neuroscience Research, 8*, 221-254.

Jepson, O. (1963) Middle ear muscle reflexes in man. In J. Jerger (Ed.), *Modern developments in audiology.* Academic Press, New York, pp. 193-239.

Jerger, J. (1960) Bekesy audiometry in analysis of auditory disorders. *Journal of Speech and Hearing Research, 3*, 275-287.

Jerger, J. (1973) Audiological Findings in Aging. *Advances in Oto-Rhino-Laryngology, 20*, 115-124.

Jerger, J. and Hall, J. (1980) Effects of age and sex on auditory brainstem response. *Archives of Otolaryngology, 106*, 387-391.

Jerger, J. and Hayes, D. (1977) Diagnostic speech audiometry. *Archives of Otolaryngology, 103*, 216-222.

Jerger, J. and Hayes, D. (1979) Hearing and aging. In S.S. Han and D.H. Coons (Eds.), *Special senses in aging.* University of Michigan Press, Ann Arbor, pp. 109-118.

Jerger, J., Hayes, D. and Anthony, L. (1978) Effect of age on prediction of sensorineural hearing level from the acoustic reflex. *Archives of Otolaryngology, 104*, 393-394.

Jerger, J., Hayes, D., Anthony, L., and Mauldin, L. (1978) Factors influencing prediction of hearing levels from the acoustic reflex. *Monographs in Contemporary Audiology, 1*.

Jerger, J. and Jerger, S. (1971) Diagnostic significance of PB word functions. *Archives of Otolaryngology, 93*, 573-580.

Jerger, J. and Jerger, S. (1975) A simplified tone decay test. *Archives of Otolaryngology, 101*, 403-407.

Jerger, J., Jerger, S., and Mauldin, L. (1972) Studies in impedance audiometry. I. Normal and sensorineural ears. *Archives of Otolaryngology, 96*, 513-523.

Jerger. J., Jerger, S., Oliver, T., and Pirozzolo, F. (1989) Speech understanding in the elderly. *Ear and Hearing, 10*, 79-89.

Jerger, J. and Johnson, K. (1988) Interactions of age, gender, and sensorineural hearing loss on ABR latency. *Ear and Hearing, 9*, 168-176.

Jerger, J., Johnson, K., and Jerger, S. (1988) Effect of response criterion on measures of speech understanding in the elderly. *Ear and Hearing, 9*, 49-56.

Jerger, J. and Oliver, T. (1987) Interaction of age and intersignal interval on acoustic reflex amplitude. *Ear and Hearing, 8*, 322-325.

Jerger, J., Oliver, T., and Chmiel, R. (1988) Auditory middle latency response: A perspective. *Seminars in Hearing, 9*, 75-85.

Jerger, J., Shedd, J., and Harford, E. (1959) On the detection of extremely small changes in sound intensity. *Archives of Otolaryngology, 96*, 513-523.

Jerger, J., Stach, B., Pruitt, J., Harper, R., and Kirby, H. (1989) Comments on "Speech understanding and aging." *Journal of the Acoustical Society of America, 85*, 1352-1354.

Jerger, J., Tillman, T.W., and Peterson, J.L. (1960) Masking by octave bands of noise in normal and impaired ears. *Journal of the Acoustical Society of America, 32*, 385-390.

Jerger, S. (1980) Diagnostic applications of impedance audiometry: Central auditory disorders. In J. Jerger and J.L. Northern (Eds.), *Clinical impedance audiometry.* American Electromedics, Acton, Massachusetts, pp. 128-141.

Johannsen, H.S. and Lehn, T. (1984) The dependence of early acoustically evoked potentials on age. *Archives of Oto-Rhino-Laryngology, 240*, 153-158.

Johnsson, L.-G. (1973) Reissner's membrane in the human cochlea. *Annals of Otology Rhinology and Laryngology, 80,* 425-438.

Johnsson, L.-G. (1974) Sequence of degeneration of Corti's organ and its first-order neurons. *Annals of Otology Rhinology and Laryngology, 83,* 294-303.

Johnsson, L.-G., Felix, H., Gleeson, M., and Pollak, A. (1990) Observations on the pattern of sensorineural degeneration in the human cochlea. *Acta Oto-Laryngologica Supplement, 470,* 88-96.

Johnsson, L.-G. and Hawkins, J.E. (1972a) Sensory and neural degeneration with aging, as seen in microdissections of the human inner ear. *Annals of Otology Rhinology and Laryngology, 81,* 179-193.

Johnsson, L.-G., and Hawkins, J.E., Jr. (1972b) Vascular changes in the human inner ear associated with aging. *Annals of Otology Rhinology and Laryngology, 81,* 364-376.

Johnsson, L.-G. and Hawkins, J.E., Jr. (1972c) Strial atrophy in clinical and experimental deafness. *Laryngoscope, 82,* 1105-1125.

Johnsson, L.-G., and Hawkins, J.E., Jr. (1976) Degeneration patterns in human ears exposed to noise. *Annals of Otology Rhinology and Laryngology, 85,* 725-739.

Johnsson, L.-G., and Hawkins, J.E. (1979) Age-related degeneration of the inner ear. In S.S. Han and D.H. Coons (Eds.), *Special senses in aging.* Institute of Gerontology, Ann Arbor, pp. 119-135.

Jokinen, K. (1969) Presbycusis. I. Comparison of manual and automatic thresholds. *Acta Oto-Laryngologica, 68,* 327-335.

Jokinen, K. (1970) Presbyacusis. III. Perstimulatory threshold adaptation. *Acta Oto-Laryngologica, 69,* 324-328.

Jokinen, K. (1973) Presbyacusis: VI. Masking of speech. *Acta Oto-Laryngologica, 76,* 426-430.

Jokinen, K. and Karja, J. (1970) Presbycusis. IV. Forward vs. reverse frequency sweep audiometry. *Acta Oto-Laryngologica, 70,* 227-231.

Jorgensen, B.M. (1961) Changes of aging in the inner ear. *Archives of Otolaryngology, 70,* 154-170.

Jorgensen, M.B. and Kristensen, H.K. (1967) Frequency of otosclerosis. *Annals of Otology Rhinology and Laryngology, 76,* 83-88.

Kalikow, D.N., Stevens, K.N., and Elliott, L.L. (1977) Development of a test of speech intelligibility in noise using sentence materials with controlled word predictability. *Journal of the Acoustical Society of America, 61,* 1337-1351.

Kaplan, H. and Pickett, J.M. (1981) Effects of dichotic/diotic versus monotic presentation on speech understanding in noise in elderly hearing-impaired listeners. *Ear and Hearing, 2,* 202-207.

Kaplan, H. and Pickett, J.M. (1984) Release from first-formant masking in presbyacusis. *Audiology, 23,* 165-180.

Kasden, S.D. (1970) Speech discrimination in two age groups matched for hearing loss. *Journal of Auditory Research, 10,* 210-212.

Katz, J. (1962) The use of staggered spondaic words for assessing the integrity of the central auditory nervous system. *Journal of Auditory Research, 2,* 327-337.

Keay, D.G. and Murray, J.A. (1988) Hearing loss in the elderly: a 17-year longitudinal study. *Clinical Otolaryngology, 13,* 31-35.

Keithley, E.M. (1989) Auditory nerve fibers within the cochlear nucleus of young and old Fischer 344 rats. *Association for Research in Otolaryngology Abstracts, 12,* 8-9.

Keithley, E.M. (1990) Single-unit responses in the cochlear nucleus of young and aged rats. *Society for Neuroscience Abstracts, 16,* 796.

Keithley, E.M. and Croskrey, K.L. (1990) Spiral ganglion cell endings in the cochlear nucleus of young and old rats. *Hearing Research, 49,* 169-178.

Keithley, E.M. and Feldman, M.L. (1979) Spiral ganglion cell counts in an age-graded series of rat cochleas. *Journal of Comparative Neurology, 188,* 429-442.

Keithley, E.M. and Feldman, M.L. (1982) Hair cell counts in an age-graded series of rat cochleas. *Hearing Research, 8,* 249-262.

Keithley, E.M. and Feldman, M.L. (1983) The spiral ganglion and hair cells of Bronx waltzer. *Hearing Research, 12,* 381-391.

Keithley, E.M. and Feldman, M.L. (1991) Cochlear degeneration in aged pigmented versus albino rats. *Association for Research in Otolaryngology Abstracts, 14,* 16.

Keithley, E.M., Ryan, A.F., and Woolf, N.K. (1988) Spiral ganglion cell density in young and old gerbils. *Hearing Research, 38,* 125-134.

Kell, R.L., Pearson, J.C.G., Acton, W.I., and Taylor, W. (1971) Social effects of hearing loss due to weaving noise. In D.W. Robinson (Ed.), *Occupation hearing loss.* Academic Press, London, pp. 179-191.

Kelley, N.H. (1939) A study in presbycusis. Auditory loss with increasing age and its effect on the perception of music and speech. *Archives of Otolaryngology, 29,* 506-513.

Kelly-Ballweber, D. and Dobie, R.A. (1984) Binaural interaction measured behaviorally and electrophysiologically in young and old adults. *Audiology, 23,* 181-194.

Kemp, D.T. (1978) Stimulated acoustic emissions from within the human auditory system. *Journal of the Acoustical Society of America, 64,* 1386-1391.

Khanna, S.M. and Leonard, D.G.B. (1986) Relationship between basilar membrane tuning and hair cell condition. *Hearing Research, 23,* 55-70.

Kiang, N.Y.S., Moxon, E.C. and Levine, R.A. (1970) Auditory-nerve activity in cats with normal and abnormal cochleas. In G.E.W. Wolstenholme and T. Knight (Eds.), *Sensorineural hearing loss.* Churchill, London, pp. 241-273.

Kim, D.O. (1984) Functional roles of inner and outer hair cell subsystems in the cochlea and brainstem. In C.I. Berlin (Ed.), *Hearing science: Recent advances.* College-Hill Press, San Diego, pp. 241-262.

Kimura, R.S. (1973) Cochlear vascular lesions. In A.J.D. de Lorenzo (Ed.), *Vascular disorders and hearing defects.* University Park Press, Baltimore, pp. 205-218.

Kirikae, I., Sato, T., and Shitara, T. (1964) A study of hearing in advanced age. *Laryngoscope, 74,* 205-220.

Kirikae, L. (1969) Auditory function in advanced age with reference to histological changes in the central auditory system. *International Audiology, 8,* 221-230.

Kirkwood, T.B.L. (1985) Comparative and evolutionary aspects of longevity. In C.E. Finch and E.L. Schneider (Eds.), *Handbook of the biology of aging.* Van Nostrand, New York, pp. 27-44.

Kisiel, D.L. and Bobbin, R.P. (1981) Miscellaneous ototoxic agents. In R.D. Brown and E.A. Daigneault (Eds.), *Pharmacology of hearing: Experimental and clinical bases.* Wiley, New York, pp. 231-270.

Kjaer, M. (1980) Recognizability of brain stem auditory evoked potential components. *Acta Neurologica Scandinavica, 62,* 20-33.

Klein, A.J., Mills, J.H., and Adkins, W.Y. (1990) Upward spread of masking, hearing loss, and speech recognition in young and elderly listeners. *Journal of the Acoustical Society of America, 87,* 1266-1271.

Klotz, R.E. and Kilbane, M. (1962) Hearing in an aging population. *New England Journal of Medicine, 266,* 277-280.

Knight, K.K. and Margolis, R.H. (1984) Magnitude estimation of loudness II: Loudness perception in presbycusic listeners. *Journal of Speech and Hearing Research, 27,* 28-32.

Knowles, K., Blauch, B., Leipold, H., Cash, W., and Hewett, J. (1989) Reduction of spiral ganglion neurons in the aging canine with hearing loss. *Zentralblatt Veterinaermedzin, 36,* 188-199 (Medline abstract).

Kobrak, F. (1952) Altersschwerhorigkeit, eine schwache der "hortonus" (hypotonia senilis acustica). *Zeitschrift fuer Laryngologie, Rhinologie, Otologie, 31,* 232-235, (cited in Proctor, 1960).

Koerber, K.C., Pfeiffer, R.R., Warr, W.B., and Kiang, N.Y.S. (1966) Spontaneous spike discharges from single units in the cochlear nucleus after destruction of the cochlea. *Experimental Neurology, 16,* 119-130.

Koitchev, K., Aran, J.-M., Ivanov, E., and Cazals, Y. (1986) Progressive degeneration in the cochlear nucleus after chemical destruction of the cochlea. *Acta Oto-Laryngologica, 102,* 31-39.

Konig, E. (1957) Pitch discrimination and age. *Acta Oto-Laryngologica, 48,* 475-489.

Konig, E. (1969) Audiological tests in presbyacusis. *International Audiology, 8,* 240-259.

Konigsmark, B.W. and Murphy, E.A. (1970) Neuronal populations in the human brain. *Nature, 228,* 1335-1336.

Konigsmark, B. W. and Murphy, E. A. (1972) Volume of the ventral cochlear nucleus in man: Its relationship to neuronal population and age. *Journal of Neuropathology and Experimental Neurology, 31,* 304-316.

Konigsmark, B.W. (1971) Hereditary deafness syndromes with onset in adult life. *Audiology, 10,* 257-283.

Konigsmark, B.W. (1972) Genetic hearing loss with no associated abnormalities: A review. *Journal of Speech and Hearing Disorders, 37,* 89-99.

Konkle, D.F., Beasley, D.S., and Bess, F.H. (1977) Intelligibility of time-altered speech in relation to chronological aging. *Journal of Speech and Hearing Research, 20,* 108-115.

Korabic, E.W., Freeman, B.A., and Church, G.T. (1978) Intelligibility of time-expanded speech with normally hearing and elderly subjects. *Audiology, 17,* 159-164.

Korsan-Bengtsen, M. (1973) Distorted speech audiometry. *Acta Oto-Laryngologica Supplement, 310.*

Kraus, H. (1970) Quantitativ-cytochemische untersuchungen am innenohr junger und seniler meerschweinchen. *Acta Oto-Laryngologica Supplement 278.*

Krmpotic-Nemanic, J. (1969) Presbycusis and retrocochlear structures. *International Audiology, 8,* 210-220.

Krmpotic-Nemanic, J. (1971) A new concept of the pathogenesis of presbycusis. *Archives of Otolaryngology, 93,* 161-166.

Krmpotic-Nemanic, J., Nemanic, D., and Kostovic, I. (1972) Macroscopical and microscopical aging changes of the internal auditory meatus and its consequences on the auditory nerve and vessels. *Acta Oto-Laryngologica 73,* 254-258.

Kryter, K.D. (1983) Presbycusis, sociocusis and nosocusis. *Journal of the Acoustical Society of America, 73,* 1897-1916.

Kryter, K.D. (1985) *The effects of noise on man.* Academic Press, New York.

Kryter, K.D. (1988) *Definitions: Presbycusis, sociocusis, and nosiocusis.* The Aging Ear (conference), St. Louis.

Krzanowski, J.J., Jr. and Matschinsky, F.M. (1975) Adenosine triphosphate and phosphocreatinine levels in cochlear structures: Use rate and effect of salycilates.

Journal of Histochemistry and Cytochemistry, 23, 766-773.

LaCroix, P.G. and Harris, J.D. (1979) Effects of high-frequency cue reduction on the comprehension of distorted speech. *Journal of Speech and Hearing Disorders, 44,* 236-246.

Lakatta, E.G. (1985) Heart and circulation. In C.E. Finch and E.L. Schneider (Eds.), *Handbook of the biology of aging.* Van Nostrand, New York, pp. 377-413.

Lambert, P.R. and Schwartz, I.R. (1982) A longitudinal study of changes in the cochlear nucleus in the CBA mouse. *Otolaryngology Head Neck Surgery, 90,* 787-794.

Lange, W. (1937) Horleistung und patologisch-anatomischer befund in ductus cochlearis. *Archiv fuer Ohren-, Nasen-, und Kehlkopfheilkunde, 41,* 209 (cited in Bredberg, 1968).

Lawrence, M. (1958) Audiometric manifestations of inner ear physiology: The aural overload test. *American Ophthalmological Otolaryngological Society Transactions, 62,* 104-119.

Lawrence, M. (1966) Histological evidence for localized radial flow of endolymph. *Archives of Otolaryngology, 83,* 406-412.

Lawrence, M. (1979) Cochlear physiology and the aging process. In S.S. Han and D.H. Coons (Eds.), *Special senses in aging.* Institute of Gerontology, Ann Arbor, pp. 136-142.

Lawrence, M., Nuttall, A.L., and Burgio, P.A. (1975) Cochlear potentials and oxygen associated with hypoxia. *Annals of Otology Rhinology and Laryngology, 84,* 499-513.

Lawrence, M. and Yantis, P.A. (1956) Onset and growth of aural harmonic in the overloaded ear. *Journal of the Acoustical Society of America, 28,* 852-858.

Leisti, T.J. (1949) Audiometric studies of presbyacusis. *Acta Oto-Laryngologica, 37,* 555-562.

Lenzi, A., Chiarelli, G., and Sambataro, G. (1989) Comparative study of middle-latency responses and auditory brainstem responses in elderly subjects. *Audiology, 28,* 144-151.

Leshowitz, B. (1977) *Speech intelligibility in noise for listeners with sensorineural hearing damage.* IPO Annual Progress Report No. 12, 11-23, Institute for Perception Research, Eindhoven (cited in Tyler, 1986).

Leshowitz, B. and Lindstrom, R. (1979) Masking and the speech-to-noise ratio. *Audiology Deaf Education, 6,* 5-8.

Leske, M.C. (1981) Prevalence estimates of communicative disorders in the U.S.: Language, hearing and vestibular disorders. *American Speech and Hearing Association, 23,* 229-237.

Levine, M.S., Lloyd, R.L., Hull, C.D., Fisher, R.S., and Buchwald, N.A. (1987) Neurophysiological alterations in caudate neurons in aged cats. *Brain Research, 401,* 213-230.

Liang, C.T., Barnes, J., Takamato, S., and Sacktor, B. (1989) Effect of age on calcium uptake in isolated duodenum cells: Role of, 1, 25-dihydroxyvitamin D3. *Endocrinology, 124,* 2830-2836.

Liberman, A.M. (1970) The grammar of speech and language. *Cognitive Psychology, 1,* 301-323.

Liberman, A.M. (1989) *The relation of speech to other specializations.* Presidential Special Lecture, Meeting of the Society for Neuroscience, Phoenix.

Liberman, M.C. (1984) Single-neuron labeling and chronic cochlear pathology. I. Threshold shift and characteristic-frequency shift. *Hearing Research, 16,* 33-41.

Liberman, M.C. and Dodds, L.W. (1984a) Single-neuron labeling and chronic cochlear pathology. II. Stereocilia damage and alterations of spontaneous discharge rates.

Hearing Research, 16, 43-53.

Liberman, M.C. and Dodds, L.W. (1984b) Single-neuron labeling and chronic cochlear pathology. III. Stereocilia damage and alterations of threshold tuning curves. *Hearing Research, 16*, 55-74.

Liberman, M.C. and Kiang, N.Y.S. (1978) Acoustic trauma in cats: Cochlear pathology and auditory-nerve activity. *Acta Oto-Laryngologica Supplement 358*, 1-63.

Liberman, M.C. and Kiang, N.Y.S. (1984) Single-neuron labeling and chronic cochlear pathology. IV. Stereocilia damage and alterations in rate-and phase-level functions. *Hearing Research, 16*, 75-90.

Liberman, M.C. and Beil, D.G. (1979) Hair cell condition and auditory nerve response in normal and noise-damaged cochleas. *Acta Oto-Laryngologica, 88*, 161-176.

Liden, G., Engstrom H. and Hall, J. (1973) Audiological and morphological assessment of the effect of noise on cochlea and brain stem in cat. *Acta Oto-Laryngologica, 75*, 325-328.

Lindsay, J.R. (1985) Otosclerosis. In M.M. Paparella and D.A. Shumrick (Eds.), *Otolaryngology, 2*. W. B. Saunders, Philadelphia, pp. 1617-1644.

Lindsay, J.R. and Beal, D.D. (1966) Sensorineural deafness in otosclerosis. *Annals of Otology Rhinology and Laryngology, 75*, 436-457.

Linthicum, F.H. (1966) Correlation of sensorineural hearing impairment and otosclerosis. *Annals of Otology Rhinology and Laryngology, 75*, 512-524.

Linthicum, F. H., Filipo, R., and Brody, S. (1975) Sensorineural hearing loss due to cochlear otospongiosis: theoretical considerations of etiology. *Annals of Otology Rhinology and Laryngology, 84*, 544-551.

Lloyd, L.L. and Kaplan, H. (1978) *Audiometric interpretation: A manual of basic audiometry*. University Park Press, Baltimore.

Lonsbury-Martin, B.L., Harris, F.P., Stagner, B.B., Hawkins, M.D., and Martin, G.K. (1990) Distortion product emissions in humans. I. Basic properties in normally hearing subjects. *Annals of Otology Rhinology and Laryngology Supplement, 147*, 3-14.

Lowell, S.H. and Paparella, M.M. (1977) Presbyacusis: what is it? *Laryngoscope, 87*, 1710-1717.

Ludlow, C.L., Cudahy, E.A., and Bassich, C.J. (1982) Developmental, age, and sex effects on gap detection and temporal order. *Journal of the Acoustical Society of America, 71*, S47.

Luscher, E. and Zwislocki, J. (1948) A simple method for indirect monaural determination of the recruitment phenomenon *Acta Oto Laryngologica Supplement 78*, 156-172.

Luterman, D. M., Welsh, O.L., and Melrose, J. (1966) Responses of aged males to time-altered speech stimuli. *Journal of Speech and Hearing Research, 9*, 226-230.

Lutman, M.E. (1991) Degradations in frequency and temporal resolution with age and their impact on auditory function. *Acta Oto-Laryngologica Supplement 476*, 120-126.

Lutman, M.E., Gatehouse, S., and Worthington, A.G. (1991) Frequency resolution as a function of hearing threshold level and age. *Journal of the Acoustical Society of America, 89*, 320-328.

Luxon, L.M. (1981) The anatomy and pathology of the central auditory pathways. *British Journal of Audiology, 15*, 31-40.

Macrae, J.H. (1971) Noise-induced hearing loss and presbyacusis. *Audiology, 10*, 323-333.

Makishima, K. (1967) Clinicopathological studies in presbycusis. *Otologia Fukuoka, 3*, 333-364.

Makishima, K. (1978) Arteriolar sclerosis as a cause of presbycusis. *Otolaryngology, 86*, 322-326.

Malmo, H.P. and Malmo, R.B. (1982) Multiple unit activity recorded longitudinally in rats from pubescence to old age. *Neurobiology of Aging, 3*, 43-53.

Manasse, P. (1906) Uber chronische, progressive labyrinthare taubheit. *Zeitschrift fuer Ohrenheilkunde, 52*, 1 (cited in Bredberg, 1968).

Marcus, D.C. (1986) Nonsensory electrophysiology of the cochlea: Stria vascularis. In R.A. Altschuler, R.P. Bobbin, and D.W. Hoffman (Eds.), *Neurobiology of hearing: The cochlea*. Raven, New York, pp. 123-138.

Margolis, R.H. and Goldberg, S.M. (1980) Auditory frequency selectivity in normal and presbycusic subjects. *Journal of Speech and Hearing Research, 23*, 603-613.

Margolis, R.H., Popelka, G.R., Handler, S.D., and Himelfarb, M.Z. (1981) The effects of age on acoustic-reflex thresholds in normal-hearing subjects. In G.R. Popelka (Ed.), *Hearing assessment with the acoustic reflex*. Grune and Stratton, New York, pp. 85-95.

Marks, M.G. (1982) The effects of noise, age, sensorineural hearing loss and speakers upon word recognition. *Dissertation Abstracts International, 42*, 3181-3182.

Marshall, L. (1981) Auditory processing in aging listeners. *Journal of Speech and Hearing Disorders, 46*, 226-240.

Marshall, L., Martinez, S.A., and Schlaman, M.E. (1983) Reassessment of high-frequency air-bone gaps in older adults. *Archives of Otolaryngology, 109*, 601-606.

Marshall, L. and Bacon, S.P. (1981) Prediction of speech discrimination scores from audiometric data. *Ear and Hearing, 2*, 148-155.

Marston, L.E. and Goetzinger, C.P. (1972) A comparison of sensitized words and sentences for distinguishing nonperipheral auditory changes as a function of aging. *Cortex, 8*, 213-223.

Martin, E.M. and Pickett, J.M. (1970) Sensorineural hearing loss and upward spread of masking. *Journal of Speech and Hearing Research, 13*, 426-437.

Martini, A., Bovo, R., Agnolitto, M., DaCol, M., Drusian, A., Liddeo, M., and Morra, B. (1988) Dichotic performance in elderly Italians with Italian stop consonant-vowel stimuli. *Audiology, 27*, 1-7.

Matschke, R.G. (1991) Frequency selectivity and psychoacoustic tuning curves in old age. *Acta Oto-Laryngologica Supplement, 476*, 114-119.

Matthies, M.L., Bilger, R.C., and Rzeczkowski, C. (1983) SPIN as a predictor of hearing-aid use. *American Speech and Hearing Association, 25*, 61, (cited in WGSUA, 1988).

Matzker, J. and Springborn, E. (1958) Directional hearing and age. *Zeitschrift fuer Laryngologie, 37*, 739-745 (cited in Proctor, 1960).

Maurer, J.F. and Rupp, R.R. (1979) *Hearing and aging: Tactics for intervention*. Grune & Stratton, New York.

Maurizi, M., Altissimi, G., Ottaviani, F., Paludetti, G., and Bambini, M. (1982) Auditory brainstem Responses (ABR) in the aged. *Scandinavian Audiology, 11*, 213-221.

Mayer, C. L. (1975) The effects of aging on the discrimination of speech in noise. *American Speech and Hearing Association, 17*, 653.

Mayer, O. (1920) Das anatomische substrat der altersschwerhorigkeit. *Archiv fur Ohrenheilkunde, 105*, 1-13.

Mayer, O. (1930) Uber die entstehung der spontanfrakturen der labyrinthkapsel und ihre bedeutung fur die otosklerose. *Zeitschirft fuer Hals,-Nasen-,und Ohrenheilkunde, 26*, 261-279 (cited in Covell, 1952).

McCoy, C., Butler, M., and Broekhoff, J. (1977) Effects of age and sex on dichotic listening: The SSW test. *Journal of Auditory Research, 17,* 263-268.

McCroskey, R.L. and Davis, S.M. (1976) *Auditory fusion: Developmental trends.* American Speech and Hearing Association.

McCroskey, R.L. and Kasten, R.N. (1980) Assessment of central auditory processing. In R. Rupp and K.C. Stockwell (Eds.), *Speech protocols in audiology.* Grune and Stratton, New York, pp. 339-390.

McCroskey, R.L. and Kasten, R.N. (1982) Temporal factors and the aging auditory system. *Ear and Hearing, 3,* 124-127.

McGinn. M.D. and Faddis, B.T. (1987) Auditory experience affects degeneration of the ventral cochlear nucleus in mongolian gerbils. *Hearing Research, 31,* 235-244.

McGinn, M.D., Henry, K.R., and Coss, R.G. (1984) Age-related hearing loss affects dendritic spine density in mouse neocortex: A Golgi study. *Society for Neuroscience Abstracts, 10,* 451.

Melrose, J., Welsh, O.L., and Luterman, D.M. (1963) Auditory responses in selected elderly men. *Journal of Gerontology, 18,* 267-270.

Meurman, O.H. (1954) The difference limen of frequency in tests of auditory function. *Acta Oto-Laryngologica Supplement, 118,* 144-155.

Meyerhoff, W.L. and Liston, S.L. (1980) Metabolism and hearing loss. In M.M. Paparella and D.A. Shumrick (Eds.), *Otolaryngology, 2,* (2nd ed.). W. B. Saunders, Philadelphia, pp. 1828-1845.

Mikaelian, D.O. (1979) Development and degeneration of hearing in the C57/b16 mouse: Relation of electrophysiologic responses from the round window and cochlear nucleus to cochlear anatomy and behavioral responses. *Laryngoscope, 34,* 1-15.

Miller, G.D. (1981) Comparisons of the critical ratios for two different age groups. *Dissertation Abstracts International, 42,* 555.

Miller, J.D. (1970) Audibility curve of the chinchilla. *Journal of the Acoustical Society of America, 48,* 513-523.

Miller, M.H. and Ort, R.G. (1965) Hearing problems in a home for the aged. *Acta Oto-Laryngologica, 59,* 33-44.

Mills, J.A. and Ryals, B.M. (1985) The effects of reduced cerebrovascular circulation on the auditory brain stem response (ABR). *Ear and Hearing, 6,* 139-143.

Mills, J.H., Kulish, L.F., and Adkins, W.Y. (1989) Noise-induced hearing loss and age-related hearing loss in mongolian gerbil. *Association for Research in Otolaryngology Abstracts, 12,* 42-43.

Mills, J.H. and Schmiedt, R.A. (1989) Age-related hearing loss in quiet-reared mongolian gerbils. *Association for Research in Otolaryngology Abstracts, 12,* 44.

Mills, J.H., Schmiedt, R.A., and Kulish, L.F. (1990) Age-related changes in auditory potentials of *Mongolian gerbil. Hearing Research, 46,* 201-210.

Milne, J.S. (1976) Hearing loss related to some signs and symptoms in older people. *British Journal of Audiology, 10,* 65-73.

Milne, J.S. (1977a) The air-bone gap in older people *British Journal of Audiology, 11,* 1-6.

Milne, J.S. (1977b) A longitudinal study of hearing loss in older people *British Journal of Audiology, 11,* 7-14.

Milne, J.S. and Lauder, I.J. (1975) Pure tone audiometry in older people. *British Journal of Audiology, 9,* 50-58.

Minaker, K.L., Meneilly, G.S., and Rowe, J.W. (1985) Endocrine systems. In C.E. Finch and E.L. Schneider (Eds.), *Handbook of the biology of aging.* Van Nostrand, New York,

pp. 433-458.

Mitchell, C., Phillips, D.S., and Trune, D.R. (1989) Variables affecting the auditory brainstem response: Audiogram, age, gender, and head size. *Hearing Research, 40,* 75-86.

Moller, M.B. (1981) Hearing in 70 and 75 year old people: Results from a cross sectional and longitudinal population study. *American Journal of Otolaryngology, 2,* 22-29.

Moller, M.B. (1983) Changes in hearing measures with increasing age. In R. Hinchcliffe (Ed.), *Hearing and balance in the elderly.* Churchill Livingstone, Edinburgh, pp. 97-122.

Mollica, V. (1969) Acoustic trauma and presbyacusis. *International Audiology, 8,* 305-311.

Moore, B.C.J. and Glasberg, B.R. (1986) The role of frequency selectivity in the perception of loudness, pitch, and time. In B.C.J. Moore (Ed.), *Frequency selectivity in hearing.* Academic Press, New York, pp. 251-308.

Moore, J.K. (1986) Cochlear nuclei: Relationship to auditory nerve. In R.A. Altschuler, R.P. Bobbin, and D.W. Hoffman (Eds.), *Neurobiology of hearing: The cochlea.* Raven, New York, pp. 283-302.

Morest, D.K. and Bohne, B.A. (1983) Noise-induced degeneration in the brain and representation of inner and outer hair cells. *Hearing Research, 9,* 145-151.

Morest, D.K. and Jean-Baptiste, M. (1975) Degeneration and phagocytosis of synaptic endings and axons in the medial trapezoid nucleus of the cat. *Journal of Comparative Neurology, 162,* 135-156.

Moscicki, E.K., Elkins, E.F., Baum, H.M., and McNamara, P. (1985) Hearing loss in the elderly: An epidemiologic study of the Framingham heart study cohort. *Ear and Hearing, 6,* 184-190.

Mountain, D.C. (1980) Changes in endolymph potential and crossed olivocochlear bundle stimulation alter cochlear mechanics. *Science, 210,* 71-72.

Musiek, F.E. and Baran, J. A. (1987) Central auditory assessment: thirty years of challenge and change. *Ear and Hearing, 8,* 22S-35S.

Musiek, F.E., Kibbe, K., Rackliffe, L., and Weider, D.J. (1984) The auditory brain stem response I-V amplitude ratio in normal, cochlear, and retrocochlear ears. *Ear and Hearing, 5,* 52-55.

Nabelek, A.K. (1988) Identification of vowels in quiet, noise, and reverberation: Relationships with age and hearing loss. *Journal of the Acoustical Society of America, 84,* 476-484.

Nabelek, A.K. and Robinson, P.K. (1982) Monaural and binaural speech perception in reverberation for listeners of various ages. *Journal of the Acoustical Society of America, 71,* 1242-1248.

Nadol, J.B., Jr. (1979) Electron microscopic findings in presbycusic degeneration of the basal turn of the human cochlea. *Otolaryngology Head and Neck Surgery, 87,* 818-836.

Nadol, J.B., Jr. (1981) The aging peripheral hearing mechanism. In D.S. Beasley and G.A. Davis (Eds.), *Aging: Communication processes and disorders.* Grune & Stratton, New York, pp. 63-85.

Nadol, J.B., Jr. (1989) Survival of spiral ganglion cells in profound sensorineural hearing loss: Implications for cochlear implantation. *Annals of Otology Rhinology and Laryngology, 98,* 411-416.

Nadol, J.B., Jr. (1990) Degeneration of cochlear neurons as seen in the spiral ganglion of man. *Hearing Research, 49,* 141-154.

Nadol, J.B., Jr., Young, Y.S., and Glynn, R.S. (1989) Survival of spiral ganglion cells in profound sensorineural hearing loss. Implications for cochlear implantation. *Annals of Otology Rhinology and Laryngology 98*, 411-416.

Nager, F.R. and Fraser, J.S. (1938) On bone formation in the scala tympani of otosclerosis. *Journal of Laryngology and Otology, 53*, 173-180.

Nager, G.T. (1966) Sensorineural deafness and otosclerosis. *Annals of Otology Rhinology and Laryngology, 75*, 481-511.

Nager, F.R. (1947) Pathology of the labyrinthine capsule and its clinical significance. In E.P. Fowler (Ed.), *Nelson's loose-leaf medicine of the ear*. Thomas Nelson and Sons, New York (cited in Covell, 1952).

NCHS (U.S. Department of Health, Education and Welfare, National Center for Health Statistics), Rowland, M. (1980) *Basic data on hearing levels of adults, 25-75, U.S., 1971-1975*, USDHEW Publ No. (PHS), 80-1663, Office of Health Research, Statistics, and Technology, Series, 11, No., 215, Hyattsville, MD.

Neff, W.D. (1947) The effects of partial section of the auditory nerve. *Journal of Comparative Neurology, 40*, 203-215.

Nemecek, S., Parizek, J., Spacek, J. (1969) *Folia morphologica* (Warszawa), *17*, 171 (cited in Hansen, 1973).

Nerbonne, M.A., Bliss, A.T., and Schow, R.L. (1978) Acoustic impedance values in the elderly. *Journal of the American Audiological Society, 4*, 57-59.

Newman, C.W. and Spitzer, J.B. (1981) Eustachian tube efficiency of geriatric subjects. *Ear and Hearing, 2*, 103-107.

Nielsen, D.W. and Slepecky, N. (1986) Stereocilia. In R.A. Altschuler, R.P. Bobbin, and D.W. Hoffman (Eds.), *Neurobiology of hearing: The cochlea*. Raven, New York, pp. 23-46.

Nienhuys, T.G.W. and Clark, G.M. (1978) Frequency discrimination following the selective destruction of cochlear inner and outer hair cells. *Science, 199*, 1356-1358.

Nienhuys, T.G.W. and Clark, G.M. (1979) Critical bands following the selective destruction of cochlear inner and outer hair cells. *Acta Oto-Laryngologica, 88*, 350-358.

Nittrouer, S. and Boothroyd, A. (1990) Context effects in phoneme and word recognition by young children and older adults. *Journal of the Acoustical Society of America, 87*, 2705-2715.

Nixon, J., Glorig, A. and High, W. (1962) Changes in air and bone conduction thresholds as a function of age. *Annals of Otology Rhinology and Laryngology, 74*, 288-298.

Noffsinger, P.D. and Kurdziel, S.A. (1979) Assessment of central auditory lesions. In W.F. Rintelmann (Ed.), *Hearing assessment*. University Park, Baltimore, pp. 351-377.

Nomura, Y. (1970) Lipidosis of the basilar membrane. *Acta Oto-Laryngologica, 69*, 352-357.

Nomura, Y. (1976) Nerve fibers in the human organ of corti. *Acta Oto-Laryngologica, 82*, 317-324.

Nomura, Y. and Kirikae, I. (1967) Innervation of the human cochlea. *Annals of Otology Rhinology and Laryngology, 76*, 57-68.

Nomura, Y. and Kirikae, I. (1968) Presbycusis: A histological-histochemical study of the human cochlea. *Acta Oto-Laryngologica, 66*, 17-24.

Nordlund, B. (1964) Directional audiometry. *Acta Oto-Laryngologica, 57*, 1-18.

Novak, R.E. and Anderson, C.V. (1982) Differentiation of types of presbycusis using the masking-level difference. *Journal of Speech and Hearing Research, 25*, 504-508.

Novotny, Z. (1975a) Age factor in auditory fatigue in occupational hearing disorders due to noise. *Ceskoslovenska Otolaryngologie, 24*, 5-9 (cited in Humes, 1984).

Novotny, Z. (1975b) Development of occupational deafness after entering into a noisy job at an advanced age. *Ceskoslovenska Otolaryngologie, 24*, 151-154 (cited in Humes, 1984).

Obler, L.K. and Albert, M.L. (1985) Language skills across adulthood. In J.E. Birren and K.W. Schaie (Eds.), *Handbook of the psychology of aging*. Van Nostrand Reinhold, New York, pp. 463-473.

Olpe, H.R. and Steinmann, M.W. (1982) Age-related decline in the activity of noradrenergic neurons of the rat locus coeruleus. *Brain Research, 251*, 174-176.

Olsen, W.O. and Noffsinger, D. (1974) Comparison of one new and three old tests of auditory adaptation. *Archives of Otolaryngology, 99*, 94-99.

Olsen, W.O., Noffsinger, D., and Carhart, R. (1976) Masking level differences encountered in clinical populations. *Audiology, 15*, 287-301.

Orchik, D.J. and Burgess, J. (1977) Synthetic sentence identification as a function of the age of the listener. *Journal of the American Audiological Society, 3*, 42-46.

Osterhammel, D. and Osterhammel, P. (1979a) Age and sex variations for the normal stapedial reflex thresholds and tympanometric compliance values. *Scandinavian Audiology, 8*, 153-158.

Osterhammel, D. and Osterhammel, P. (1979b) High-frequency audiometry. Age and sex variations. *Scandinavian Audiology, 8*, 73-81.

Ota, C.Y. and Kimura, R.S. (1980) Ultrastructural study of the human spiral ganglion. *Acta Oto-Laryngologica, 89*, 53-62.

Ottaviani, F., Maurizi, M., D'Alatri, L., and Almadori, G.. (1991) Auditory brainstem responses in the aged. *Acta Oto-Laryngologica Supplement 476*, 110-113.

Otte, J., Schuknecht, H.F., and Kerr, A.G. (1978) Ganglion cell populations in normal and pathological human cochleae. Implications for cochlear implantation. *Laryngoscope, 38*, 1231-1246.

Otto, W. and McCandless, G.A. (1982a) Aging and auditory site of lesion. *Ear and Hearing, 3*, 110-117.

Otto, W.C. and McCandless, G.A. (1982b) Aging and the auditory brain stem response. *Audiology, 21*, 466-473.

Oyer, H.J. and Oyer, E.J. (1976) *Aging and communication*. University Park, Baltimore.

Paludetti, G., Maurizi, M., D'Alatri, L., and Galli, J. (1991) Relationships between middle latency auditory responses (MLR) and speech discrimination tests in the elderly. *Acta Oto-Laryngologica Supplement, 476*, 105-109.

Palva, A. and Jokinen, K. (1970) Presbyacusis: V. Filtered speech test. *Acta Oto-Laryngologica, 70*, 232-241.

Papanicolaou, A.C., Loring, D.W., and Eisenberg, H.M. (1984) Age-Related differences in recovery cycle of auditory evoked potentials. *Neurobiology of Aging, 5*, 291-295.

Paparella, M.M., Hanson, D.G., Rao, K.N., and Ulvestad, R. (1975) Genetic sensorineural deafness in adults. *Annals of Otology Rhinology and Laryngology, 84*, 459-472.

Paparella, M.M. (1978) Differential diagnosis of hearing loss. *Laryngoscope, 88*, 952-959.

Parham, K. and Willott, J.F. (1988) Acoustic startle response in young and aging C57BL/6J and CBA/J mice. *Behavioral Neuroscience, 102*, 881-886.

Park, J.C., Cook, K.C., and Verde, E.A. (1990) Dietary restriction slows the abnormally rapid loss of spiral ganglion neurons in C57BL/6 mice. *Hearing Research, 48*, 275-280.

Parnell, M.M. and Amerman, J.D. (1979) Age and the

decoding of coarticulatory cues. *Journal of Speech and Hearing Research, 22,* 433-445.

Parving, A., Ostri, B., Poulsen, J. and Gyntelberg, F. (1983) Epidemiology of hearing impairment in male adult subjects at 49-69 years of age. *Scandinavian Audiology, 12,* 191-196.

Patterson, J.V., Michalewski, H.J., Thompson, L.W., Bowman, T.E. and Litzelman, D.K. (1981) Age and sex differences in the human auditory brainstem response. *Journal of Gerontology, 36,* 455-462.

Patterson, R.D., Nimmo-Smith, I., Weber, D.L., and Milroy, R. (1982) The deterioration of hearing with age: Frequency selectivity, the critical ratio, the audiogram, and speech threshold. *Journal of the Acoustical Society of America, 72,* 1788-1804.

Patuzzi, R.B. and Sellick, P.M. (1983) The alteration of the low frequency response of the primary auditory afferents by cochlear trauma. *Hearing Research, 11,* 125-132.

Patuzzi, R.B., Yates, G.K., and Johnstone, B.M. (1989) Outer hair cell receptor current and sensorineural hearing loss. *Hearing Research, 42,* 47-72.

Pauler, M., Schuknecht, H.F., and Thornton, A.R. (1986) Correlative studies of cochlear neuronal loss with speech discrimination and pure-tone thresholds. *Archives of Oto-Rhino-Laryngology, 243,* 200-206.

Pauler, M., Schuknecht, H.F., and White J.A. (1988) Atrophy of the stria vascularis as a cause of sensorineural hearing loss. *Laryngoscope, 98,* 754-759.

Pedersen, C.B. (1973) Brief tone audiometry in patients with acoustic trauma. *Acta Oto-Laryngologica, 75,* 332-333.

Pedersen, C.B. and Elberling, C. (1973) Temporal integration of acoustic energy in patients with presbycusis. *Acta Oto-Laryngologica, 75,* 32-37.

Pedersen, K.E., Rosenhall, U., and Moller, M.B. (1989) Changes in pure-tone thresholds in individuals aged 70-81: Results from a longitudinal study. *Audiology, 28,* 194-204.

Pestalozza, G. and Shore, J. (1955) Clinical evaluation of presbycusis on the basis of different tests of auditory function. *Laryngoscope, 65,* 1136-1163.

Pestalozza, G., Davis, H., Eldredge, D.H., Covell, W.P., and Rogers, J.B. (1957) Decreased bio-electric potentials in the ears of senile guinea pigs. *Laryngoscope, 67,* 1113-1122.

Peters, A. and Vaughan, D.W. (1981) Central nervous system. In Johnson, J.E. (Ed.), *Aging and cellstructure,* Plenum Press, New York, pp. 1-34..

Peterson, J.L. and Liden, G. (1972) Some static characteristics of the stapedial muscle reflex. *Audiology, 11,* 97-114.

Pfefferbaum, A., Ford, J., Roth, W., Hopkins, III, W.F., and Kopell, B. (1979) Event-related potential changes in healthy aged females. *Electroencephalography and Clinical Neurophysiology, 46,* 81-86.

Pfefferbaum, A., Ford, J., Roth, W., and Kopell, B. (1980a) Age differences in P3-reaction time associations. *Electroencephalography and Clinical Neurophysiology, 49,* 257-265.

Pfefferbaum, A., Ford, J.M., Roth, W.T., and Kopell, B. (1980b) Age related changes in auditory event-related potentials. *Electroencephalography and Clinical Neurophysiology, 49,* 266-276.

Pfefferbaum, A., Wenegrat, B.G., Ford, J., Roth, W., and Kopell, B. (1984) Clinical applications of the P3 component of event-related potentials. II. Dementia, depression, and schizophrenia. *Electroencephalography and Clinical Neurophysiology, 59,* 104-124.

Pfeiffer, R.R. (1966) Classification of response patterns of

spike discharges for units in cochlear nucleus: Tone burst stimulation. *Experimental Brain Research, 1,* 220-235.

Pick, G.F., Evans, E.F., and Wilson, J.P. (1977) Frequency resolution in patients with hearing loss of cochlear origin. In E.F. Evans and J.P. Wilson (Eds.), *Psychophysics and physiology of hearing.* Academic Press, London.

Pickett, J.M., Bergman, M., and Levitt, H. (1979) Aging and speech understanding. In J.M. Ordy and K.R. Brizzee (Eds.), *Sensory systems and communication in the elderly.* Raven Press, New York, pp. 167-186.

Picton, T.W., Stuss, D.T., Champagne, S.C., and Nelson, R.F. (1984) The effects of age on human event-related potentials. *Psychophysiology, 21,* 312-326.

Plath, P. (1991) Speech recognition in the elderly. *Acta Oto-Laryngologica Supplement 476,* 127-130.

Plomp, R. and Mimpen, A.M. (1979) Speech-reception threshold for sentences as a function of age and noise level. *Journal of the Acoustical Society of America, 66,* 1333-1342.

Pokotilenko, A.K. (1965) Patho-histological changes of the internal auditory artery in hypertension. *Vrachebnoe Delo, 7,* 64 (cited in Fisch, 1972).

Polich, J., Howard, L., and Starr, A. (1985) Effects of age on the P300 component of the event-related potential from auditory stimuli: Peak definition, variation, and measurement. *Journal of Gerontology, 40,* 721-726.

Politzer, A. (1926) *Diseases of the ear.* Lea and Febiger, Philadelphia.

Pollak, A., Felix, H., and Schrott, A. (1987) Methodological aspects of quantitative study of spiral ganglion cells. *Acta Oto-Laryngologica, 436,* 37-42.

Pollock, V.E. and Schneider, L.S. (1989) Effects of tone stimulus frequency on late positive component activity (P3) among normal elderly subjects. *International Journal of Neuroscience, 45,* 127-32.

Poon, L.W. (1985) Differences in human memory with aging: Nature, causes, and clinical implication. In J.E. Birren and K.W. Schaie (Eds.), *Handbook of the psychology of aging.* Van Nostrand Reinhold, New York, pp. 427-462.

Popelar, J. and Syka, J. (1982) Noise impairment in the guinea pig. II. Changes of single unit responses in the inferior colliculus. *Hearing Research, 8,* 273-283.

Powell, T.P.S. and Cowan, W.M. (1962) An experimental study of the projection of the cochlea. *Journal of Anatomy, 96,* 269-284.

Powell, T.P.S. and Erulkar, S.D. (1962) Transneuronal cell degeneration in the auditory relay nuclei of the cat. *Journal of Anatomy, 96,* 249-268.

Prazma, J., Carrasco, V.N., Butler, B., Waters, G., Anderson, T., and Pillsbury, H.C. (1990) Cochlear microcirculation in young and old gerbils. *Archives of Otolaryngology Head Neck Surgery, 116,* 932-936.

Price, G.R. (1976) Age as a factor in susceptibility to hearing loss: young versus adult ears. *Journal of the Acoustical Society of America, 60,* 886-891.

Price, P.J. and Simon, H.J. (1984) Perception of temporal differences in speech by "normal-hearing" adults: Effects of age and intensity. *Journal of the Acoustical Society of America, 76,* 405-410.

Prince, J.B. (1982) The relationship between age and auditory temporal processing. *Dissertation Abstracts International, 42,* 3182.

Preibisch-Effenberger, R. (1966) Zur methodik der richtungsaudiometrie: Prufung der schallokalisationsfahigkeit durch elekroakustische verzogerungskette oder messungen im freien schallfeld? *Archiv fuer Ohren,*

Nasen-, und Kehlkopfheilkunde, 187, 588-592 (cited in Konig, 1969).

Proctor, B. (1960) *Chronic progressive deafness.* Wayne State University Press, Detroit.

Proctor, B. (1977) Diagnosis, prevention, and treatment of heredity sensorineural hearing loss. *Laryngoscope, 87,* Supplement 7.

Prosser, S., Turrini, M., and Arslan, E. (1991) Effects of different noises on speech intelligibility in the elderly. *Acta Oto-Laryngologica Supplement 476,* 136-142.

Psatta, D.M. and Matei, M. (1988) Age-dependent amplitude variation of brain-stem auditory evoked potentials. *Electroencephalography and Clinical Neurophysiology, 71,* 27-32.

Pujol, R., Reibillard, G., Puel, J.-L., Lenoir, M., Eybalin, M., and Recasens, M. (1991) Glutamate neurotoxicity in the cochlea: A possible consequence of ischemic or anoxic conditions occurring in aging. *Acta Oto-Laryngologica Supplement, 476,* 32-36.

Punch, J.L. (1978) Masking of spondees by interrupted noise in hearing-impaired listeners. *Journal of the American Audiological Society, 3,* 245-252.

Punch, J.L. and McConnell, F. (1969) The speech discrimination function of elderly adults. *Journal of Auditory Research, 9,* 159-166.

Pyykko, I., Koskimies, K., Strack, J., Pekkarinen, J., and Inaba, R. (1988) Evaluation of factors affecting sensory neural hearing loss. *Acta Oto-Laryngologica Supplement, 449,* 155-158.

Quaranta, A., Amoroso, C. and Cervellera, G. (1978) Remote masking in presbycusis. *Journal of Auditory Research, 18,* 125-129.

Quaranta, A., Cassano, P., and Amoroso, C. (1980) Presbyacousie et reflexometrie stapedienne (Acoustic reflexometry in presbyacusis). *Audiology, 19,* 310-315.

Quaranta, A., Salonna, I., and Longo, G. (1991) Subclinical changes in auditory function in the aged. *Acta Oto-Laryngologica Supplement 476,* 91-96.

Rabbitt, P. (1991) Mild hearing loss can cause apparent memory failures which increase with age and reduce with IQ. *Acta Oto-Laryngologica Supplement 476,* 167-176.

Ramadan, H.H. and Schuknecht, H. F. (1989) Is there as conductive type of presbycusis? *Otolaryngology Head and Neck Surgery, 100,* 30-34.

Randolph, L.J. and Schow, R.L. (1983) Threshold inaccuracies in an elderly clinical population: Ear canal collapse as a possible cause. *Journal of Speech and Hearing Research, 26,* 54-58.

Rasmussen, A.T. (1940) Studies of the VIIIth cranial nerve of man. *Laryngoscope, 50,* 67-83.

Rastatter, M., Watson, M., and Strauss-Simmons, D. (1989) Effects of time-compression on feature and frequency discrimination in aged listeners. *Perceptual and Motor Skills, 68,* 367-372.

Rawool, V.W. (1989) Speech recognition scores and ABR in cochlear impairment. *Scandinavian Audiology, 18,* 113-117.

Reed, G.F. (1960) An audiometric study of two hundred cases of subjective tinnitus. *Archives of Otolaryngology, 71,* 84-94.

Reff, M.E. (1985) RNA and protein metabolism. In C.E. Finch and E.L. Schneider (Eds.), *Handbook of the biology of aging.* Van Nostrand, New York, pp. 225-254.

Rintelmann, W.F. and Schumaier, D. (1974) Five experiments on speech discrimination utilizing CNC monosyllables (N.U. Auditory Test No. 6). Experiment III: Factors affecting speech discrimination in a clinical setting: List

equivalence, hearing loss, and phonemic regression. *Journal of Auditory Research Supplement, 2,* 12-15.

Rittmanic, P.A. (1962) Pure-tone masking by narrow-noise bands in normal and impaired ears. *Journal of Auditory Research, 2,* 287-304.

Robertson, D. (1983) Functional significance of dendritic swelling after loud sounds in the guinea pig cochlea. *Hearing Research, 9,* 263-278.

Robertson, D. and Johnstone, B.M. (1979) Aberrant tonotopic organization in the inner ear damaged by kanamycin. *Journal of the Acoustical Society of America, 66,* 466-469.

Robinson, D.W. and Sutton, G.J. (1979) Age effect in hearing: A comparative analysis of published threshold data. *Audiology, 18,* 320-334.

Rodriguez, G.P., DiSarno, N.J., and Hardiman, C.J. (1990) Central auditory processing in normal-hearing elderly adults. *Audiology, 29,* 85-92.

Rogers, J. and Bloom, F.E. (1985) Neurotransmitter metabolism and function in the aging central nervous system. In C.E. Finch and E.L. Schneider (Eds.), *Handbook of the biology of aging.* Van Nostrand, New York, pp. 645-691.

Rogers, J., Silver, M.A., Shoemaker, W.J., and Bloom, F.E. (1980) Senescent changes in a neurobiological model system: Cerebellar Purkynje cell electrophysiology and correlative anatomy. *Neurobiology of Aging, 1,* 3-11.

Roosa, D.B. St. J. (1885) Presbykousis. *American Otological Society Transactions, 3,* 449-460 (cited in Hawkins and Johnsson, 1985).

Rosen, J.K. (1979) Psychological and social aspects of the evaluation of acquired hearing impairment. *Audiology, 18,* 238-252.

Rosen, S. (1966) Hearing studies in selected urban and rural populations. *New York Academy of Science Transactions, 29,* 9-21.

Rosen, S., Bergman, M., Plester, D., El-Mofty, A., and Satti, M.H. (1962) Presbycusis study of a relatively noise-free population in the Sudan. *Annals of Otology Rhinology and Laryngology, 71,* 727-743.

Rosen, S. and Olin, P. (1965) Hearing loss and coronary heart disease. *Archives of Otolaryngology, 82,* 236-243.

Rosen, S., Plester, D., El-Mofty, A., and Rosen, H.V. (1964) High frequency audiometry in presbycusis: A comparative study of the Mabaan tribe in the Sudan with urban populations. *Archives of Otolaryngology, 79,* 18-32.

Rosen, S., Preobrajensky, N., Khechinashvili, S., Glazunov, I., Kipshidze, N., and Rosen, H.V. (1970) Epidemiologic hearing studies in the USSR. *Archives of Otolaryngology, 91,* 424-428.

Rosen, S.M. and Fourcin, A. (1986) Frequency selectivity and the perception of speech. In B.C.J. Moore (Ed.), *Frequency selectivity in hearing.* Academic Press, New York, pp. 373-487.

Rosenhall, U. (1985) The influence of hearing loss on directional hearing. *Scandinavian Audiology, 14,* 187-189.

Rosenhall, U., Bjorkman, G., Pedersen, K., and Kall, A. (1985) Brain-stem auditory evoked potentials in different age groups. *Electroencephalography and Clinical Neurophysiology, 62,* 426-430.

Rosenhall, U., Pedersen, K., and Dotevall, M. (1986) Effects of presbycusis and other types of hearing loss on auditory brainstem responses. *Scandinavian Audiology, 15,* 179-185.

Rosenhamer, H.J., Lindstrom, B., and Lundborg, T. (1980) On the use of click-evoked electric brainstem responses in audiological diagnosis. II. The influence of sex and age upon the normal response. *Scandinavian Audiology, 9*, 93-100.

Rosenwasser, H. (1964) Otitic problems in the aged. *Geriatrics, 19*, 11-17.

Ross, M., Huntington, D.A., Newby, H.A., and Dixon, R.F. (1965) Speech discrimination of hearing-impaired individuals in noise. *Journal of Auditory Research, 5*, 47-72.

Rowe, M.J., III. (1978) Normal variability of the brain-stem auditory evoked response in young and old adult subjects. *Electroencephalography and Clinical Neurophysiology, 44*, 459-470.

Rowe, M.J., III. (1981) The brainstem auditory evoked response in neurological disease: A review. *Ear and Hearing, 2*, 41-51.

Royster, L.H., Driscoll, D.P., Thomas, W.G., and Royster, J.D. (1980) Age effect hearing levels for a black non industrial-noise-exposed population (ninep.). *American Industrial Hygene Association Journal, 41*, 113 (cited in Erlandsson et al., 1982).

Rubinstein, M., Hildesheimer, M. Zohar, S. and Chilarovitz, T. (1977) Chronic cardiovascular pathology and hearing loss in the aged. *Gerontology, 23*, 4-9.

Ruah, C.B., Schachern, P.A., and Paparella, M.M. (1991) The development and change of the normal human tympanic membrane with age. *Association for Research in Otolaryngology Abstracts, 14*, 54.

Ruedi, L. (1965) Histopathologic confirmation of labyrynthine otosclerosis. *Laryngoscope, 75*, 1582-1609.

Ruedi, L. and Spoendlin, H. (1966) Pathogenesis of sensorineural deafness in otosclerosis. *Annals of Otology Rhinology and Laryngology, 75*, 525-552.

Rupp, R.R. (1970) Understanding the problems of presbycusis. *Geriatrics, 25*, 100-107.

Ryals, B.M. and Westbrook, E.W. (1988) Ganglion cell and hair cell loss in Coturnix quail associated with aging. *Hearing Research, 36*, 1-8.

Ryan, A.F., Axelsson, A., Myers, R., and Woolf, N.K. (1988) Changes in cochlear blood flow during acoustic stimulation as determined by 14C-iodoantipyrine autoradiography. *Acta Oto-Laryngologica, 105*, 232-241.

Ryan, J.N. (1989) *Middle latency auditory evoked potentials as a function of age.* Doctoral dissertation, University of Texas at Dallas.

Rybak, L.P. (1986) Ototoxic mechanisms. In R.A. Altschuler, R.P. Bobbin, and D.W. Hoffman (Eds.), *Neurobiology of hearing: The cochlea.* Raven, New York, pp. 441-454.

Salomon, G. (1991) Hearing in the aged. *Acta Oto-Laryngologica Supplement, 476.*

Salthouse, T.A. (1985) Speed of behavior and its implications for cognition. In J.E. Birren and K.W. Schaie (Eds.), *Handbook of the psychology of aging.* Van Nostrand Reinhold, New York, pp. 400-426.

Salvi, R.J., Hamernik, R.P., and Henderson, D. (1978) Discharge patterns in the cochlear nucleus of the chinchilla following noise induced asymptotic threshold shift. *Experimental Brain Research, 32*, 301-320.

Salvi, R.J., Henderson, D., and Hamernik, R.P. (1979) Single auditory nerve fiber and action potential latencies in normal and noise-treated chinchillas. *Hearing Research, 1*, 237-251.

Salvi, R., Henderson, D., Hamernik, R.P., and Parkins, C. (1980) VIII Nerve response to click stimuli in normal and pathological cochleas. *Hearing Research, 2*, 335-342.

Sandridge, S. (1988) *The event-related potential "P3"; A central auditory test for the older adult?* Doctoral dissertation, University of Florida.

Santi, P.A. Ruggero, M.A., Nelson, D.A., and Turner, C.W. (1982) Kanamycin and bumetanide ototoxicity: Anatomical, physiological and behavioral correlates. *Hearing Research, 7*, 261-279.

Sataloff, J., Farb, S., Menduke, H., and Vassallo, L. (1964) Sensorineural hearing loss in otosclerosis. *American Academy of Opthalmology and Otolaryngology Transactions, 68*, 243-250.

Sataloff, J. and Vassallo, L. (1966) Hard-of-hearing senior citizens and the physician. *Geriatrics, 21*, 182-185.

Sataloff, J., Vassallo, L., and Menduke, H. (1965) Air and bone conduction thresholds. *Laryngoscope, 75*, 889-901.

Saunders, J.C. and Hirsch, K.A. (1976) Changes in cochlear microphonic sensitivity after priming C57BL/6J mice at various ages for audiogenic seizures. *Journal of Comparative and Physiological Psychology, 90*, 212-220.

Saxen, A. (1952) Inner ear in presbyacusis. *Acta Oto-Laryngologica, 41*, 213-237.

Scheibel, M.E., Lindsay, R.D., Tomiyasu, U., and Scheibel, A.B. (1975) Progressive dendritic changes in aging human cortex. *Experimental Neurology, 47*, 392-403.

Schmiedt, R.A., Hellstrom, L.I., and Lee, F.S. (1990) Comparisons of compound action potential thresholds and endocochlear potentials in aged gerbils. *Association for Research in Otolaryngology Abstracts, 13*, 150.

Schmiedt, R.A. and Mills, J.H. (1991) Spontaneous rates of auditory-nerve fibers in quiet-and noise-aged gerbils. *Association for Research in Otolaryngology Abstracts, 14*, 80.

Schmiedt, R.A., Mills, J.H., and Adams, J.C. (1987) Endocochlear potentials decrease with age in gerbils. *Society for Neuroscience Abstracts, 13*, 1260.

Schmiedt, R.A., Mills, J.H., and Adams, J.C. (1989) Auditory nerve fiber activity in aged gerbils raised in quiet or in noise. *Association for Research in Otolaryngology Abstracts, 12*, 41-42.

Schmiedt, R.A., Mills, J.H., and Adams, J.C. (1990) Tuning and suppression in auditory nerve fibers of aged gerbils raised in quiet or noise. *Hearing Research, 45*, 221-236.

Schmiedt, R.A., Zwislocki, J.J., and Hamernik, R.P. (1980) Effects of hair cell lesions on responses of cochlear nerve fibers. I. Lesions, tuning curves, two-tone inhibition, and responses to trapezoidal-wave patterns. *Journal of Neurophysiology, 43*, 1367-1389.

Schmiedt, R.A. and Zwislocki, J.J. (1980) Effects of hair cell lesions on responses of cochlear nerve fibers. II. Single- and two-tone intensity functions in relation to tuning curves. *Journal of Neurophysiology, 43*, 1390-1405.

Schmidt, P.H. (1969) Presbyacusis and noise. *International Audiology, 8*, 278-280.

Schmitt, J.F. (1981) Sentence comprehension in elderly listeners: The factor of rate. *Journal of Gerontology, 36*, 441-445.

Schmitt, J. F. (1983) The effects of time compression and time expansion on passage comprehension by elderly listeners. *Journal of Speech and Hearing Research, 26*, 373-377.

Schmitt, J.F. and Carroll, M. R. (1985) Older listeners' ability to comprehend speaker-generated rate alteration of passages. *Journal of Speech and Hearing Research, 28*, 309-312.

Schon, T.D. (1970) The effects on speech intelligibility of time-compression and-expansion on normal-hearing, hard of hearing, and aged males. *Journal of Auditory Research, 10*, 263-268.

Schorn, K. and Zwicker, E. (1990) Frequency selectivity and temporal resolution in patients with various inner ear disorders. *Audiology, 29*, 8-20.

Schow, R.L., Christensen, J.M., Hutchinson, J.M., and Nerbonne, M.A. (1978) *Communication disorders of the aged.* University Press, Baltimore.

Schow, R.L. and Goldbaum, D.E. (1980) Collapsed ear canals in the elderly nursing home population. *Journal of Speech and Hearing Disorders, 45*, 259-267.

Schow, R.L. and Nerbonne, M.A. (1980) Hearing levels among elderly nursing home residents. *Journal of Speech and Hearing Disorders, 45*, 124-132.

Schuknecht, H.F. (1953) Lesions of the organ of Corti. *American Academy of Otolaryngology Transactions, 57*, 366-383.

Schuknecht, H.F. (1955) Presbycusis. *Laryngoscope, 65*, 407-419.

Schuknecht, H.F. (1964) Further Observations on the pathology of presbycusis. *Archives of Otolaryngology, 80*, 369-382.

Schuknecht, H. (1967) The effect of aging on the cochlea. In A.B. Graham (Ed.), *Sensorineural hearing processes and disorders.* Little Brown, Boston, pp. 393-401.

Schuknecht, H.F. (1974) *Pathology of the ear.* Harvard University Press, Cambridge.

Schuknecht, H.F. (1989) Pathology of presbycusis. In J.C. Goldstein, H.K. Kashima, and C.F. Koopmann (Eds.), *Geriatric otolaryngology.* B.C. Decker, Inc., Toronto, pp. 40-44.

Schuknecht, H.F. and Gross, C.W. (1966) Otosclerosis and the inner ear. *Annals of Otology Rhinology and Laryngology, 75*, 423-435.

Schuknecht, H.F. and Igarashi, M. (1964) Pathology of slowly progressive sensori-neural deafness. *Otolaryngology, 68*, 222-242.

Schuknecht, H.F., Watanuki, K., Takahashi, T., Belal, A., Kimura, R.S., Jones, D.D., and Ota, C.Y. (1974) Atrophy of the stria vascularis, a common cause for hearing loss. *Laryngoscope, 84*, 1777-1821.

Schuknecht, H. and Woellner, R. (1953) Hearing losses following partial section of the cochlear nerve. *Laryngoscope, 63*, 441-465.

Schulte, B.A. and Adams, J.C. (1989) Degeneration of the stria vascularis and stromal cells in the spiral ligament of aging gerbils as assessed by loss of Na+,K+ ATPase immunoreactivity. *Association for Research in Otolaryngology Abstracts, 12*, 47.

Schum, D.J. and Matthews, L.J. (1990) SPIN test performance of elderly, hearing-impaired listeners. *Association for Research in Otolaryngology Abstracts, 13*, 183-184.

Sercer, A. and Krmpotic, J. (1958) Uber die ursache der porgressiven altersschwerhorigkeit. *Acta Oto-Laryngologica, 143*, 6-36 (cited in Proctor, 1960).

Shadden, B.B. (1988) *Communication behavior and aging: A sourcebook for clinicians.* Williams and Wilkins, Baltimore.

Shambaugh, G.E. (1989) Zinc: The neglected nutrient. *American Journal of Otology, 10*, 156-160.

Shanon, E., Gold, S., and Himelfarb, M. (1981) Assessment of functional integrity of brain stem auditory pathways by stimulus stress. *Audiology, 20*, 65-71.

Shapiro, A.M., Strominger, R.N., Arbabzadeh, H., Cacace, A.T., Parnes, S.M., and Strominger, N.L. (1990) Age-related temporary threshold shifts and cochlear microphonic alterations after calcitonin infusion in a macaque monkey model. *Society for Neuroscience Abstracts, 16*, 876.

Shapiro, M.J., Purn, J.M., and Raskin, C. (1981) A study of the effects of cardiopulmonary bypass surgery on auditory function. *Laryngoscope, 91*, 2046-2052.

Sheldon, J.H. (1948) *The social medicine of old age.* Oxford University Press, London.

Shirane, M. and Harrison, R.V. (1987) The effects of deferoxamine mesylate and hypoxia on the cochlea. *Acta Oto-Laryngologica, 104*, 99-107.

Shirinian, M.J. and Arnst, D.J. (1982) Patterns in the performance-intensity functions for phonetically balanced word lists and synthetic sentences in aged listeners. *Annals of Otology Rhinology and Laryngology, 108*, 15-20.

Shone, G., Miller, J.M., Nuttall, A.L., and Altshuler, R.A. (1991) Noise induced cochlear sensitivity change in the aged mice. *Association for Research in Otolaryngology Abstracts, 14*, 27.

Shubert, K. (1958) *Sprachhorprufmethoden. Grundlagen, wurdigung und anwendung bei betutachtung und horgerateanpassung.* Thieme, Stuttgart (cited in Bergman, 1971).

Sidman, J.D., Prazma, J., Pulver, S.H., and Pillsbury, H.C. (1988) Cochlea and heart as end-organs in small vessel disease. *Annals of Otology Rhinology and Laryngology, 97*, 9-13.

Siegel, J.H. and Kim, D.O. (1982) Efferent neural control of cochlear mechanics? Olivocochlear bundle stimulation affects cochlear biomechanics nonlinearity. *Hearing Research, 6*, 171-182.

Siegel, J.H., Kim, D.O., and Molnar, C.E. (1982) Effects of altering organ of corti on cochlear distortion products f2-f1 and 2f1 f2. *Journal of Neurophysiology, 47*, 303-327.

Sillman, J.S., LaRouere, M.J., Nuttall, A.L., Lawrence, M., and Miller, J.M. (1988) Recent advances in cochlear blood flow measurements. *Annals of Otology Rhinology and Laryngology, 97*, 1-8.

Silman, S. (1979a) The effects of aging on the stapedius reflex thresholds. *Journal of the Acoustical Society of America, 66*, 735-738.

Silman, S. (1979b) The acoustic reflex, aging, and the distortion product: A reply to Jerger. *Journal of the Acoustical Society of America, 66*, 909-910.

Silman, S. and Gelfand, S.A. (1979) Prediction of hearing levels from acoustic reflex thresholds in persons with high-frequency hearing losses. *Journal of Speech and Hearing Research, 22*, 697-707.

Silman, S. and Gelfand, S.A. (1981) Effect of sensorineural hearing loss on the stapedius reflex growth function in the elderly. *Journal of the Acoustical Society of America, 69*, 1099-1106.

Silman, S., Popelka, G.R., and Gelfand, S.A. (1978) The effect of sensori-neural hearing loss on acoustic stapedius reflex growth functions. *Journal of the Acoustical Society of America, 64*, 1406-1411.

Silverman, C.A., Silman, S., and Miller, M.H. (1983) The acoustic reflex threshold in aging ears. *Journal of the Acoustical Society of America, 73*, 248-255.

Simpson, G.V., Knight, R.T., Brailowsky, S., Prospero-Garcia, O., and Scabini, D. (1985) Altered peripheral and brainstem auditory function in aged rats. *Brain Research, 348*, 28-35.

Sjostrom, B. and Anniko, M. (1990) Variability in genetically induced age-related impairment of auditory brainstem response thresholds. *Acta Oto-Laryngologica, 109*, 353-360.

Smith, R.A. (1969) A study of phoneme discrimination in older versus younger subjects as a function of various listening conditions. *Dissertation Abstracts International, 30*, 2456.

Smith, R.A. and Prather, W.F. (1971) Phoneme discrimination in older persons under varying signal-to-noise conditions. *Journal of Speech and Hearing Research, 14*, 630-638.

Smits, J.T.S. and Duifhus, H. (1982) Masking and partial masking in listeners with a high-frequency hearing loss. *Audiology, 21*, 310-324.

Sohmer, H., Freeman, S., and Schmuel, M. (1989) ABR threshold is a function of blood oxygen level. *Hearing Research, 40*, 87-91.

Soucek, S. and Mason, S.M. (1990) Investigation of stimulus rate effects in the elderly using non-invasive electrocochleography and auditory brainstem response. *Association for Research in Otolaryngology Abstracts, 13*, 218.

Soucek, S. and Michaels, L. (1991) Hearing loss in the elderly: An audiometric study, with special reference to the significance of intra-and extracochlear factors. *Association for Research in Otolaryngology Abstracts, 14*, 102.

Soucek, S., Michaels, L., and Frohlich, A. (1987) Pathological changes in the organ of Corti in presbycusis as revealed by microslicing and staining. *Acta Oto-Laryngologica Supplement, 436*, 93-102.

Soucek, S., Michaels, L., and Mason, S.M. (1988) Old age hearing loss: An endogenous disorder of cochlear hair cells. *Association for Research in Otolaryngology Abstracts, 11*, 120.

Spencer, J.T. (1973) Hyperlipoproteinemias in the etiology of inner ear disease. *Laryngoscope, 83*, 639-678.

Spilich, G.J. (1985) Discourse comprehension across the lifespan. In N. Charness (Ed.), *Aging and human performance*. Wiley, New York, pp. 143-190.

Spoendlin, H. (1970) Changes due to aging. In A. Bischoff (Ed.), *Ultrastructure of the peripheral nervous system and sense organs*. Thieme, Stuttgart, pp. 260-261.

Spoendlin, H. (1971) Primary structural changes in the organ of Corti after acoustic overstimulation. *Acta Oto-Laryngologica, 71*, 166-176.

Spoendlin, H. (1984) Factors inducing retrograde degeneration of the cochlear nerve. *Annals of Otology Rhinology and Laryngology Supplement 112*, 76-82.

Spoendlin, H. and Gacek, R.R. (1963) Electronmicroscopic study of the efferent and afferent innervation of the organ of Corti in the cat. *Annals of Otology Rhinology and Laryngology, 72*, 660-686.

Spoendlin, H. and Schrott, A. (1989) Analysis of the human auditory nerve. *Hearing Research, 43*, 25-38.

Spoendlin, H. and Schrott, A. (1990) Quantitative evaluation of the human cochlear nerve. *Acta Oto-Laryngologica Supplement, 470*, 61-70.

Spoor, A. (1967) Presbycusis values in relation to noise induced hearing loss. *International Audiology, 6*, 48-57.

Squires, K.C. and Hecox, K.E. (1983) Electrophysiological evaluation of higher level auditory processing. *Seminars in Hearing, 4*, 415-433.

Stach, B.A. (1987) The acoustic reflex in diagnostic audiology from Metz to present. *Ear and Hearing, 8*, 36S-42S.

Stach, B.A., Jerger, J.F., and Fleming, K.A. (1985) Central presbycusis: A longitudinal case study. *Ear and Hearing, 6*, 304-306.

Steel, K., Niaussat, M.M., and Bock, G.R. (1983) The genetics of hearing. In J.F. Willott (Ed.), *Auditory psychobiology of the mouse*. Charles Thomas, Springfield, Illinois, pp. 341-394.

Stelmachowicz, P.G., Beauchaine, K.A., Kalberer, A., and Jesteadt, W. (1989) Normative thresholds in the 8-to 20-kHz range as a function of age. *Journal of the Acoustical Society of America, 86*, 1384-1391.

Stephens, S.D.G. and Hinchcliffe, R. (1968) Studies on temporary threshold drift. *International Audiology, 7*, 267-279.

Steurer, O. (1926) Degenerative und verwandte prozesse des innerven ohres. In Henke and Lubarsch (Eds.), *Handbuch der speziellen pathologischen anatomie und histologie*. Springer-Verlag, Berlin (cited in Jorgensen, 1961).

Stevenson, P.W. (1975) Responses to speech audiometry and phonemic discrimination patterns in the elderly. *Audiology, 14*, 185-231.

Sticht, T.G. and Gray, B.B. (1969) The intelligibility of time compressed words as a function of hearing loss. *Journal of Speech and Hearing Research, 12*, 443-448.

Stover, L. and Norton, S.J. (1990) Age associated changes in cochlear mechanics. *Association for Research in Otolaryngology Abstracts, 13*, 235.

Stucker, N. (1908) Uber die unterschiedsempfindlichkeit fur tonhohen in verschiedenen tonregionen. *Sinnesphysiologie, 42*, 392-408 (cited in Konig, 1969).

Sturzebecher, E., Kevanishvili, Z., Werbs, M., Meyer, E., and Schmidt, D. (1985) Interpeak intervals of auditory brainstem response, interaural differences in normal-hearing subjects and patients with sensorineural hearing loss. *Scandinavian Audiology, 14*, 83-87.

Sturzebecher, E. and Werbs, M. (1987) Effects of age and sex on auditory brain stem response. *Scandinavian Audiology, 16*, 153-157.

Sturzebecher, E. and Werbs, M. (1988) Influence of age, sex, and hearing loss on auditory brain stem response (ABR) latencies. *Scandinavian Audiology, 17*, 248-250.

Suga, F. and Lindsay, J.R. (1976) Histopathological observations of presbycusis. *Annals of Otology Rhinology and Laryngology, 85*, 169-184.

Suga, N. (1990) Subsystems for processing different types of auditory information: Speculations on speech-sound processing. *Association for Research in Otolaryngology Abstracts, 13*, 111-112.

Surr, R.K. (1977) Effect of age on clinical hearing aid evaluation results. *Journal of the American Audiological Society, 3*, 1-5.

Susmano, A. and Rosenbush, S.W. (1988) Hearing loss and ischemic heart disease. *American Journal of Otology, 9*, 403-408.

Suzuka, Y. and Schuknecht, H.F. (1988) Retrograde cochlear neuronal degeneration in human subjects. *Acta Oto-Laryngologica Supplement 450*.

Sweet, R.J., Price, J.M. and Henry, K.R. (1988) Dietary restriction and presbyacusis: Periods of restriction and auditory threshold losses in the CBA/J mouse. *Audiology, 27*, 305-312.

Sweitzer, R.S. (1964) *A comparison of acoustic impedance of young and aged subjects*. Master's thesis, State University of Iowa.

Syndulko, K., Hansch, E.C., Cohen, S.N., Pearce, J.W., Goldberg, Z., Monton, B., Tourtellotte, W.W., and Potvin, A.R. (1982) Long-latency event-related potentials in normal aging and dementia. In J. Courjon, F. Mauguiere, and M. Revol (Eds.), *Clinical applications of evoked potentials in neurology*. Raven, New York, pp. 279-285.

Takahashi, T. (1971) The ultrastructure of the pathologic stria vascularis and spiral prominence in man. *Annals of Otology Rhinology and Laryngology, 80*, 721-735.

Takahashi, T. and Kimura, R.S. (1970) The ultrastructure of the spiral ligament of the rhesus monkey. *Acta Oto-Laryngologica, 69*, 46-60.

Talland, G.A. (1968) *Human aging and behavior*. Academic Press, New York.

Tamir, L.M. (1979) *Communication and the aging process*. Pergamon, New York.

Terracol, J., Corone, A., and Guerrier, Y. (1949) *La trompe d'eustache*. Masson et Cie, Editeurs, Paris (cited in Covell, 1952).

Thalmann, R., Miyoshi, T., and Thalmann, I. (1972) The influence of ischemia upon the energy reserves of inner ear tissues. *Laryngoscope, 82*, 2249-2272.

Theopold, H.M. (1975) Degenerative alterations in the ventral cochlear nucleus of the guinea pig after impulse noise exposure: A preliminary light and electron microscopic study. *Archives of Oto-Rhino-Laryngology, 209*, 247-262.

Thompson, D.J., Sills, J.A., Recke, K.S., and Bui, D.M. (1979) Acoustic admittance and the aging ear. *Journal of Speech and Hearing Research, 22*, 29-36.

Thompson, D.J., Sills, J.A., Recke, K.S. and Bui, D.M. (1980) Acoustic reflex growth in the aging adult. *Journal of Speech and Hearing Research, 23*, 405-418.

Thomsen, J., Terkildsen, K., and Osterhammel, P. (1978) Auditory brainstem responses in patients with acoustic neuromas. *Scandinavian Audiology, 7*, 179-183.

Tice, R.R. and Setlow, R.B. (1985) DNA repair and replication in aging organisms and cells. In C.E. Finch and E.L. Schneider (Eds.), *Handbook of the biology of aging*. Van Nostrand, New York, pp. 173-224.

Tillman, T.W., Carhart, R., and Nicholls, S. (1973) Release from multiple maskers in elderly persons. *Journal of Speech and Hearing Research, 16*, 152-160.

Tillman, T.W., Carhart, R., and Olsen, W.O. (1970) Hearing aid efficiency in a competing speech situation. *Journal of Speech and Hearing Research, 13*, 789-811.

Tonndorf, J. (1976) Relationship between the transmission characteristics of the conductive system and noise-induced hearing loss. In D. Henderson, R.P. Hamernik, D.S. Dosanjh, and J.H. Mills (Eds.), *Effects of noise on hearing*. Raven Press, New York, pp. 159-178.

Townsend, T.H. and Bess, F.H. (1980) Effects of age and sensorineural hearing loss on word recognition. *Scandinavian Audiology, 9*, 245-248.

Toyoda, K. and Yoshisuke, G. (1969) Speech discrimination in presbyacusis. *International Audiology, 12*, 135-139.

Tsai, H.-K., Fong-Shyong, C., and Tsa-Jung, C. (1958) On changes in ear size with age, as found among Taiwanese-Formosans of Fulienese extraction. *Journal of the Formosan Medical Association, 57*, 105-111 (cited in Maurer and Rupp, 1979).

Turner, C.W. and Nelson, D.A. (1982) Frequency discrimination in regions of normal and impaired sensitivity. *Journal of Speech and Hearing Research, 25*, 34-41.

Turnock, M.T. and Harrison, J.M. (1975) Effects of age on hearing in rats. *Journal of the Acoustical Society of America Supplement 1, 58*, S90.

Tyler, R.S. (1986) Frequency resolution in hearing-impaired listeners. In B.C.J Moore (Ed.), *Frequency selectivity in hearing*. Academic Press, New York, pp. 309-372.

Tyler, R.S., Fernandes, M.A., and Wood, E.J. (1982) Masking of pure tones by broad-band noise in cochlear-impaired listeners. *Journal of Speech and Hearing Research, 25*, 117-124.

Ulehlova, L. (1975) Ageing and the loss of neuroepithelium in the guinea pig. *Advances in Experimental Medicine and Biology, 53*, 257-264.

U.S. National Health Survey *Hearing status and ear examination. Findings among adults, 1960-1962 Vital and Health Statistics*. Series 11, Number, 32, U.S. Department of Health, Education, and Welfare, Washington, D.C.

Uziel, A., Baldy-Moulinier, M., Marot, M., Abboudi, C., and Passouant, P. (1980) Les potentiels evoques auditifs du tronc cerebral chez le sujet age. Correlation avec l'E.E.G. *Revue d'Electroencephalographie et de Neurophysiologie Clinique, 10*, 153-160.

Van Heusden, E. and Smoorenburg, G.F. (1983) Responses from AVCN units in the cat before and after inducement of acute noise trauma. *Hearing Research, 11*, 295-326.

van Rooij, J.C.G.M. and Plomp, R. (1990) Auditive and cognitive factors in speech perception by elderly listeners. II. Mulitvariate analyses. *Journal of the Acoustical Society of America, 88*, 2611-2624.

Van Rooij, J.C.G.M. and Plomp, R. (1991) Auditive and cognitive factors in speech perception by elderly listeners. *Acta Oto-Laryngologica Supplement 476*, 177-181.

Van Rooij, J.C.G.M., Plomp, R., and Orlebeke, J.F. (1989) Auditive and cognitive factors in speech perception by elderly listeners. I. Development of a test battery. *Journal of the Acoustical Society of America, 86*, 1294-1309.

Vaughan, D.W, and Peters, A. (1974) Neuroglial cells in the cerebral cortex of rats from young adulthood to old age: an electron microscope study. *Journal of Neurocytology, 3*, 405-429.

Vaughan, D.W. (1977) Age-related deterioration of pyramidal cell basal dendrites in rat auditory cortex. *Journal of Comparative Neurology, 171*, 501-515.

Ventry, I.M., Chaiklin, J.B., and Boyle, W.F. (1961) Collapse of the ear canal during audiometry. *Archives of Otolaryngology, 73*, 727-731.

Vertes, D., Nilsson, P., Wersall, J., Axelsson, A., and Bjorkroth, B. (1982) Cochlear hair cell and vascular changes in the guinea pig following high level pure-tone exposures. *Acta Oto-Laryngologica, 94*, 403-411.

Vestal, R.E. and Dawson, G.W. (1985) Pharmacology and aging. In C.E. Finch and E.L. Schneider (Eds.), *Handbook of the biology of aging*. Van Nostrand, New York, pp. 744-819.

Walsh, E.J. and McGee, J. (1986) The development of function in the auditory periphery. In R.A. Altschuler, R.P. Bobbin, and D.W. Hoffman (Eds.), *Neurobiology of hearing: The cochlea*. Raven, New York, pp. 247-270.

Walton, J.P., Meierhans, L.R., Farcich, K.J., and Frisina, R.D. (1991) Recovery of forward masking in a young and middle-aged mouse model of presbycusis. *Association for Research in Otolaryngology Abstracts, 14*, 25.

Wang, S.Y. (1990) [Changes in hearing threshold in the elderly] *Chung Hua Ko Tsa Chih, 25*, 6-8 (Medline abstract).

Ward, W.D. (1976) A comparison of the effects of continuous, intermittent, and impulse noise. In D. Henderson, R.P. Hamernik, D.S. Dosanjh, and J.H. Mills (Eds.), *Effects of noise on hearing*. Raven Press, New York, pp. 407-420.

Ward, W.D. and Duvall, A.J. (1971) Behavioral and ultrastructural correlates of acoustic trauma. *Annals of Otology Rhinology and Laryngology, 80*, 881-896.

Warr, W.B., Guinan, J.J., and White, J.S. (1986) Organization of the efferent fibers: The lateral and medial olivocochlear systems. In R.A. Altschuler, R.P. Bobbin, and D.W. Hoffman (Eds.), *Neurobiology of hearing: The cochlea*. Raven, New York, pp. 333-348.

Warren, L.R., Wagener, J.W., and Herman, G.E. (1978) Binaural analysis in the aging auditory system. *Journal of*

Gerontology, 33, 731-736.

Waudby, C. (1984) Hearing threshold levels according to age. *British Journal of Audiology, 18,* 55-57.

Wedel, H. von (1979) Differences in brainstem response with age and sex. *Scandinavian Audiology Supplement 9,* 205-209.

Wedel, H. von, von Wedel, U.-Ch., and Streppel, M. (1991) Selective hearing in the aged with regard to speech perception in quiet and in noise. *Acta Oto-Laryngologica Supplement, 476,* 131-135.

Wedel, H. von, von Wedel, U.-Ch., and Zorowka, P. (1991) Tinnitus diagnosis and therapy in the aged. *Acta Oto-Laryngologica Supplement 476,* 195-201.

Welleschik, B. and Raber, A. (1978) Einfluss von expositionzeit und alter auf den iarmbedingten horverlust. *Laryngologie Rhinologie Otologie, 57,* 1037-1048 (cited in Humes, 1984).

Welsh, L.W., Welsh, J.J., and Healy, M.P. (1985) Central presbycusis. *Laryngoscope, 95,* 128-136.

Wenngren, B. and Anniko, M. (1988a) A frequency-specific auditory brainstem response technique exemplified in the determination of age-related auditory thresholds. *Acta Oto-Laryngologica, 106,* 238-243.

Wenngren, B. and Anniko, M. (1988b) Age-related auditory brainstem response (ABR) threshold changes in the dancer mouse mutant. *Acta Oto-Laryngologica, 106,* 386-392.

Weston, T.E.T. (1964) Presbycusis: A clinical study. *Journal of Laryngology and Otology, 78,* 273-286.

Wever, E.G. and Bray, C.W. (1930) Present possibilities for auditory theory. *Psychological Review, 37,* 365-380.

WGSUA (Working Group on Speech Understanding and Aging of the Committee on Hearing, Bioacoustics, and Biomechanics, Commission on Behavioral and Social Sciences and Education, National Research Council, Washington, D.C.) (1988) Speech understanding and aging, *Journal of the Acoustical Society of America, 83,* 859-895.

Wharton, J.A. and Church, G.T. (1990) Influence of menopause on the auditory brainstem response. *Audiology, 29,* 196-201.

White, R.F. (1978) Aging effects on lateralized auditory function in the human brain. *Dissertation Abstracts International, 39,* 1507-1508.

Wiederhold, M.L. (1986) Physiology of the olivocochlear system. In R.A. Altschuler, R.P. Bobbin, and D.W. Hoffman (Eds.), *Neurobiology of hearing: The cochlea.* Raven, New York, pp. 349-370.

Wilkins, L.T. (1947) *Survey of the prevalences of deafness in the population of England, Scotland, and Wales.* Central Office of Information, London (cited in Davis, 1983).

Willott, J.F. (1981) Comparison of response properties of inferior colliculus neurons of two inbred mouse strains differing in susceptibility to audiogenic seizures. *Journal of Neurophysiology, 45,* 35-47.

Willott, J.F. (Ed.), (1983) *The auditory psychobiology of the mouse.* Charles C. Thomas, Springfield, Illinois.

Willott, J.F. (1986) Effects of aging, hearing loss, and anatomical location on thresholds of inferior colliculus neurons in C57BL/6 and CBA mice. *Journal of Neurophysiology, 56,* 391-408.

Willott, J.F. (1990) Neurogerontology: The aging nervous system. In K. Ferraro (Ed.), *Perspectives and issues in gerontology.* Springer Publishing, New York, pp. 58-86.

Willott, J.F. (1991) Central physiological correlates of aging and presbycusis in mice. *Acta Oto-Laryngologica*

Supplement, 476, 153-156.

Willott, J.F., Bross, L.S., and McFadden, S.L. (1991) Morphology of the dorsal cochlear nucleus in young and aging C57BL/6J and CBA/J mice. Manuscript submitted for publication.

Willott, J.F. and Mortenson, V. (1991) Age-related cochler histopathology in C57BL/6J and CBA/J mice. *Association for Research in Otolaryngology Abstracts, 14,* 16.

Willott, J.F. and Bross, L. (1990) Morphology of the octopus cell area of the ventral cochlear nucleus in young and aging C57BL/6J and CBA/J mice. *Journal of Comparative Neurology, 300,* 61-81.

Willott, J.F., Hunter, K.P., and Coleman, J.R. (1988) Aging and presbycusis: Effects on, 2-deoxy-D-glucose uptake in the mouse auditory brainstem in quiet. *Experimental Neurology, 99,* 615-621.

Willott, J.F., Jackson, L.M., and Hunter, K.P. (1987) Morphometric study of the anteroventral cochlear nucleus of two mouse models of presbycusis. *Journal of Comparative Neurology, 260,* 472-480.

Willott, J.F. and Lu, S.-M. (1982) Noise-induced hearing loss can alter neural coding and increase excitability in the central nervous system. *Science, 216,* 1331-1332.

Willott, J.F., Pankow, D., Hunter, K.P., and Kordyban, M. (1985) Projections from the anterior ventral cochlear nucleus to the central nucleus of the inferior colliculus in young and aging C57BL/6 mice. *Journal of Comparative Neurology, 237,* 545-551.

Willott, J.F., Parham, K., and Hunter, K.P. (1988a) Response properties of inferior colliculus neurons in young and very old CBA/J mice. *Hearing Research, 37,* 1-14.

Willott, J.F., Parham, K., and Hunter, K.P. (1988b) Response properties of inferior colliculus neurons in middle-aged C57BL/6J mice with presbycusis. *Hearing Research, 37,* 15-28.

Willott, J.F., Parham, K., and Hunter, K.P. (1988c) Response properties of cochlear nucleus neurons in young and middle aged C57BL/6J mice with presbycusis. *Society for Neuroscience Abstracts, 14,* 646.

Wilson, R.H. (1981) The effects of aging on the magnitude of the acoustic reflex. *Journal of Speech and Hearing Research, 34,* 406-414.

Wingfield, A., Poon, L.W., Lombardi, L. and Lowe, D. (1985) Speed of processing in normal aging: Effects of speech rate, linguistic structure, and processing time. *Journal of Gerontology, 40,* 579-585.

Winslow, R.L. and Sachs, M.B. (1987) Effect of electrical stimulation of the crossed olivocochlear bundle on auditory nerve response to tones in noise. *Journal of Neurophysiology, 57,* 1002-1021.

Wittmaack, K. (1916) Uber die pathologische-anatomischen und pathologisch-physiologis-chen grundlagen der neicheitrigen erkankungsprozesse des inneren ohres und hornerven. *Archiv fuer Ohren Nasen Kehlkopfheilkunde, 99,* 71-136 (cited in Johnsson and Hawkins, 1973b).

Woods, D.L. and Clayworth, C.C. (1986) Age-related changes in human middle latency auditory evoked potentials. *Electroencephalography and Clinical Neurophysiology, 65,* 297-303.

Woolf, N.K. and Ryan, A.F. (1985) Ventral cochlear nucleus neural discharge characteristics in the absence of outer hair cells. *Brain Research, 342,* 205-218.

Woolf, N.K., Ryan, A.F., and Bone, R.C. (1981) Neural phase-locking properties in the absence of cochlear outer hair cells. *Hearing Research, 4,* 335-346.

Woolf, N.K., Ryan, A.F., Silva, E.J., Keithley, E.M., and

Schwartz, I.R. (1987) Physiology and anatomy in the aging mongolian gerbil auditory system. *Society for Neuroscience Abstracts, 13,* 1260.

Wright, C.G. (1976) Neural damage in the guinea pig cochlea after noise exposure. *Acta Oto-Laryngologica, 82,* 82-94.

Wright, J.L. and Schuknecht, H.F. (1972) Atrophy of the spiral ligament. *Archives of Otolaryngology, 96,* 16-21.

Wright, A., Davis, A., Bredberg, G., Ulehlova, L., and Spencer, H. (1987) Hair cell distributions in the normal human cochlea. *Acta Oto-Laryngologica Supplement, 444.*

Yellin, H.W., Jerger, J., and Fifer, R.C. (1989) Norms for disproportionate loss of speech intelligibility. *Ear and Hearing, 10,* 231-234.

Yoo, T.-J. (1986) Autoimmune disorder of the cochlea. In R.A. Altschuler, R.P. Bobbin, and D.W. Hoffman (Eds.), *Neurobiology of hearing: The cochlea.* Raven, New York, pp. 425-440.

Yoon, T.H., Paparella, M.M., Schachern, P.A., Giebink, G.S., Le, C.T., and Evans, K.E. (1990) Age related histopathological characteristics of human middle ear mucosa in otitis media. *Association for Research in Otolaryngology Abstracts, 13,* 131-132.

Young, I.M. and Harbert, F. (1967) Significance of the SISI test. *Journal of Auditory Research, 7,* 303-311.

Zallone, A.Z., Teti, A., Balle, V., and Iurato, S. (1987) Degeneration patterns in the organ of Corti and spiral lamina. *Acta Oto-Laryngologica Supplement 436,* 126-132.

Zanzucchi, D.G. (1938) Sulle modificanzioni delle fibre elastiches della membrana timpanica in rapporto coll'eta. *Archives Italiennes de Otologie, 50,* 203-224 (cited in Covell, 1952).

Zechner, G. and Altmann, F. (1969) Ground substance of the otic capsule. *Archives of Otolaryngology, 90,* 418-428.

Zwaardemaker, H. (1893) Das presbyacusische gesetz. *Zeitschrift fuer Ohrenheilkunde, 24,* 280-287 (cited in Hawkins and Johnsson, 1985).

Zwicker, E. (1976) and Schorn, K. Psychoacoustical tuning curves in audiology. *Audiology, 17,* 120-140.

AUTHOR INDEX

SUBJECT INDEX